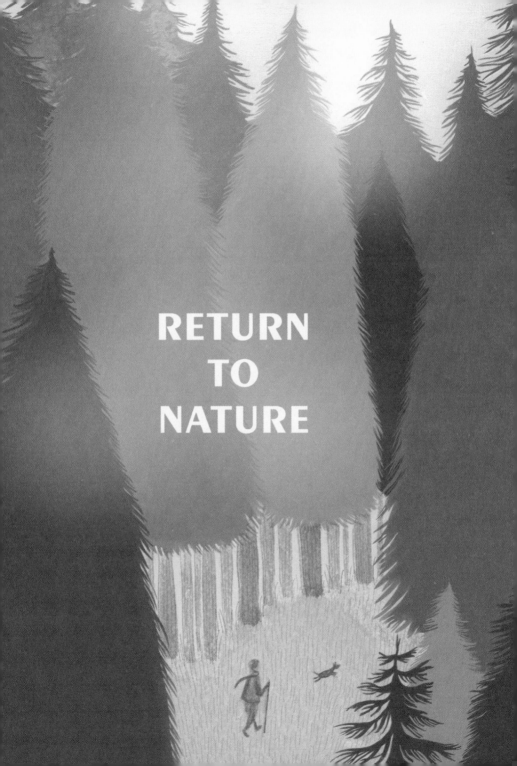

RETURN
TO
NATURE

Also by Emma Loewe

THE SPIRIT ALMANAC

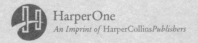

HarperOne
An Imprint of HarperCollins*Publishers*

RETURN TO NATURE

THE NEW SCIENCE OF HOW NATURAL LANDSCAPES RESTORE US

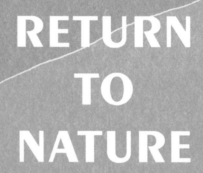

EMMA LOEWE

FIRST EDITION

Designed by Janet Evans-Scanlon

Illustrations by Harriet Lee-Merrion

Library of Congress Cataloging-in-Publication Data is available upon request.

ISBN 978-0-06-306127-9

22 23 24 25 26   PNB   10 9 8 7 6 5 4 3 2 1

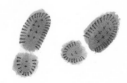

To nature—my favorite muse

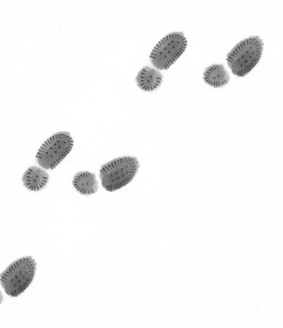

CONTENTS

INTRODUCTION 1

CHAPTER ONE
PARKS & GARDENS
21

CHAPTER TWO
OCEANS & COASTS
51

CHAPTER THREE
MOUNTAINS & HIGHLANDS
79

CHAPTER FOUR
FORESTS & TREES
105

CHAPTER FIVE
ICE & SNOW
133

CHAPTER SIX
DESERTS & DRYLANDS
159

CHAPTER SEVEN
RIVERS & STREAMS
183

CHAPTER EIGHT
CITIES & BUILT ENVIRONMENTS
209

EPILOGUE 241

Acknowledgments 245

Notes 248

Further Reading
by Landscape 275

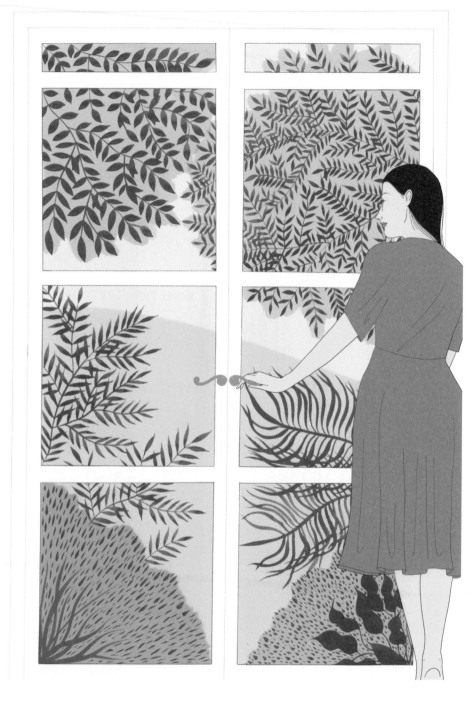

INTRODUCTION

The tree was a third parent. It was the first thing I saw when I begrudgingly opened my eyes for the early morning school bus, the last to hold my gaze before bed. Always up for entertaining, its long-lived web of branches was a jungle gym for the local squirrels and birds. It creaked and cawed with age but stayed young at heart, ready to referee backyard games or chaperone barbecues at a moment's notice. From my bed pressed against a second-story window, the tree took up the entire view. It was, quite literally, my whole world.

As my memories of my childhood home fade, that maple has stayed with me. The color of the fireplace bricks, the material of the kitchen cabinets—those details are fuzzy. But the way the tree glowed when the sunlight crept over our roof to hit it just right? That's clear as day, ingrained to the point that it's now just another part of me.

Most people have their own tree—or rock, or patch of grass, or beach—a part of nature in which they reached some epiphany, had a new joy or pain, or simply grew up. Our experiences in the outdoors have a funny way of sticking with us long after we head back inside, and we, rightfully so, feel some instinct to make more of them.

Signs of this desire to head outside are everywhere: in our technologies (preprogrammed with backgrounds of sugar-glazed Yosemite sunsets, the painterly whoosh of waves, sunlight cutting through tree canopy), in our language ("I had a mountain to climb"; "I'm riding the wave"; "The grass is always greener"), in our living spaces (the most desirable homes, after all, always have the best views of the natural world).

And yet, humans are increasingly indoor creatures. According to a survey sponsored by the Environmental Protection Agency in the 1990s,[1] the average American spent 87 percent of the day indoors (and an additional 6 percent in enclosed vehicles like cars or public transit). A more recent 2017 report on "the nature of Americans" concluded that "Americans face a significant gap between their interests in nature and their efforts, abilities, and opportunities to pursue those interests."[2] Barriers that respondents said kept them inside included competing priorities for their time and attention, lack of access to nearby nature, and, of course, the distraction of technology. (We may have only a few hours to spend outdoors a week, but we pass upward of seventy-seven of them in front of screens, according to Nielsen data.)[3]

These days, stepping outside for some air can feel like an act of resistance— a blatant disregard for the emails that need to be sent, the projects that need tending to, the family that needs taking care of. Those who can afford to travel get their nature fix on weekends away or faraway vacations, then return for another indoor stint until burnout hits again.

We've evolved to feel safer, more comfortable, and more productive inside, on our devices—even though the outdoors is where many of us are our most calm, creative, and captivated. Is it any surprise, then, that levels of stress, anxiety, and overwhelm have reached soaring heights? The World Health Organization has called stress the health epidemic of the twenty-first century and considers depression a leading cause of disability worldwide.[4] As of 2019, nearly one in five adults in the United States lived with a diagnosable mental illness, with anxiety disorders being the most common.[5]

And as our mental health suffers and stress levels climb, the nature we used to turn to for reprieve is disappearing before our eyes. As I'm writing this, millions in Texas are without power and water following a once-in-a-century winter blast thought to be exacerbated by warming conditions in the Arctic.[6] In Pew Research polling done within the last year, 63 percent of Americans surveyed said they felt like climate change was affecting their community.[7] There's no denying it: human-caused emissions are fundamentally changing Earth's climate, and they're already forging an ugly and alarming new world.

I've spent the last six years watching the climate conversation pick up from behind my computer, as the sustainability editor at mindbodygreen, a health website. In that time, I've come to believe that these dual emergencies—the mental health crisis and the climate crisis—are intricately connected. Removing ourselves from nature is making us sick, stressed, and profoundly out of sync. And it's doing the same thing to our environment. As we've lost touch with nature, we've lost touch with ourselves, and we've hurt our planet in the process. The good news? It doesn't have to be this way.

Return to Nature provides a framework for reconnecting with the outdoors for the sake of our health and the planet's. This book proposes a new definition of wellness—one that's rooted in simplicity, self-awareness, and meaningful exchange with the wise and healing world all around.

While it's easy to fully immerse in nature when you're on an extended hike or beach getaway, I'm more interested in sharing ways to do it every single day, no matter where you live or how much vacation time you have. How can we continue to live in developed cities and the burbs without completely severing ourselves from the natural world? How can we convince ourselves that backing away from our screens and stepping outside is not a luxury but an essential part of being human? How can we see nature not as a place to escape to on the weekends but as a refuge that is always sitting outside our front door? These are some of the questions we'll be unpacking in the coming pages. And any time we discuss how to get more out of nature, we need to consider what we're giving back to it in return, so expect plenty of ideas on how to conserve natural environments near and far along the way. Ready? Our landscape-to-landscape return to nature starts now.

I believe that soon, neuroscientists will tell us that being in the presence of nature lights up our brains the same way as the faces of those we love. . . . When we step outside, nose to nose, eye to eye, fully immersed in the wild, we are the best versions of ourselves.

—WALLACE J. NICHOLS
TED Talk "Neuroconservation—
Your Brain on Nature"

The Big Wide World of Research on Nature and Mental Health

If this book were to take the form of my beloved maple, its trunk would be the increasingly sturdy research on the mental health benefits of nature.

Environmental psychology is a field of study that explores the relationship between individuals and the natural and built environment, and it's one I'll be referencing often. Since its early days in the 1980s, coalitions of researchers have taken the question "Why does spending time outside make us feel so good?" and run with it—sometimes to parks and beaches, other times to laboratories and VR simulator centers.

At this point, you might be wondering why we need science to reinforce what we already know to be true: that getting outside is healthy. The idea that nature is good for us is nothing new, but reinforcing it with sturdy science can help it spread farther and wider. This research can, for example, be leveraged to protect more natural areas around the world, encourage those in power to invest in nature for the sake of population health, and show physicians that getting outdoors can be an essential health intervention, on par with eating healthily and exercising. By encouraging human-nature interactions, this research can also lead to potentially transformative outdoor experiences. After years of interviewing those on the front lines of the climate movement, I've noticed that most of them can trace their work back to a memory they or a loved one had outdoors. If I had a solar panel for every time a climate-focused scientist or activist, entrepreneur or engineer, told me a story about a landscape that fueled their work, the US would have met its renewable energy goals already. These experiences in nature have a special way of pushing people to act against climate change from a place of love, reverence, and respect—not fear. I believe that those are the kinds of actions that prove the most effective and enduring.

Like most reporters covering climate change, I've written my share of terrifying stories about terrifying things (and felt terrified afterward). But I'm increasingly convinced that fear alone won't elicit the changes we need. Love might. So with this book, I'm taking a different approach. I'm choosing to explore what a more loving and reciprocal relationship with nature can look like, starting with the science of what makes this relationship special.

It is, as you can imagine, challenging to study the health effects of out-door experiences within the confines of a randomized placebo-controlled double-blind trial. Nature is dynamic and ever-changing. It's not a pill that you can easily administer or withhold—certainly not without people knowing that you're doing it. This means that researchers in this field have had to get creative with the way they design and carry out their work.

For some, that looks like finding groups of people who have similar life experiences save for the amount of nature they are exposed to, and tracking their health outcomes—usually psychological (mood, cognition, etc.) or physiological (blood pressure, heart rate, etc.). Whatever differences come up between the groups could potentially be attributable to that nature component. Other researchers work more qualitatively: they ask people to describe their experiences in nature, looking out for trends and patterns in their responses. Wider-lensed studies use global satellite images to see how green a neighborhood is and compare the health of its residents with that of those living in an area that is less green. Smaller-scale studies distill nature into its component parts and administer them in a lab to a few people at a time. High-tech studies can simulate and monitor a community's outdoor spaces in Sims-like computer universes, or ping people on their cellphones to ask how their mood is now that they're in that lush park. The type of health information collected in these studies is equally varied. Mental health can be measured in different ways: parasympathetic nervous system activity, cortisol levels, and heart-rate variability can all tell you how revved up a person's system is and how much stress that person feels. People can usually tell you about this themselves too, and self-reported data are common.

Clearly, this field of research can take on many forms. While this means that studies can be difficult to compare, replicate, and verify, it also means that we now have a thick tapestry of findings on what happens to us when we step outside, both consciously and subconsciously.

Though they approach this topic using a slightly different framework, the vast majority of studies so far have come to the same general conclusion: compared with human-made structures (buildings, roads, etc.), natural spaces tend to make most people feel more positive and less stressed. The fact that so many different kinds of studies have similar findings tells us that there is, indeed, reason to seek out green over gray. But why?

For decades, researchers have leaned on two theories to explain it: the first and most widely cited is attention restoration theory (ART), presented by a husband-and-wife team of environmental psychologists, Rachel Kaplan and Stephen Kaplan, in the 1980s. ART states that, in such a distracting world, we use up a lot of our cognitive resources trying to stay focused on the tasks at hand. Constantly needing to actively direct our attention this way leaves us mentally fatigued. After years of studying people's perceptions of nature both near and far, the Kaplans theorized that nature is one place we can go to restore our attention, given that it has four key qualities: extent (there's enough of it to explore to keep us occupied), being away (it feels removed from whatever is draining our cognitive resources), compatibility (it's in line with what we expect and supports our goals), and fascination (it's a place for the attention to rest). As their theory goes, natural scenes provide a place for our attention to recharge, so we can go back to cognitively draining activities feeling a little more rejuvenated and alert. Emails, pings, and other distractions empty our mental cups, so to speak, and nature fills them back up.

The other explanation is stress reduction theory (SRT), which was proposed by the architect Roger Ulrich around the same time as ART. While ART focuses on how nature influences our cognition, SRT is more concerned with its effects on our emotional lives—namely, our stress levels. SRT says that humans are hardwired to relax while looking at environments that have extensive views, areas to retreat, and essential resources like shade and water. Since these are the places that our primitive ancestors sought out for survival, it would make sense that they still feel innately welcoming to us. When our stress response—another vestige from the early days of humanity—is activated and our bodies go into fight-or-flight mode, these natural settings can subtly remind us that we are, in fact, safe.

No experiment has directly compared the theories, so the relative importance of these two relaxation mechanisms (attention restoration and stress reduction) isn't completely understood. Regardless, these dual hypotheses have provided a jumping-off point for researchers to work from for decades.

But as environmental psychologists continue to ask more-nuanced questions about what exactly it is about the outdoors that we find so inherently soothing, which aspects of nature are most restorative, and what kinds of people stand to gain the most from time outside, they're realizing that there's room to expand on these two landmark ideas. While ART and SRT give us a sense of why we prefer green over gray, they don't say much about how the other colors in nature can make us feel: the blues of the ocean, the reds and oranges of leaves changing colors, the browns of the desert, the whites of snowy scenes. This more personal, colorful approach is the one I'm fascinated by, and it's what we'll be exploring in this book.

In *Return to Nature*, we'll traverse eight landscapes—parks, oceans, mountains, forests, ice, deserts, rivers, and cities to—unpack the latest research on how each one makes us feel, see, and think a little differently. Along the way, we'll hear from dozens of researchers around the globe who have their own creative approaches to examining this topic. A British scientist streaming forest soundtracks on BBC to study how people react to nature's acoustics, a Canadian nurse seeing what happens when people get the chance to visit their favorite spots in nature at the end of life, and a Swedish researcher creating a new type of nature meditation out of his campus greenhouse are just some of the experts you'll meet in these pages.

After weaving together their findings, landscape by landscape, we'll be left with a rich ecosystem of knowledge about the health benefits of various types of nature contact. From there, we'll drop the science cap and put on a more spiritual one. There are, after all, some things about our connection to the natural world that can't be neatly explained, only felt.

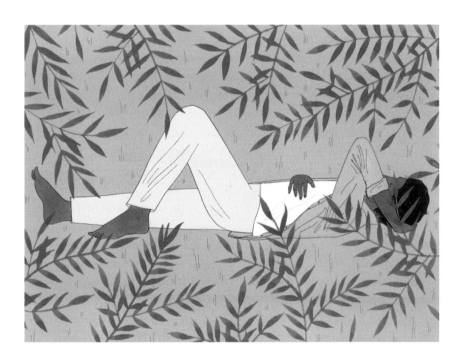

For several centuries, the rational mind has been ascendant, even though science, its finest expression, can still in
all its brilliance answer only the question of how but never
come close to addressing the ultimate question—why.

—WADE DAVIS,
in *Ecopsychology: Science, Totems,
and the Technological Species*

The Spiritual Potential That Lives
Where Humans and Nature Meet

Science plays an integral role in explaining the impact of nature experience
on humans—but it can only go so far. The scientific process studies all that
can be measured. And though it casts a wide net, it will always fall a little
short when attempting to define something as vast as "the health benefits
of nature." Where it leaves off, a type of spirituality picks up. I think of spirituality as a connection that has some degree of randomness to it. It can't
be completely explained or predicted, but we know it when we feel it. In
the outdoors, it might look like a moment of ecstasy, a feeling of total
peace, or an unexplainable serenity and clarity in the presence of a new
view. For me, it can come when I'm walking on the beach near where I
grew up, running along the Hudson River in Manhattan, or standing under
a really big tree.

   While Western philosophies of expansion, growth, and profit have
physically separated us from nature, our innate spiritual connection to it
remains. In their work, the Kaplans found that *wholeness, oneness*, and
purity were words that people often used to describe their wilderness

experience.[8] It's easy to draw parallels between this nature vernacular and that of a church, temple, or place of worship for some higher power.

With this in mind, I wanted to carry this book beyond the quantifiable and into the realm of the unproved and unprovable: to, as the ecological scientist and member of Citizen Potawatomi Nation Robin Wall Kimmerer writes in *Braiding Sweetgrass: Indigenous Wisdom, Scientific Knowledge, and the Teachings of Plants*, "be bilingual between the lexicon of science and the grammar of animacy."[9] So, alongside measures of heart-rate variability and brain waves, you'll find descriptions of archetypes, fables, and spiritual and religious philosophies that further probe how nature makes us feel in body and mind. I present these side by side not to conflate faith and science or discount the significance of rigorous research (or religion, for that matter). I do it because I believe that together, the two can form a more complete picture of what happens when we step outside.

I am less important than I thought, the human race is less important than I thought. I rejoice in that. My mind loses its urgings, senses its nature, and is free.

—WENDELL BERRY,
"A Native Hill" in *Think Little: Essays*

To tell this side of the story, I recruited some help—as spirituality is, by definition, deeply personal. And, it turns out, so is nature. The beliefs, lived experiences, and memories we carry into the outdoors inevitably shape how relaxed and receptive we feel in it. Take, for example, the ocean on a big-wave day: someone who grew up surfing might find this a lovely, almost divine scene. Someone who has never been to the beach would find the same view completely foreign and potentially terrifying. Or a mountain peak: experienced hikers will feel drawn to it, while Indigenous populations whose gods are said to live on the mountains will see it as a sacred place where they are not to set foot. (This is another reason to look beyond scientific research when exploring this topic: much of it is conducted in Western, developed nations on white subjects who can't necessarily stand in for the global population.)

With this in mind, it was important for me to invite as many voices into this book as possible. As we travel from landscape to landscape, expect to hear from Himalayan mountaineers and city hikers, big-wave surfers and professional cloudspotters, deep-sea divers and forest bathing guides, all reflecting on the role that nature has played in their self-discovery.

Weaving It All Together:
Science- and Spirit-Backed Nature Excursions
for a Burned-Out Age

Come the second half of each chapter, I hope that you'll close this book and begin putting it into practice. That's when I'll turn science and story into activities that can help you get the most out of your time in that landscape. This is your opportunity to take some of the research and run with it, incorporating it into a life that feels nourishing, restorative, and true to you.

These activities come in many forms. Some take hours, others minutes. Some are more prescriptive routines (take a trek through the forest that engages all five senses), while some are simple mindset shifts (sit in the grass taking on the perspective of an artist looking for the next muse). Each chapter also provides ideas for tapping into the themes and lessons of that landscape from afar, even from indoors. The variation is meant to help everyone find an activity to latch onto and continue to practice daily, weekly, monthly, or as needed during times of stress, sadness, or upheaval.

Feel free to take liberties with how you define each landscape: these activities can be done anywhere there is a hint of the natural world. Grasslands can be your own backyard; forests can be small clusters of trees in your neighborhood.

This might take some unlearning. These days, so many of us think that nature has to be some grand, distant place without a hint of the human: a national park, a secluded beach, a mountain summit. In the report *The Nature of Americans* referenced earlier, when nearly twelve thousand Americans of all ages were asked to define nature, respondents "overwhelmingly regarded nature as something separated from and independent of human influence or activity." Unlike the children polled, adults tended to "set a high and even impossible standard for what they perceived to be 'authentic' and unforgettable nature, believing that it requires solitude and travel to faraway places, which reinforces their perceptions of the relative inaccessibility of nature."

This viewpoint is to be expected, as it has deep roots in environmental theory. The 1964 Wilderness Act defines wilderness as "an area where the earth and its community of life are untrammeled by man, where man himself is a visitor who does not remain."[10] A 1999 paper in the *Journal of Environmental Psychology* defines it similarly as "a region which contains no permanent inhabitants, no possibility for motorized travel, and is spacious enough so that a traveler crossing it by foot must have the experience of sleeping out of doors."[11]

I'd argue that wilderness is not the same as nature, and confusing the two is problematic on many levels: for one, untamed wilderness areas are not available—or necessarily appealing—to everyone. Many people don't have the money or physical ability to go to them, don't feel safe in them, or feel unwelcome in them because of their gender, their physical ability, or the color of their skin. (Long-standing oppression, control, and institutional racism have historically robbed people of color of many liberties in America—and access to outdoor spaces is one of them.) There's also the concern that, as one researcher put it to me, when we all flock to the relatively few pristine natural places left, we will "love them to death." When everyone chooses to fly to national parks over their own neighborhood na-

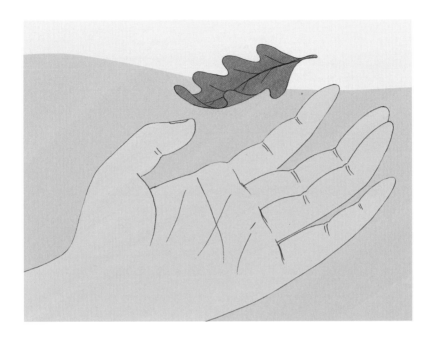

ture, we're left with a lot of carbon emissions—and some overrun national parks. The more we see nature as something untouched and far away, the more it will become impossible to find.

Thankfully, as you'll see in the coming chapters, the science is clear: we don't need to take that expensive trip off the grid to experience the well-being benefits of nature. Instead, with a little guidance and practice, we can—for lack of a better word—"microdose" on nature and feel a similar sense of awe, clarity, and gratitude on a morning commute that we would in the backcountry.

To reflect this, we need a new definition for what nature can be. For that, I'm drawn to a response that researchers got in a qualitative study on how listening to bird sounds makes us feel. The study participant noted that when she connects to nature, she's connecting with something "more

> In my capacity as an artist, I have always thought about attention, but it's only now that I fully understand where a life of sustained attention leads. In short, it leads to awareness, not only of how lucky I am to be alive, but to ongoing patterns of cultural and ecological devastation around me—and the inescapable part that I play in it, should I choose to recognize it or not. In other words, simple awareness is the seed of responsibility.
>
> —JENNY ODELL,
> *How to Do Nothing:*
> *Resisting the Attention Economy*

real than some of the stressful things that happen in life."[12] Nature is, simply put, something real—more real than the indoor lives we have constructed for ourselves.

To brush against this reality, you don't need to be an avid hiker, surfer, or climber. I myself am none of these things. While I love being outside, my anxious personality and not-insignificant fear of heights means that my ideal nature excursion is a day in the park or an afternoon walk through the woods—not a weeklong backcountry trip or whitewater rafting journey. This used to make me feel slightly ashamed: How could I write about loving nature without ever having experienced it in these more traditionally "outdoorsy" ways? But over time, I've started to embrace the idea that everyone—myself included—is outdoorsy, in the sense that we all have the capacity to tap into the best parts of ourselves outdoors. My hope is that this book will be a source of ideas to help you do so, no matter what outdoor experience you opened it with.

Paying It Forward with Personal, Meaningful Climate Actions

Given the current climate crisis, it feels wrong to send people out to reap the gifts of nature without reminding them to give something back in return. Like any healthy relationship, this one needs to be reciprocal. That's why I end every chapter by describing the threats that a particular landscape faces and how you can get involved in combating them.

I preface this in saying that there is no one way to be an environmental citizen. Though I've written my fair share of "X Things You Can Do to Stop Climate Change" articles, I'm no longer sure that this prescriptive approach is the way to go. For one, it doesn't acknowledge that we all come to the problem with varying abilities to take action. The advice to compost at home or bike to work will ring hollow if you don't have a backyard or live in an area with safe bike lanes. Beating too hard on the individual action drum can also distract us from the larger changes that need to happen in order to bring down global emissions in a significant way. According to one 2017 report from a global carbon monitoring data set, upward of 70 percent of human-caused greenhouse gas emissions can be attributed to one hundred fossil fuel companies—many of which have tried to shift blame onto citizens in order to distract from their own responsibility.[13] Our energy is better spent banding together to support policies and systems that force these companies to reduce their emissions than it is worrying about avoiding plastic straws (as annoying as they may be). Individual action isn't pointless, but it's not the whole point either. Systemic shifts are needed too.

You might find that these shifts are a little easier to support once you've spent some time outside. Several studies show that those who visit nature more often are also more likely to engage in pro-environmental behaviors.[14] Those who have more access to natural green or blue (the ocean) spaces in their neighborhood have also been found to adopt more eco-friendly behaviors than those who have less access—regardless of their socioeconomic status.[15] This has caused researchers to conclude that "improving access to, and contact with, nature, e.g., through better urban planning, may be one approach for meeting sustainability targets."[16]

This makes intuitive sense when we consider one of the truths that the outdoors teaches us again and again: we are a small part of a much larger world. This can both ease some stress (by helping us zoom out on our problems) and increase feelings of communion (with the world around us and the people who live in it). While an insular, me-centric view can lead to equally insular and me-centric behavior, a wider one might free up some room to consider the greater good. In this way, going into nature is an opportunity to fuel our spirits for sustainable action ahead.

"Are you hopeful?" is one question that people working in climate change are asked constantly. I'll always remember the environmentalist David Orr's response to it during a conference I attended with him: Orr told the room that he had to stay hopeful because "hope is a verb with its sleeves rolled up. If you're optimistic, you don't have to do anything. If you're in despair, you can't do anything. But if you're hopeful, you have to do something."

At the end of the day, the most effective climate action we can take is the one that we can sustain into the future. We have to come to it on our own, through a curious consideration of our skills, interests, and capabilities. It's less told than it is found. For this reason, I don't offer many specific actions to take in this book. Instead, I offer mindset shifts that might help you approach these problems from a new perspective, and a more hopeful one at that.

Returning to Nature, Together

Whether you're an avid hiker with easy access to trails or a city dweller whose view is more of a concrete jungle, I hope you'll walk away from this book with an arsenal of new ideas about how to engage with the world around you for the sake of your health.

Time in nature can help us shed a lot—unhealthy reactions to stress, repetitive negative thoughts, and so forth—but I've found that each landscape also gives us something special to gain. In chapter 1, we'll stroll through green parks and gardens to see how they can help us become more mindful and establish our place in community. In chapter 2, we'll travel beachside to learn how the ocean and its waves can be portals to memory. Chapter 3 heads to the hills to explore how mountains are gateways to awe and breakthrough. Chapter 4 is set in the forest, and it unpacks why being around trees can help us relax into our intuitive wisdom. In chapter 5's deep freeze, we'll study how snow, ice, and cold can connect us with our inner resilience. Chapter 6 considers how the desert's sun and heat evoke creativity and personal discovery. Chapter 7 traces how life's journey can play out alongside winding rivers. And finally, chapter 8 finds the big restorative potential in the tiny pockets of nature tucked into cities.

> What we're living through is deeply, deeply personal. And emotional. It's heartbreakingly human.
>
> —MARY ANNAÏSE HEGLAR,
> "The Fight for Climate Justice
> Requires a New Narrative" in *Inverse*

While you might feel drawn to one landscape right off the bat, I suggest reading all the chapters in order, as their themes blend and build off one another. Mountains often have forests, and ice and snow blanket many a park and city. As they do in nature, these landscapes make the most sense when considered together, in the context of the whole system.

I encourage you to get creative when thinking about what each landscape could look like in your area: if you don't get much in the way of snow where you live, picture rain or storms as you read that chapter. If you don't dwell near the desert, home in on the sunshine discussed in those pages. And if there's one landscape that you feel a strong initial attraction to—maybe you've always been a beach person or enjoyed spending time among the trees—notice if your preference changes at all over the course of this reading. You might find that when you enter a new landscape, it invites you into a new part of yourself—and holds a lesson you need to internalize the most.

I have always felt a strong pull to the forest, probably because of my childhood spent among the canopy. But as I sit typing this on the twentieth story of my New York apartment building, looking out onto no less than six other apartment buildings, I wonder if, with a shift in attention and deepening of awareness, I can find the same sparkles of delight and comfort in this view as I did with my maple tree all those years ago. I open the window, close my eyes, and trust it's possible.

CHAPTER ONE

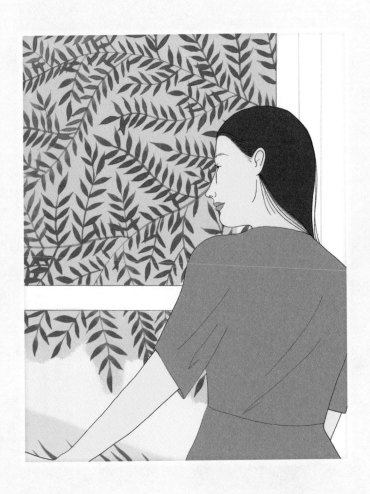

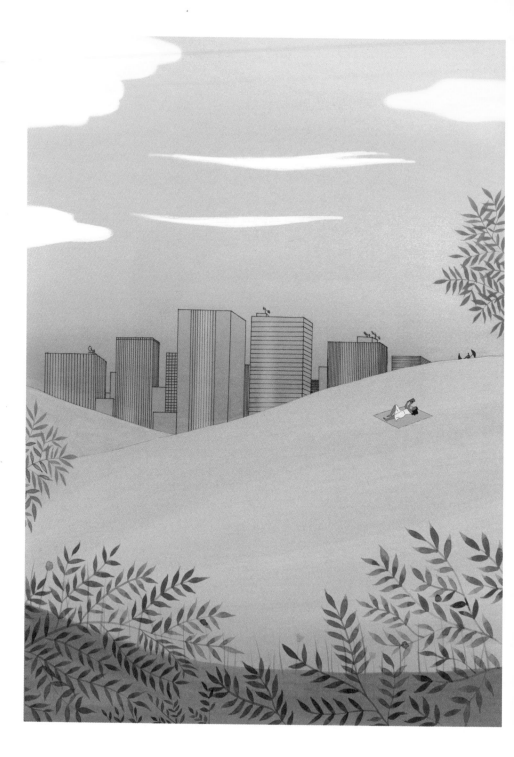

PARKS & GARDENS

community, mindfulness, discovery

I t's busy in the park today. I sit down and feel the humbling. My fellow Brooklynites seem to feel it too—that sense of smallness that happens when you're closer to the earth. Some are reading, others chatting or looking up at the clouds. There is such peace and pleasure here on the edge of city life that it makes me wonder if humanity's problems are simply the result of us feeling too big.

Running my fingers through the million little worlds tangled in the grass below, resting my back on the wrinkled tree behind, I close my eyes and listen to the noises of people and nature mixing, and feel right at home. Opening them up again is like coming out of a dream that I'm not ready to have end—not quite yet.

The Remedy

Natural grasslands form in subhumid climates where there's too much rain for a desert but not enough for a forest. Sometimes called prairies, savannahs, and rangelands, these wide-open spaces offer fertile soil and enough grass and plants to keep grazing animals happy. In the US we've converted many of our grasslands for industrialization and agriculture,[1] but we've come up with something to take their place: the public park.

While humans can't build a mountain or ocean from scratch, we can create a park relatively easily. You can now find open expanses of grass, smattered with trees here and there, in most urban and suburban areas across the country. It makes sense, then, that this landscape is the most widely studied for its impact on human health—which has been shown to be overwhelmingly positive.

How Parks Promote Longer, Healthier Lives

In short, people who live near green spaces live longer. That's what one World Health Organization–funded research review, the largest of its kind, found after analyzing results from nine large-scale longitudinal studies (conducted over a period of years) in 2019.[2] These studies captured data on all-cause mortality and neighborhood greenness for 8,324,652 individuals across seven countries. Each one quantified greenness using satellite data, so forests fell into the green bucket, as did parks. After adjusting their findings by socioeconomic status (less affluent areas tend to have less green space, and less access to quality medical care), seven of the nine studies "found a significant inverse relationship between an increase in surrounding greenness and the risk of all-cause mortality," leading reviewers to conclude that "interventions to increase and manage green spaces should therefore be considered as a strategic public health intervention." These findings extend across generations, and smaller research studies have even linked exposure to green space during pregnancy to higher birth weights[3] and healthier births[4] overall.

As for why people with access to greenery tend to be healthier and live longer, researchers think part of it probably has to do with the activities that green space allows for: exercise, social interaction, and so forth, which have longevity benefits of their own. Green parks can also help regulate surrounding temperatures, reduce pollution, and stifle noise. In turn, they improve air quality and can reduce citizens' risk of developing conditions like heart disease.[5]

Then there are the psychological benefits of parks, gardens, and other public green spaces, which we'll focus on in this chapter. Studies have found that those who live near green space have lower levels of the stress hormone cortisol,[6] reduced rates of anxiety disorder and depression,[7] and better overall mood—all of which can decrease one's likelihood of getting sick.

Why We Love Parks: Two Schools of Thought on Their Universal Appeal

There are two theories to explain why parks and green spaces make us feel mentally at ease: the evolutionary and the cultural. Evolutionary scholars, who fall more in line with stress reduction theory, think humans feel more relaxed in parks, and more tense in cities, because grasslands mimic the areas where most early humans evolved.

In prehistoric times, settling in grassy plains scattered with a few trees, hills, and water features gave us a better chance of survival. They provided clear views of predators, shady places to rest, landmarks to guide us in case we got lost, and opportunities to find food and water.

While enclosed forests and sky-high mountains can stoke fears of being attacked by a bear or falling to our death, grassy landscapes are low stakes by comparison. This type of landscape may be where many of our ancestors learned how to relax in the first place—a life-giving skill in itself. "If you can run away from a saber-toothed tiger, your survival is enhanced. But if after running away, you can get to a peaceful place, relax, and gather your strength, that may further enhance your survival," the epidemiologist Howard Frumkin writes in *Ecopsychology*.[8]

The other argument for why we find peace in parks is more cultural: in "Do Humans Really Prefer Semi-Open Natural Landscapes? A Cross-Cultural Reappraisal,"[9] Caroline Hägerhäll, a landscape architect and professor at the Swedish University of Agricultural Sciences, questioned whether evolution alone drives our unconscious longing for this landscape.

"It's a consensus assumption that all humans have similar preferences for that natural environment. And that might be. But of course, we haven't tested very many types of environments—or people," she tells me of the motivation for this study. "We have a very limited range of environments that have been studied. Most of them are Western types of planned nature like parks. And when it comes to the people, we mainly asked students in Western countries or at least industrialized, well-off countries."

To test this assumption on a new participant pool, Hägerhäll and her team linked up with members of five non-Western Indigenous communities— the Jahai from the Malay Peninsula, the Lokono from Suriname, the Makalero and Makasae from Timor, and the Wayuu in Colombia. The team presented members of these communities with digital renderings of different landscapes and asked them questions about their preferred landscape, comparing their answers with those of Swedish university students. In general, those in the Indigenous communities said they preferred to live in flatter landscapes that had a higher density of vegetation, while the university students would rather live in more hilly, less-forested areas, consistent with the savannah-like landscape of evolutionary theory. The fact that some of the Indigenous communities believed that gods lived on raised ground could have made the hilly scenes register as off-limits to them, causing the difference in preference.

Though Hägerhäll is quick to say that this study has a small sample size and is in no way conclusive, it challenges the notion that landscape preference is purely the result of human evolution. Culture and upbringing probably play a role too.

I see room for both theories to coexist. Listening to Matthew J. Wichrowski, a horticultural therapist at the Department of Rehabilitation Medicine at NYU Grossman School of Medicine, describe what we know about the Hanging Gardens of Babylon, constructed in the sixth century BC, it's hard not to draw parallels between the prehistoric paradise and the parks we frequent today. The gardens contained local flowers, water features, and expansive views of the surrounding land. They were a retreat from the desert beyond, as neighborhood parks are a respite from the demands of technology, work, and other challenges of modern life. Thousands of years later, these gardens still sound like a paradise, indicating that some of our preference for grassland is innate and eternal.

But the more researchers learn about outdoor experiences, the more they see that what people bring to nature matters just as much as what nature brings to them. The reason that our shoulders drop and we take a big exhale when we enter flat, grassy expanses can't always be explained by some unconscious longing alone. "So much of it," Catharine Ward Thompson, a professor of landscape architecture at the University of Edinburgh, tells me, "is about stories you're told and your own experience and how familiar you are with a place."

Relaxing in grassland may be in our nature, but we have to nurture that feeling too. Looking around a neighborhood park on a sunny Saturday afternoon can give us some ideas on how to do that. The various activities we tend to do in public green spaces—walking, cloud gazing, and so forth—all tap into something unique that this landscape has to offer.

The Friends Who Picnic Together: Green Space Grows Community

It's no wonder that families and friend groups flock to parks; green space fosters social interactions. Multiple studies have found that people who live in greener areas tend to socialize more and feel a greater sense of community. Even in urban environments, features like grassy parks and clusters of trees can boost camaraderie among neighbors.

Take one 1997 experiment conducted in two public housing complexes in Chicago.[10] Landscape researchers mapped where the complexes' residents assembled and found that the greater the number of trees that surrounded a unit, the greater the likelihood that people would gather there.

Following this initial observation,[11] those who lived in the apartments surrounded by greenery and those surrounded by concrete sat through interviews on the strength of their social ties. Sure enough, the density of the vegetation was a strong positive predictor of the answers, recalls William C. Sullivan, a professor in the Department of Landscape Architecture at the University of Illinois who worked on the study. The greater the number of trees, the stronger the social bonds.

Upon further investigation,[12] more-vegetated areas were also found to have less graffiti and crime and a greater sense of safety. Frances E. Kuo, another researcher involved, reflected on these findings in a 2003 paper: "If stronger social ties among neighbors are key to creating more effective, safer neighborhoods, and treed spaces help promote ties among neighbors, perhaps the greenness of neighborhood landscape ultimately affects levels of safety and security in a neighborhood."[13]

Some twenty years later, studies continue to show that small green patches of parks can profoundly affect public health—especially in poor neighborhoods with a large BIPOC population, which have previously been neglected on the green front.

So why can green spaces feed the collective? It probably starts with their impact on the individual. We know that spending time in nature can boost mood and ease stress, and happier people tend to make better companions. "When you're mentally fatigued, you're more likely to be irritable. You're more likely to be distracted and miss portions of the conversation or subtle social cues," Sullivan says. Natural scenes also seem to light up the parts of the brain associated with empathy,[14] hinting that it might be easier for us to relate to others when greenery surrounds us.

These resulting social ties are good for more than just your mood; the rest of your body thanks you for them too. We now have reason to believe that people who have rich social lives tend to live longer than those who don't,[15] and healthy relationships have been associated with health markers like reduced inflammation[16] and healthier immune function.[17]

The Bird-Watchers:
Observing Wildlife Is a Shortcut to Mindfulness

Urban green spaces and parks don't just give us a comfortable place to gather with other humans: they also provide an arena for animal watching. For both amateur and avid birders, the practice inspires wonder, mindfulness, relaxation, and joy—and a park with running water and the possibility of scraps from someone's picnic is an ideal place for it.

Walking slowly, ears open and binoculars at the ready, birders demonstrate how going out into nature to look for something can boost the experience. Richard Fuller, a conservation biologist and professor at the University of Queensland in Australia, is a self-proclaimed "obsessive bird-watcher." "When I go out to a natural landscape, I'm often bird-watching," he tells me from the other side of the world. "For me it's absolute mindfulness. When you're bird-watching, you're entirely focused on what's happening right there in the present. Nothing in the past, in the future, or elsewhere really matters."

To root us in the immediate present, birds first engage our senses. Before you see one, you might hear its song, which the acoustic ecologist Gordon Hempton says is the primary indicator that a habitat is safe and hospitable. "We have a very discreet bandwidth of supersensitive hearing, and that's between 2.5 and 5 kilohertz in the resident frequencies of the auditory canal. Is there something in our ancestors' environment that matches our peak hearing human sensitivity?," he asks Krista Tippett, a journalist and author, during an episode of her podcast, *On Being*.[18] "Indeed, there's a perfect match: birdsong."

This harks back to the evolutionary hypothesis. The high-pitched call of a robin and the melodic chirp of a goldfinch register as relaxing to us because, on some level, they signal that our surroundings contain the resources we need to survive. Eleanor Ratcliffe, a lecturer in environmental psychology at the University of Surrey, put this theory to the test when she asked twenty people to describe the nature experiences they felt would be

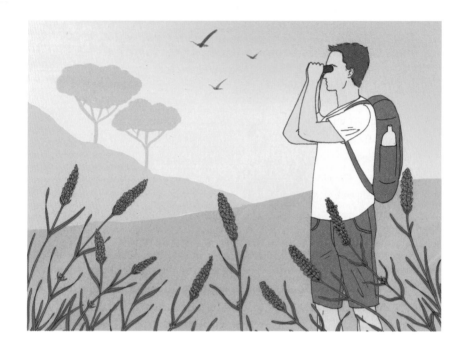

psychologically restorative when they were stressed or mentally fatigued or both. Birdsongs and calls played a prominent role in many of their narratives and "were found to be the type of natural sound most commonly associated with perceived stress recovery and attention restoration."[19]

The songs also evoked positive memories during some interviews. "For several participants these associations related to the enjoyment of childhood," her study continues. This ties into an idea we'll explore more in the ocean chapter: certain natural sounds can provide a gateway to a rich vault of memories. Though not all birdsongs were rated positively (Ratcliffe recalls that smooth, melodic songs from birds like wrens were preferred to aggressive, staccato ones from magpies), on average people considered them welcome distractions from everyday stressors, new features on which to latch their attention.

The Cloudspotters:
Even the Park's "Mundanities" Are Engaging

Visit any busy park on a warm day, and you're bound to spot at least one kid horizontal on the grass, eyes to the sky. A popular childhood pastime, cloudspotting can be valuable for adults too, as it connects us to what Sir John Lubbock described in his nineteenth-century book *The Pleasures of Life* as "a succession of glorious pictures in never-ending variety." Even in 1887, Lubbock lamented that it was "remarkable how few people seem to derive any pleasure from the beauty of the sky."[20]

Over time, we've only become even more indifferent to the ever-evolving performance above our heads. With an infinite amount of television to watch and an entire internet's worth of content to consume, one doesn't need to look up to be entertained. Instead, these days most of us just see the rolling clouds as a hindrance to the sun or a foreboding sign of rain to come. But as the climate scientist Kate Marvel points out in her TED talk, "every sunny day is the same. Every cloudy day is cloudy in its own way."[21]

Gavin Pretor-Pinney has made it his mission to encourage more people to slow down long enough to watch the clouds pass by. The founder of the Cloud Appreciation Society, a network of self-identified cloud enthusiasts, Pretor-Pinney considers cloudspotting a fast track to restoration—one that is completely free and available to nearly everyone, for a few hours a day at least.

"We think that clouds are Nature's poetry, and the most egalitarian of her displays, since everyone can have a fantastic view of them," reads the society's "manifesto" in Pretor-Pinney's book *The Cloudspotter's Guide.*[22] "We seek to remind people that clouds are expressions of the atmosphere's moods, and can be read like those of a person's countenance."

He considers clouds the most democratic of nature's forms. While you might need to spend hours driving to a mountain vista or shell out money for an ocean view, clouds are almost always accessible, and they can prompt similar feelings of serenity. "Doing something like cloudspotting is a way of actively putting yourself into that sort of idle mode of the brain," Pretor-Pinney tells me over video from the Cloud Appreciation Society's UK headquarters. "There's a little Zen-like thing about finding shapes in the clouds—you have to let yourself go. It's more of a subconscious level of the brain that's at work when you're cloud gazing." This theory tracks with the attention restoration hypothesis: clouds, especially ones that hang low in the sky and take on distinct shapes, hold our attention without draining our mental resources.

As for the best place to do the restorative practice, Pretor-Pinney says it's your backyard or public park—somewhere familiar where you can return to splay out on the lawn or take to a bench with your neck awkwardly bent in awe again and again.

The Strollers:
Walking Is a Route to Better Health

Perhaps the most obvious health perk of a park is that it gets people exercising. People who live near parks tend to be more avid walkers than those who don't,[23] likely because most parks have well-maintained, relatively quiet designated walking trails. Studies on park walks show that they can engage our parasympathetic (rest and digest) response, and quell our negative emotions and anxieties[24]—no matter the weather. Even on drizzly days, their psychological benefits are clear.

Park walking is such a promising medicine that doctors around the world are starting to actively prescribe it. Networks like Parks Victoria in Australia and Park Rx in America are getting the word out about how it can be a low-cost and side-effect-free health intervention.

When you walk out of a doctor's office in the Park Rx network, you might have a prescription for an afternoon nature excursion in hand instead of a traditional script. In place of the name of a pharmaceutical, you'd see a directive to take a walk around your local park for thirty minutes, three times a week. You could then check back with your doctor about how you're progressing toward the goal, whether during your next appointment or in real time via an app. This level of accountability makes the somewhat flimsy recommendation to "move outside more" feel more like a necessity, as essential as taking your blood pressure medication in the morning or sleeping pills at night.

> There's something about the rhythm of walking . . . It's a natural human rhythm. If you want to get a baby to sleep, walking it up and down is much more effective than standing still. But there's also something therapeutic about the rhythm of walking—something I've noticed often with families in difficult circumstances is that talking about things while walking is actually very different from sitting across the table. The combination of physical activity, the rhythm, and the natural environment offers something particularly valuable.
>
> —CATHARINE WARD THOMPSON,
> professor of landscape architecture,
> University of Edinburgh

In his cardiology practice in Ohio, Dr. David Sabgir takes a more social approach to nature prescribing. After years of being discouraged by his inability to help patients get more active, he wondered if it would help if he offered to go on scheduled walks through the park with them. Ever since his first outing in 2005, Sabgir has been steadily building a program that makes it easy for other physicians to do the same. There are now 574 chapters of Walk with a Doc spread across thirty-seven countries, and medical professionals of all stripes are heading outside with their patients. When surveyed,[25] walkers in the program consistently said it improves their mood, boosts their energy level, increases their confidence to continue being active, and gives them a chance to socialize. As for why he encourages nature walks and not urban strolls or treadmill sessions, Sabgir says it's simple: most people inherently love to get outdoors. Sometimes they just need a reason to do it.

Considering the state of our current medical system, he foresees programs like Walk with a Doc becoming more common in the future. "I think that the docs overall share the same frustrations that I have," he tells me. "Just writing more Lipitor or insulin shots, you have the feeling you're paying off interest instead of paying down on the principal."

Indeed, in some US states, health care companies are beginning to take note of lifestyle prescriptions. Kaiser Permanente, for example, has invested in the Healthy Parks Healthy People initiative in California's Bay Area,[26] which connects doctors with programs designed to get infrequent park visitors outside more and break down any barriers to entry. Partnerships like this show that the health benefits of nature are starting to be recognized by the mainstream medical establishment and could signal an influx of park strollers to come.

The Ones Watching the World Go By: If You're Having Trouble Meditating, Take It Outside

In parks, you'll also find those people who take to a bench or patch of grass to close their eyes and look within.

While most structured mindfulness programs are conducted indoors in relatively bland environments, Freddie Lymeus, a clinical psychologist specializing in health psychology and environmental psychology at Sweden's Uppsala University, recently studied how meditating outdoors in a greenhouse garden setting could enhance people's ability to drop into mindfulness.

After some trial and error, he created a five-week outdoor mindfulness course, called restoration skills training (ReST),[27] that harnessed the elements of nature as guides and motivators instead of distractions. Over the course of the nature-based outdoor training, he found that participants' performance on attention tests improved—an indication of restoration. Those who took part in a traditional mindfulness program didn't see the same restored attention performance as the outdoor program participants.

And after comparing the participation in ReST to traditional programs,[28] Lymeus saw that ReST participants were also less likely to drop out and more likely to complete the assigned mindfulness homework over the five weeks.

Another study found that even though the ReST program seemed to require less effort,[29] its participants left with the same mindful skill set as those who graduated from the indoor program. "ReST is a promising alternative for otherwise healthy people with stress or concentration problems who would be less likely to complete more effortful CMT (conventional mindfulness training)," the study concludes.

When I asked Lymeus why meditating outdoors might be easier for people, he said that by helping to restore our attention, natural environments can, in a sense, get us halfway into a calm, meditative state: "In a high-quality natural setting, there is less need to specifically instruct participants in how to deal with difficult thoughts, emotions, and physical sensations. Spontaneous processes in the person-environment interaction already support a more open, accepting, and unattached relationship with yourself."

This mirrors an observation that Stephen Kaplan, the creator of ART, had at the turn of the century: in a 2001 research article,[30] he wrote that there are inherent similarities between his theory and Eastern meditation, which can also quiet the mind of strenuous thought so that we can enter a more relaxed and receptive state.

It seems that if you're looking to tune out noise and enter a place of stillness, nature can help. And the nice thing is that you don't need to head to a picturesque meadow or impressive beach to use this method. A quiet patch of grass is enough.

This is a good reminder that nature doesn't always need to be grand. While Googling "parks in America" serves up links to the National Park Service and striking photos of Yellowstone and the Great Smoky Mountains, your local pocket park can deliver the benefits we've touched on just as well as these faraway places.

"You can experience euphoria and deep reflection in those very intense natural away experiences—but they're not enough for a healthy life," William Sullivan from the University of Illinois explains to me. "What we need to do is find ways to have easy access to nature at every doorstep."

On the topic of green space and health research, he says that a little bit of the outdoors is so much better than none. With that in mind, here are some ideas for how to connect with any bit of green space you have access to—be it a large neighborhood park, modest backyard, or patch of city grass.

The Practice

IF YOU HAVE 5–10 MINUTES:

Take a tech-free microbreak.

If the sight of grass and the sound of birds immediately put us at ease, our tech does the opposite. Even though scrolling through social media or reading an article online seems like a relaxing enough way to spend a few minutes, the psychologists I've talked to agree that it drains cognitive resources. "People use those activities as a break—as a way to relax or destress. And what's actually happening is that those activities are putting them at an even greater attentional deficit," Jason Duvall, a lecturer at the University of Michigan Program in the Environment, tells me. "If you have people take cognitive functioning tests before and after those activities, it's very likely they would perform worse afterwards."

On the other hand, looking at greenery for as little as forty seconds at a time seems to improve mental capacity, based on findings from Australia.[31] In that research, 150 university students took cognition tests after looking over a computer image of a bare patch of roof or a green roof covered in a garden for forty-second spurts. On average, the students who looked at the green roof image made fewer errors after their microbreaks than those who looked at the bare roof: proof that sometimes letting yourself rest (with nature in sight) is the most productive thing you can do.

So instead of mindlessly scrolling (which might not be so mindless after all), take your next short break from work, chores, childcare, and so forth in a park or patch of grass if you have one near home. If you can't get outside, look out the window for a minute or so and just let the mind settle on any green you can see. Whatever you do, leave the phone behind.

Do an open-monitoring meditation.

See if meditating outside makes the practice any easier for you to stick with by heading to a local park or quiet grassy area where you feel safe enough to close your eyes or soften your gaze for a few minutes. In an environment as engaging and dynamic as a park, the point isn't to tune out your surroundings. Instead of telling yourself to focus on your breath or only pay attention to how your exhale feels on your upper lip, feel free to let your attention latch onto whatever comes its way.

Say you see a drop of water fall onto a surface, for example. You might allow yourself to consider how its ripples are a metaphor for the benefits of mindfulness expanding out and out and out into the rest of your life. This type of open-monitoring (versus focused-attention) meditation lends nature room to attract your attention in its signature effortless way—and in doing so, help you relax into the moment and shed stress.

Get your head in the clouds.

There's no need to wait for a clear day to head to the park. When's the last time you ventured outside for the sole purpose of cloudspotting for cloud-spotting's sake? The next opportunity you have to squeeze in some outdoor time, bring a blanket and let your eye follow the sky.

Crisp cumulus (those cotton-candy puffs that form discernable shapes) aren't the only clouds worth spotting. See what you can find in the altocumulus (the droplets of clouds that form a patterned blanket higher in the sky), or even the contrails (condensation trails left by planes). Pretor-Pinney of the Cloud Appreciation Society says that there's value in all of it: "To be a cloudspotter is to be open to what's happening in the sky," he says. "It's more about shifting a perspective and seeing what's beautiful and exotic in the mundane, the everyday that's around you."

Take your time (notice how this one gets an hour and not five minutes), and watch how the scene up above changes from one moment to the next. Let it be a practice in doing something that has no pressure attached. As Pretor-Pinney points out in *The Cloudspotter's Guide,* Aristotle was onto something when he likened clouds to dreams—they only come once expectation has been dropped.

Take a cue from kids and consider the park your playground.

Some parks include a separate area for childhood play, complete with monkey bars, slides, maybe a swing set or two. But as the cloudspotting ritual suggests, this sense of childlike wonder doesn't need to leave us once we reach adulthood—and it doesn't need to be relegated to a jungle gym.

The next time you visit a park, consider what it would mean to make it your playground. When you step into that environment, what's the first thing your body wants to do before your mind says no? Sleep in the sun?

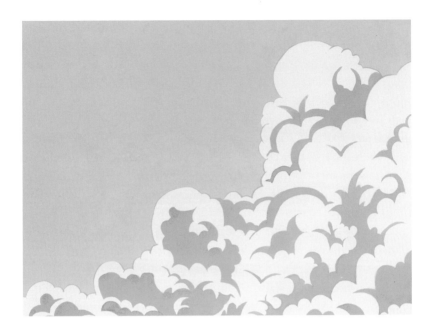

Take off your shoes and put your feet in the grass? Let yourself drop any mask and return to childhood, before you were told what to do and how to act, or the right way to play.

Collect a record of birdsongs over time.

Nature provides a break from the monotony of our indoor lives. And paying attention to the birds in your area can help you recognize its dynamic passing of time. When you go to the park, your backyard, or any other green space where you can pick up some birdsongs, listen in. Like Eleanor Ratcliffe had people do in her study, question what particular songs make you feel or remember. Are there any tunes you really love? Any that you really don't like at all?

Then, track how the music changes throughout the day, month, and year. Which birds around you migrate in the winter and return in spring? You might notice that birdsongs change with the passing of hours (they tend to reach a peak around dawn and then slowly taper until picking up again at dusk) and the shifting of weather patterns (birds don't like to sing in the rain; clouds can delay their calls; and heavy winds muddle their messages). Their songs also change based on their location, and regional dialects are as apparent in birds as they are in humans.[32] City birds need to speak up the most if they want to transcend the human noise and tend to sing at unnaturally high frequencies to make themselves heard over cars, construction, and people.[33] Human interventions like streetlamps can also throw off their sense of time, and male birds near streetlights have been shown to start singing earlier in the day than those who follow nature's lighting cues.[34]

Keeping track of these myriad changes provides a new way to connect with your environment. It also reinforces the very human lesson that things are always moving along, no matter how stagnant they can sometimes feel.

Engage with your walks in new ways.

When we head to the park equipped with curiosity, we're more likely to be rewarded with moments of wonder. One study by Jason Duvall at the University of Michigan found that people who followed "awareness plans" on outdoor walks tended to rate their environment more positively than those who walked without awareness plans.[35] These simple plans prompted the walkers to take on new personas in their environments, such as an artist on the hunt for beauty in everyday things. The results suggest that actively looking for something when you're out in green space might help you perceive your surroundings as satisfying.

You can approach park experiences with a more curious attitude by pretending you're a painter looking for your next landscape, a botanist on the hunt for a unique plant species, or a writer searching for a lively scene to put into words.

In adopting a fresh perspective, you also might find yourself noticing new details in old scenery. "You can go out and discover things that you didn't see before and see that there's richness that's available to you," Duvall says of the value of going into nature with an awareness plan of your own. "It adds another layer to the experience."

Create your own personal park . . .

Don't have any parks close to you? You can also bring the qualities of green space home by turning your yard into a personal refuge. Apply the principles of evolutionary theory to make it inherently calming: leave some grassy areas open to boost the yard's sense of expansiveness, and create retreat zones by placing seating under tree canopies. Add the sound of running water (and attract local wildlife) with a birdbath. Finally, put your own touches on it with your favorite fragrant native plants—bonus points if they transport you to a particular memory. Think of the finished product like a recharging station: the place you go to take a quick break away from it all.

Beyond delivering some of the calming, prosocial benefits outlined in this chapter, your at-home park can make way for a therapeutic new outdoor hobby: gardening. Gardening combines the innately calming qualities of nature with physical exertion, making it an effective form of exercise that you can do at any age. Improved cognitive function[36] and decreased stress[37] are just some of the reasons to garden regularly, especially as you get older. One study on 2,805 sixty-plus folks in Australia found that daily gardeners tended to have a 36 percent lower risk of hospital or nursing home admission for dementia than those who didn't tend to plants.[38]

. . . or grow a houseplant corner.

In his work as a horticultural therapist, Matthew Wichrowski rolls a cartful of greenery across NYU's Department of Rehabilitation Medicine, popping into patient rooms to allow them to plant, touch, and tend to plants of all kinds. Anecdotally, he's seen that gardening is a calming activity to do during otherwise stressful stays—and he's got some research under his belt to back this up: in his study on 107 cardiac rehabilitation inpatients,[39] those who did horticulture therapy tended to report a better mood and lower heart rate after sessions than those who did traditional rehab therapy.

Wichrowski tells me houseplants can be therapeutic outside the hospital setting too. An at-home plant corner, complete with a few different greenery varieties, can serve a similar function to a park or backyard garden. It's a place to go to take a break whenever you start yawning, reading the same text over again, or showing other signs of fatigue. Wichrowski recommends sitting with your plants and "just being with them a little bit." Notice any new growth or coloring, check out their patterns and textures, and let them bring you back to the present. If you're feeling really stressed, he adds, you can combine this with a quick meditation, breathing exercise, or visualization.

Connect to landscapes past.

Given the innate human attraction to green space, this landscape in particular lends itself to revisiting history and exploring tradition.

If you have older relatives, ask them about the parks or neighborhood spaces that they frequented growing up. Go through old photos together and see if the nature in the background reminds you of the places your family still visits today. If you're the oldest in your lineage, do this ritual with younger relatives. Consider which landscape preferences have been passed down through the generations, and which ones have shifted with the times.

Journal on the park's themes.

Parks and grasslands are inherently familiar places we can go to connect with each other and ourselves. Answer these questions and prompts to dig up how the landscape's themes of community, mindfulness, and discovery play out in your life. You won't be sharing the answers with anyone, so no need to make them eloquent or even coherent. Just let your thoughts flow through you onto the page, and notice if any new insights come through in the process.

- What do you do when you need to relax? How does doing that thing make you feel in the short and long term?

- Do you feel like you're a part of your community? If you were to choose one way to become more involved, what would it be?

- If you could take on a completely different persona, who would you be? Write it down, then consider how you could incorporate more of this imaginary life into your real life.

- When was the last time you truly did nothing? How did it feel, and when can you do it again?

The Action

Though sometimes modest in appearance, parks directly support our health and set the scene for beneficial activities. They are not a landscape to take for granted or abuse. Research confirms that people are more likely to avoid parks—and miss out on the mental, physical, and social benefits that come with them—if they consider them unsightly, damaged, or unsafe.[40] Having access to a park isn't necessarily enough to boost your health; it needs to be a clean and welcoming one. Here are a few ways to advocate for and protect green space in your community and beyond.

Habitat Loss

Humans aren't the only species that feels at home in grassy lands. Many land animals also flock to open green spaces that have food, water, and shelter—though they are increasingly becoming harder and harder to find.

According to a 2018 report by the National Wildlife Federation,[41] up to a third of America's species are vulnerable to extinction, and 1,661 species of native plants and animals are now on the endangered species list. Habitat loss is a major driver of extinction and will continue to threaten wildlife as long as grassy lands are converted to cities, suburbs, and farms.

Most of the resulting communities and farms are too developed, too fragmented, just too unnatural to support animal life. While some species can survive and adapt to these changes, others aren't able to do so quickly enough. According to the United Nations, up to one million species could go extinct in the coming decades.[42]

Designating more federal and state protected land would help us get back on track, as habitat loss is about half as likely to occur there than on private land (refer to the mountain section for information on how to advocate for protected lands).[43] In the meantime, we can take individual action to protect grassland habitats, and it starts in our own backyard.

The Mindset Shift:
"I know my yard isn't just for me."

While you might love the look of your perfectly manicured lawn, your local critters don't. Actually, they find it pretty boring.

The ideal land for wildlife like butterflies, birds, and bees has plenty of food, water, and shelter. As Susannah Lerman, a research ecologist for the US Forest Service, puts it to me, animals need a place where they can "eat and not be eaten." A yard full of short, green grass that's constantly being snipped and treated with chemical herbicides or pesticides just doesn't cut it.

Homeowners who want their yards to be more conducive to wildlife should model them after grasslands that exist in nature. Think less artificial turf and more food (nuts, pollen, berries), water (birdbaths, rain gardens), and cover (dense shrubs, evergreen trees). To find out what plant species your local wildlife will love, check out the National Audubon Society and the National Wildlife Federation websites. Choose native vegetation when you can—and encourage neighbors to do the same—as it will foster more regional habitat diversity. "If we keep on all having the same type of yard, that is, one dominated with manicured lawn, then we're going to have the same species visiting our yards across the US," Lerman explains.

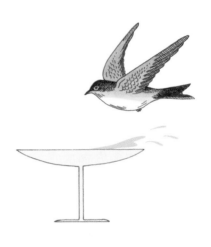

Once your yard is ready, let it get a little wild. Don't treat it with synthetics and don't mow it constantly (Lerman's research has found that mowing every two weeks instead of weekly tends to be better for bees[44]). If you're feeling really daring, embrace the "mullet effect" (short in the front, long in the back) and don't mow your backyard at all. When the ecologist Ilkka Hanski let his modest backyard in Finland grow completely wild, 375 plant species, including 2 endangered species, flocked there.[45]

The finished product can be a home base for local species and a refueling spot for critters on the go. And as discussed earlier in the chapter, having these species around to watch and observe might boost your mood too.

Neglect & Overuse

Just like local wildlife doesn't appreciate overly manicured areas, it doesn't appreciate overrun ones either. When patches of community parks and grasslands fall into disarray, the creatures who use them suffer.

We often hear about the deadly consequences of sea critters mistaking ocean plastic for food, but similar mishaps occur with land animals. When litter collects in parks, for example, birds can confuse it for nest-building materials. Conservationists have found candy wrappers, cigarette filters, and plastic packaging—as well as more peculiar items like plastic shovels, flags, and polyester hats—peeking out of nests around the world, where they have the potential to entangle or choke birds and their chicks.[46] Our waste can trap other park frequenters, like squirrels and racoons, too.

Erosion is another concern with overused and undermaintained parks. When foot traffic is so high that people trample grassland to the point of depletion, the ground underneath loses some of its ability to absorb water. Once it's prone to flooding, the land can become more damaged and less hospitable to wildlife (and humans) with each passing storm.

The Mindset Shift:
"I am aware of and concerned about
the waste around me."

Nothing opens your eyes to a litter problem like a park cleanup. While suburban folks might not have much trash to report in their parks, city dwellers may find tons in their high-trafficked green areas.

Today, I just spotted ninety-six pieces of trash (including a pencil, a Red Bull can, and a seashell?) in a block-long strip of grass along my neighborhood park. There were piles of leaves obscuring a lot of the ground, so the true tally is probably even higher.

Noticing and picking up one hundred pieces of trash may seem like a small, insignificant, and largely useless thing to do considering the scope of our planet's problems. But in my experience, cleaning up litter is an individual action that ladders up to real change. In fact, I'd credit a trash cleanup with starting my career in sustainability. I walked away from a community pickup in high school feeling so energized by the fact that I had done *something*—even if it was, in hindsight, a small thing—that I knew I wanted to keep doing more.

So, no, picking up a few pieces of trash the next time you go to the park won't solve the climate crisis. But it will remind you of your own agency and potential to do something that might.

Injustice & Inequity

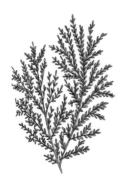

Low-income, minority neighborhoods are less likely to contain green space than high-income, white neighborhoods.[47] The parks that do exist in majority non-white areas are, on average, half as large and nearly five times as crowded as parks that serve a majority-white population.[48] The ones in primarily low-income neighborhoods are four times smaller on average—25 acres versus 101 acres—than parks that sit near high-income households, according to a report by the Trust for Public Land.

Instead of greenery, disenfranchised communities are more likely to be filled with pollution: landfills, highways, and industrial facilities disproportionately fall according to race and income.[49]

This inequity is nothing new: "There's so much historical connection to it," Jennifer D. Roberts, an assistant professor at the University of Maryland School of Public Health, tells me. If you look at redlined maps of the United States, created in the early twentieth century to break the country into zones that would help mortgage lenders identify areas of economic opportunity (often white neighborhoods), you'll notice a disturbing trend. The "green" (best) or "blue" (still desirable) zones are, to this day, the ones that have the most well-kept parks. The "red" zones areas that had a large minority population and were deemed unfit for investment, remain some of the least green areas of the country.[50] "You'll see a lot of neighborhoods that were just constantly disinvested or victimized because of urban renewal or redlining," Roberts explains. "The placement, investment, and protection of parks and other green spaces fall right along these residential settlement patterns.

"I see this in my hometown of Buffalo, New York. Our treasured Delaware Park, which was designed by Frederick Law Olmsted, is in the middle of these green and blue areas. You can constantly see these kinds of things. . . . They don't happen randomly."

Many of the parks that do exist in low-income and minority neighborhoods tend to be of poor quality—they lack greenery, are not well maintained, and are closer to threats like traffic exhaust. These "green deserts" (also known as recreation deserts or park deserts) are linked to poor health outcomes, as are more commonly known food deserts. Just like the snack aisle of a gas station can't compare to a fully stocked grocery store, a run-down and dangerous park doesn't afford the same opportunities as a pristine one. It's healthy in theory but not nourishing in practice.

This lack of quality green space is likely one reason that those in poor and minority communities are more likely to fall ill to lifestyle diseases like hypertension, obesity, and heart disease as well as pollution-related illnesses like COPD, asthma, and some cancers than those in affluent communities.[51] They are also more exposed to the threats of climate change. Rising temperatures feel even more unbearable when you don't have shady trees around your home, or a park nearby where you can escape some heat. Neighborhoods that are poor and have more residents of color can be five to twenty degrees Fahrenheit hotter in summer than wealthier, whiter parts of the same city in major US metropolises like Baltimore, Dallas, Denver, Miami, Portland, and New York.[52]

Bringing more high-quality parks into these communities could therefore be an equigenic intervention[53]—one that has a disproportionately positive effect on public health.

The Mindset Shift: "Nature is for everyone, and it's meant to be shared."

According to a report by the Trust for Public Land (TPL),[54] 11.2 million people in the one hundred most populated cities in the US didn't have a park within a ten-minute walk of their home in 2020. The nonprofit estimates that fifteen hundred strategically placed green spaces in dense US cities like Los Angeles, Houston, and Miami would solve access issues for up to 5 million of them. That number is totally achievable—with community support. "There's never a project that we make happen in a vacuum," Jeannette (Nette) Compton, director of strategy at TPL, tells me. "Nothing happens without everyday people deciding to invest in their communities and put in the time and the passion to make that happen."

If you're looking to advocate for more green in your area, a first step can be TPL's online ParkScore Index,[55] which will show you how park access in your community stacks up to the national median. The resource also maps out where existing parks are in your area and where new ones could go to serve the most people.

The next step is to build your coalition, Compton says. "Having a community that is organized around what they want and can articulate what they want is incredibly powerful." Equipped with data and supported by others, you can reach out to your local representatives to advocate for more funding to be put aside for the creation, protection, and upkeep of parks. "You don't have to let planning and land use passively happen to you," she adds. "It's for you, and it's for you to take ownership over. You have that right."

If you're not quite ready to spearhead your own movement, there are existing groups you can get involved with. Greening vacant lots, for example, is one undertaking that's becoming more popular in the US and abroad. Many large cities now have networks of folks working to convert abandoned property into public parks and gardens, so poke around to see if you can volunteer to tend to existing spaces or join a new renovation project.

Finally, keep an eye out for land conservation measures that are on the ballot. Amid the polarization and chaos of the 2020 election, Compton shares that all the twenty-six ballot measures the TPL supported—across states red and blue—were voted into law, a testament to the power of community organizing and the wide appeal of green space.

How fitting that so many of the actions we can take to protect parks are rooted in community—just the thing that these spaces help cultivate.

CHAPTER TWO

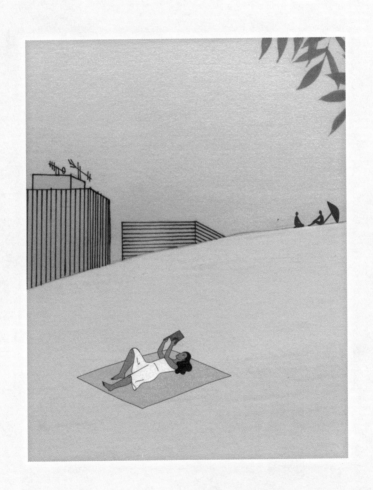

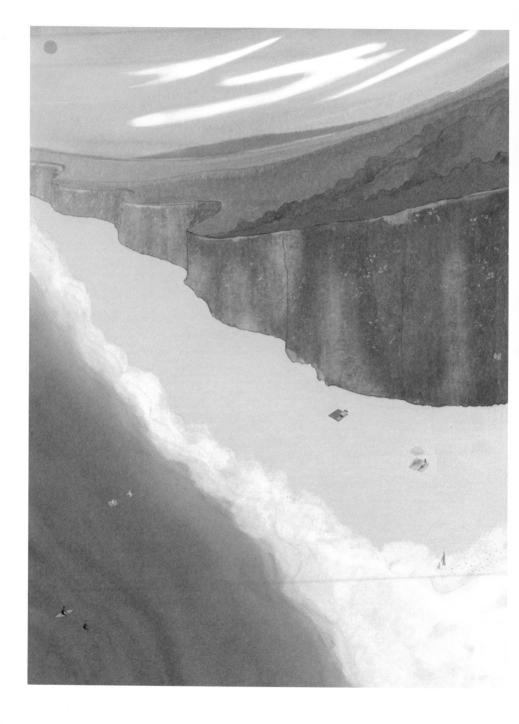

OCEANS & COASTS

memory, relaxation, surrender

I look to where the pale blue of the horizon meets its more vibrantly hued friend, the sea. The waves sound out as they come in contact with the rocky coastline, their notes building on each other like a layer cake. I feel a sudden heaviness as I listen to them, an urge to shut my eyes and lie down. The light wind coming in brings me back to the present, and I look around to see who else I'm sharing the beach with today. First, to the water, where a man sucks in a chestful of air, urgently dunks his head under the surface, and comes up a few seconds later in breathless triumph. Rinse, repeat. Closer to shore, there's a couple in beach chairs pulled just past the water's edge, their ankles cut off by the deep blue. Behind them, a group of bicyclists roll past, slowing down ever so slightly to take in the view over their shoulder.

It makes me think back to the similar cast of characters I saw during my childhood growing up in a beach community in New England. The beach was where my friends and I would meet to sprawl out and catch up—the whoosh of the waves a backdrop to our excited confessions. The sun would beat down on us, like it beats down on me today, until we'd had enough and finally felt ready to splash in.

The Remedy

More than 70 percent of our planet is covered in oceans, enchanting land-scapes that mask worlds unseen. The shore is where we can start to wade into them. As of 2007, roughly 40 percent of people on Earth lived within one hundred kilometers (sixty-two miles) of a coastline.[1] Even more un-doubtedly headed to the beach for vacation, as the coasts have long been associated with relaxation. Clearly, something happens to us when we taste salt air, hear the sound of gulls, and feel waves lap at our ankles. A relatively new field of "blue space research" is starting to uncover what exactly that something is and how we can find more of it.

For Many People, Coasts Are the Most Relaxing Landscape of Them All

Nature health research often splits the outdoors into two categories: green space, landscapes with tree cover or grass, like the parks we explored in the last chapter; and blue space, any body of water, natural or human-made. Green space caught scientists' attention first. It wasn't until the early 2000s that anyone started to look beyond the ocean's health risks (algal blooms and other pathogens, deadly deep-sea creatures, riptides) and into its potential.

BlueHealth, run out of the University of Exeter Medical School, is one group leading the way on this research. One of their more sweeping discov-eries is that England's coastal population tends to be happier on average than those who live inland. After analyzing census data on urban adults throughout England, the team found that those who lived within walking distance of the coast tended to have better self-reported general health than those who didn't.[2] And interestingly enough, after adjusting for in-come,[3] the BlueHealth team found that adults in the lowest-income house-holds were significantly less likely to report feelings of anxiety or depression if they lived within five kilometers of the coast than those in the same in-come bracket who lived over fifty kilometers from the sea. For those with higher incomes, mental health was not related to how close they lived to the coast, suggesting that coastal access could help mitigate health inequalities between socioeconomic groups.

George MacKerron, a senior lecturer in economics at the University of Sussex, also has evidence of blue space's ability to promote happiness and relieve stress. (You'll notice that much of the research in this section is happening in the UK, which is surrounded by water and run by a government that has historically been financially supportive of such work.) Throughout MacKerron's "Mappiness" study, almost sixty-six thousand people in the UK downloaded a cellphone app that randomly pinged them to check in on their self-reported happiness levels twice a day.[4] GPS data showed MacKerron's team where people were when they were pinged. About 4.5 million responses were tracked over seven years. According to preliminary data collected early in the study, respondents felt 1.8 to 2.7 notches happier on a 0–100 scale when they were in green space compared with urban environments. When they were by wetlands and estuaries, they reported feeling 6 notches happier. I asked MacKerron why these areas were happiness hotspots, and he told me he suspected that it had something to do with their mix of green space, wildlife, and blue space. A mix of green and blue seems to be inherently appealing.

More research from England on over four thousand participants found that people rated their recent visits to the coast as being more restorative than those to any other landscape.[5]

Another study out of Ireland found that simply looking at the ocean can be enough to soothe. In that research, subjects who were fifty and older who lived with the most unobstructed views of the coastline tended to report the most beneficial mental health outcomes.[6] A similar study in Japan found that those who had seaside views reported higher positive psychological effects than those who didn't.[7] These views elicited feelings of awe and peace of mind, in women and the elderly in particular. And when they put people in an fMRI machine and peeked at how different landscape images affected brain activity, researchers in Taiwan found that ocean photos tended to have the most restorative effect, by reducing activity in the mind's visual and attentional focus areas.[8]

Why Living Near (or Just Looking at) the Water Is So Soothing

There are a few theories as to why a day at the beach makes us feel more positive, hopeful, and relaxed. And like waves on the surface, they might coalesce into one explanation.

A more straightforward hypothesis is that ocean landscapes provide a nice backdrop for exercise—and physical activity of any kind releases endorphins in the body and sends more oxygen to the brain, improving cognition and enhancing mood.[9] Walking and running along the coast, swimming out into the water, and throwing a Frisbee™ in the sand are all common beach practices. One BlueHealth study lends scientific credibility to the idea that we move more when we're by the water: after analyzing survey data on how those in the UK spent their time in various natural environments,[10] researchers concluded that while visits to green space were associated with more rigorous physical activity, Brits expended more energy by the coast because they tended to stay there for longer. Separate research has found that exercising near blue space also seems to lead to a greater boost in self-esteem than exercising in green space, for reasons not entirely clear.[11]

Even when we're standing still, though, there's value to be found in the fresh ocean air. Some researchers claim that when water molecules pinball off each other, negative ions form in the air (also known as the waterfall effect[12]), and these might ease depressive feelings[13] and activate our body's natural killer cells[14] to fight infection the same way that trees in the forest do (more on that in the forest and trees chapter)—though there's some debate about this.

Others think that we can chalk up a lot of the ocean's healing touch to its high salt content. This salt therapy hypothesis traces back centuries, to when European doctors would tell patients who suffered from lung diseases to take a whiff of salty sea air or a pint of ocean water.[15] While thalassotherapy[16]—the therapeutic use of seawater and its contents—was largely phased out with the advent of antibiotics, the ocean and direct sunlight are still a legitimate medicine for those who suffer from inflammatory skin conditions like eczema and psoriasis.

Mathew White, a prolific environmental psychologist at BlueHealth who has authored dozens of studies on oceans and human health, guesses that the visual patterns of the waves—the way they invite us away from our thoughts and give us another point on which to focus—play a role too.[17] In keeping with attention restoration theory, they are dynamic enough to hold our attention but not so stimulating as to cause mental fatigue, making them a helpful tool for disengaging with some of our inner chatter, at least for a little while. Their soothing blue color, a universal favorite that encourages creativity and connectivity,[18] according to cognitive therapy, further adds to their appeal.

And then, there's the sound of the water: the gentle whoosh that, as the marine biologist Wallace J. Nichols points out in his book *Blue Mind*,[19] mimics the acoustics of the womb—fluid and rhythmic and familiar. By this logic, when we dip into the water and let ourselves float, it's not unreasonable that our bodies would feel an innate sense of coming home.

As We Wade Deeper into the Water, We Discover More of Its Benefits

In the emerging field of ocean therapy, doctors and researchers explore how a plunge in the water can heal wounds of all kinds. Case studies on group surf therapy—which layers surf lessons with elements of talk therapy and mindfulness training—have found that it can help ease symptoms of depression, anxiety, and PTSD in active duty veterans;[20] improve emotional regulation and outlook among at-risk youth in poor communities in South Africa;[21] and promote better physical health and overall fitness for children with disabilities.

Easkey Britton, an ocean health researcher and one of Ireland's first big-wave surfers, is working to measure the practice's value in more qualitative terms. Over two summers, she guided a group of children and teens with autism through surf therapy lessons paired with a unique technique known as body mapping.[22] Before each lesson, the kids completed a mindful body-scanning practice and then used sand and other items found on the beach to map out how their bodies felt that day. After surfing, the group created one large, collective body map in the sand together to show how they were all feeling post-lesson. Britton and her team found that the evolution of the kids' maps "revealed shifts in their sense of identity, self-awareness and connection to nature, improving confidence, interpersonal and communication skills for those with low self-esteem." When reflecting on their lessons, the kids reported happiness and freedom ("It makes me feel like I'm in space, I feel floaty and free," one said), a sense of community and equality ("Everyone falls off their board," another added), and pride ("I can do anything if I put my mind to it").

Natalie Small, a licensed marriage and family therapist, has found similar success working with a different group of surfers: grown women overcoming trauma. The therapists in her organization, Groundswell Community Project, use surfing as a tool to help these women reacquaint with, and ultimately reclaim, their bodies. After every wave caught, Small tells me, participants are encouraged to pause, soak in their accomplishment, and celebrate it with the group. From there, they can carry the lessons learned on the water back into their everyday lives. "It helps build new neurological pathways in the brain that build increased emotional regulation and stronger sense of self," Small says, adding that many Groundswell therapists have seen their participants make breakthroughs on the board.

Surfing isn't the only form of ocean therapy: therapeutic sailing and swimming programs are also picking up, suggesting that any kind of immersion in the water can help give us a healthier outlook on what's happening back on land.

How Memories
Shape Our Time at the Shore

In addition to promoting a positive mood and restoring the mind, the ocean can have a relaxing, almost dreamlike quality to it. After monitoring the sleep patterns of over one hundred people who walked for seven miles along either a coastal path or an inland one, Eleanor Ratcliffe (whom we met in the parks chapter) found that while both groups reported feeling significantly happier after their walks, the coastal group slept for an average of forty-seven minutes longer the night after the outing than they did the night before.[23] The inland group slept for twelve minutes longer than the night before. Both paths were a similar level of difficulty, so what was it about the coastal walk that made people more relaxed? Ratcliffe thought it might have something to do with the coast's ability to elicit memories. Those who walked next to the water said that they used the time to reflect on past stages in their life more than the inland group did. "The coast was seen as a greater opportunity for introspection and reflective thought, linking to concepts of a psychologically restorative or beneficial environment," she writes in her report. This is just one small study commissioned by a nature organization, and it wasn't peer-reviewed by other researchers, so we need to take its findings with a grain of sea salt. But the notion that the beach can recall relaxing memories and help us take a journey not just physically but in the mind too doesn't seem so far off.

But what if you don't have many coastal memories to travel back to? Anyone who is brand-new to a landscape might need time to warm up to it—and this seems especially true with the ocean. History and lived experience play a huge role in how we perceive the water and how comfortable we feel around it. Someone who grew up near the coast will have developed a stronger relationship to it than someone who has never been near the ocean before and might find its loud waves, strong pull, and frothy splash zone to be terrifyingly unfamiliar.

Alex Smalley, a PhD researcher at the University of Exeter who studies how people respond to digital re-creations of the natural world, has made an interesting discovery on this link between landscape and memory. As part of an ongoing project called Virtual Nature, Smalley broadcasted soundscapes of various abiotic sounds (generated from the landscape, such as the wind or waves), biotic sounds (which come from animals), and spoken word (poetic interpretations of nature, read aloud) as part of a BBC drama podcast series called *Forest 404*. Around eight thousand people who tuned in to the series answered questions about how these sounds made them feel, particularly how therapeutic they thought the sounds might be in times of stress or fatigue. The conclusion: "Memories really seem to matter," Smalley tells me. "Across several studies, our data suggests that people find digital representations of nature more restorative if they have lived experience of the natural world."

Smalley gives the sounds of the waves as an example: while a photo of a beach in Barbados may look beautiful, it won't necessarily remind you of your childhood visits to the coast of Rhode Island. Its sounds, though, are up for interpretation and easier to match up with your memories.

If you hear the sounds of calm waves lapping on a beach, your brain can take you to whatever beach sits in your mind—assuming one exists. Smalley's research suggests that people who didn't grow up with access to a beach wouldn't necessarily enjoy or get as much out of natural ocean soundscapes. "We think this is an immensely important argument for reconnecting people to natural spaces and places," he adds.

This isn't to say that newcomers to the coast can't reap any of its benefits. Memories alone don't need to make or break a nature experience. But if you're someone for whom the water conjures up images of Jaws and sea monsters, know that it might take you some time to warm up to this landscape and begin to form new associations with it.

Natalie Small recalls working with one woman who was new to the water and afraid to go below the surface until one of her last surf therapy ses-

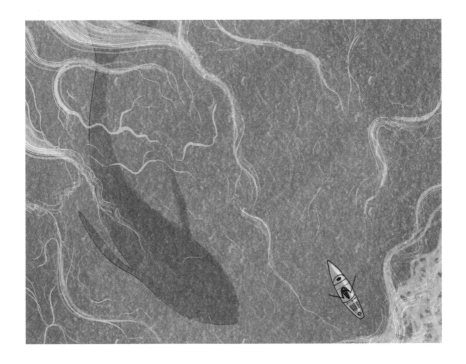

sions. When she emerged after mustering up the courage to dip her head in, her face was full of tears.

"Once she was able to speak," Small tells me, "she shared how she finally understood what was going on inside of her. Through that experience of going under a wave for her first time, she recognized that all the whitewater and chaos is just on top of the ocean. Underneath, there's depth, stillness, peace. 'That's how I am,' the woman said. 'My brain is so full of chaos and constantly reacting to triggers from my trauma, but, just like the ocean, the whitewater is only on the surface, the chaos in my brain is only on the surface. I've been stuck in the whitewater for so long. But going under that wave reminded me that I am more than whitewater. I have a deeper peace and stillness in me too. I can always dive deeper into myself. I just need to take a breath and go there.'"

This experience speaks to the ocean's more spiritual lessons. It is a teacher of duality, surrender and conquering, chaos and calm.

Roz Savage, a former management consultant who quit her desk job to reinvent herself and ended up becoming the first (and so far only) woman to row solo across the Atlantic, Pacific, and Indian Oceans, has lots of experience with rough surface waters. "I have a love-hate relationship with the ocean, having now spent 520-odd days and nights at sea," Savage tells me. Her first foray into cross-ocean rowing took place during a particularly stormy and miserable season on the Atlantic. "It seemed like the ocean knew the exact moment to send a huge wave crashing over me," she recalls to me. "I was taking it personally at the start. I tried to engage the ocean in a battle of wills, and that was my big humbling."

Practicing relinquishing control and finding small moments of surrender at sea were ultimately what made her voyage slightly more manageable. While the ocean never really calmed down, at a certain point its challenges started to show her what she was made of: "If everything had gone according to plan, I wouldn't have learned as much about myself."

The water acts as a mirror. We see ourselves reflected in it in a physical sense, and a more symbolic one too. In addition to potentially helping us stress less and feel happier, the ocean can strengthen our identity and willpower, reminding us that a little choppiness now and again is only natural.

The Practice

Luckily, you don't need to row thousands of miles to have a rich relationship with this landscape. To learn the water's lessons, you don't even need to dip your head under it if you don't want to. The following activities and rituals can help anyone—regardless of swimming skill level or access to a beach—find new ways to wade into the water's embrace.

Watch the pattern of the waves.

The ocean's surface, with its constant waves and unpredictable rips, imitates thought and emotion. While its movements can be erratic, each one eventually tapers out, just like each thought eventually leaves our consciousness. Every worry, even the ones that are six feet tall, frothing and foreboding, can someday find its end point on the shore.

With this in mind, we can take a cue from Mathew White's wave hypothesis and sit down by the coast, take a deep breath, and tune in to the pattern of the sea. As you do, turn your attention to the feeling of the surrounding moisture and wind on your skin, then the smell of the air. Try to follow one wave with your gaze. When you lose it, find another one to focus on. See if this quick break changes your perspective or allows you to leave something that was on your mind behind with the water.

Do a sit spot meditation.

Easkey Britton, the surfer and water therapy researcher, thinks that part of what makes the ocean special is the fact that it's so dynamic and ever-changing. Waves are energy you can ride only once. "Every time I engage with the ocean, it's like I'm discovering myself anew because the whole context is different," she says. The sea's charismatic nature makes it a good case study for a sensory meditation known as "sit spot."

- Choose a spot next to the water that you'll be able to access again. Then, sit down and close your eyes, taking a few moments to ground yourself in that place by listening to the sounds around you and the physical sensations on your body.

- When you're ready, open your eyes and home in on a small patch where the ocean meets the land. Notice what's coming in and out of the frame without judgment.

- Then, slowly expand your field of view, as if you're adding another layer to a bull's-eye target. Notice the sense of movement as you continue to broaden your gaze.

- Go back to your sit spot whenever you need a reminder of the ephemeral nature of our world, and our lived experience.

IF YOU HAVE AN HOUR:

Cleanse yourself.

If you feel comfortable enough in your swimming skills to take a plunge, make a mental list of things you're ready to send out to sea. Spend a few moments thinking about the habits, relationships, or thoughts that keep you stuck in some way. Then, as you enter the water, close your eyes and imagine it washing you of the items on your list. One by one, feel the waves carrying those little burdens away until they crash into the shore. If you're not as much of a swimmer, you can do this cleansing in the shallows too: wade into the water as far as you feel comfortable and wash your body and your burdens off handful by handful.

Reflect on your ocean memories.

Our early experiences of the water—positive or negative—seem to leave a strong imprint. What is your first memory of the ocean, or any body of water that felt massive to you at the time? Who were you with? Do you remember what the water looked like, what it felt like? What sorts of emotions come up when you play that memory back?

Reflecting on these questions can help you tease out how you feel about this landscape and why. Write them down in as much detail as possible and then try to play excavator: How do these memories affect how you approach the ocean today?

My earliest memory of the water was of almost drowning. I wasn't even walking yet; it was summer and my mother and I were up at a rental cottage. She was lounging on the dock, and the next thing she knew I was facedown in the water.

I just remember looking through clear water down at the sand. The way the sunlight came through the surface, creating these rainbowing ripples. It was a hot day and the water was so cool. I just remember beauty. The next image I have is of navy blue sneakers landing in front of me, this poof of silt and white shoelaces that weren't even tied, just wafting in the water.

My mom grabbed me and held me close to her. She was screaming. And then, apparently, I laughed. It was not traumatic for me. Water has been my favorite place ever since.

—JILL HEINERTH,
record-holding deep-sea cave diver

Then, visit the water again. This time, make it purely sensory. Feel into the way it looks, smells, and sounds in the now. Jill Heinerth, a record-holding cave diver who feels more comfortable in the water than on land, tells me she uses this mindfulness strategy when teaching adult swim classes to help students who have negative associations with the water separate the physical thing from the emotions they attach to it and start to discover a new appreciation for the deep blue.

Float to feel supported.

Anyone who's ever spent time floating in the ocean knows that relaxing sense of being held up, face pressed against the sky and body suddenly weightless beneath. Water is an equalizer; in it, anyone can access that transcendent, freeing feeling. It provides constant and undiscriminating support that can be hard to come by on dry land.

Flotation-REST, or reduced environmental stimulation therapy, seeks to mimic this experience indoors. When people float in Epsom salt pools enclosed in pitch-black rooms, there is anecdotal (and some scientific[24])

> My father was an ocean lifeguard, so from an early age I was exposed to the dangers of the water. He would always tell me, "You never turn your back on the ocean." He meant it in a physical sense: if you turned your back, a wave could come and take you.
>
> I treated the sea like some imaginary friend growing up, one that you've got to know how to play with. It's like a big dragon—you're not going to just run up and jump on it: you must treat it with respect. I always have what my father said in mind.
>
> And just when I start to forget, the ocean will give me a very quick reminder that it's a wild place and it's not our natural habitat. I think that deep respect brings you closer to the ocean in a way, because you treat it with dignity.
>
> —EMI KOCH,
> surfer, humanitarian, and social ecologist

evidence to show that it can relieve stress and anxiety by reducing sensory input to the nervous system. After an hour-long float session, participants in one 2018 study reported lower levels of stress, muscle tension, pain, and depression, and more serenity, relaxation, happiness, and overall well-being than they did before the session. The more anxious people were before they started floating, the more they seemed to get out of the experience.

The next time you have access to calm, salty water, hold your own therapy session by reserving time to just float. With your eyes closed and your body fully supported beneath you, free up your mind to wander.

IF YOU HAVE LONGER:

Improve your ocean literacy.

Most of us are taught the basics of on-land safety (e.g. look both ways before crossing the street) from a young age, but we might never learn ocean literacy the way that Emi Koch did. To develop a stronger relationship with the ocean, we need to backtrack and get to know it a little better first. Taking the time to learn about the tides and rip currents, the critters and plants, in our area can help make the water feel a little bit more predictable and a little bit less intimidating.

If you have a child, help them form their own friendship with the water by exposing them to it early. Whether it's a trip to the aquarium, a day by the coast, or a visit to the public pool, any positive early interaction with the water seems to be helpful down the line.

Learn a new skill in the water.

Surfing, bodyboarding, and even swimming may look like a conquest of the ocean at first glance, but in reality, these activities are a surrender to it. If you tense up or try to exert any control over the ocean as you're doing them, the water will win the fight every time. That's part of what's so rewarding about trying a new skill in this landscape: the water is a cocreator in the result. To tap into the sense of interconnectedness and accomplishment that surfers and other ocean athletes find so addictive, lean in to any opportunity to try a new water activity if you are able to do so.

Charge yourself by day . . .

To balance out the more relaxing sound quality of the ocean, imagine the sun's energy physically charging you the next time you're out on the beach. Lie down in the sand with your face to the sun and visualize yourself as a battery, collecting its charge and heat to be used at a later date. Feel into the heat of the sun as it moves up your body, starting in your toes and working its way toward your knees, then hips, then chest, and finally your head until, like a battery icon on a phone, you're fully charged. Hold on to this warmth and light, acknowledge that it is now a part of you, and consider a few ways to share with the world.

. . . and reflect by night.

This one requires some planning and access to a coastline after the sun goes down. Visit the water during an evening high tide, arriving a few minutes before the tide starts to go out. Stick your feet in the water and tune in to the feeling of the waves arriving and receding, leaving an imprint on your ankles. Notice how the tide gradually shifts and gets pulled away by the moon—how, a few inches at a time, it will eventually move down the beach.

There's a lot to be learned about flow and collaboration here. As the water moves away from your feet over the next few minutes, consider what these two forces look like in your own life. How does your mood, energy, or perspective tend to shift throughout the day? Does the transition feel free-flowing, or is it more abrupt? Does observing the water give you any kind of new perspective about how you can approach these shifts with more ease? What is your moon? In other words, what is the force that pulls you? It could be a person, a goal, an idea. What would it look like to move toward that force more effortlessly? Look to the surface of the water for support as you consider these questions.

Visit a water feature or add one to your home.

For inland dwellers, water features like fountains can be a decent stand-in for the open ocean, since they, too, carry waves and ripples that can hold our attention and potentially restore the mind.

If you have a nearby fountain, pond, or other type of water feature in your neighborhood, test out the theory by spending a few minutes sitting by it, paying special attention to its patterns and sounds. Or add a running water

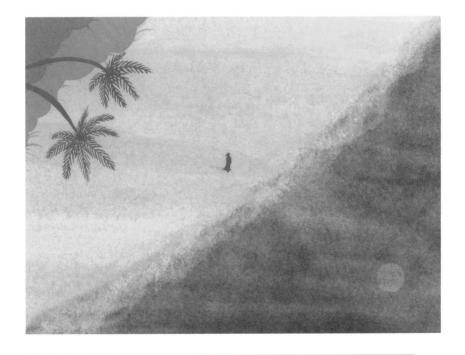

element to your home or garden—a tabletop fountain, a birdbath—to see if it makes the space feel more relaxing. Proponents of biophilic design,[25] a design philosophy that seeks to introduce nature elements in the built environment, assert that waterfalls, aquariums, reflections of water on another surface, and even imagery of water can add a soothing element to any space.

Listen to digital recordings of the coast.

Digital recordings of the hallmark whoosh of water can elicit similar feelings to the real deal. In 2017, researchers from Brighton and Sussex Medical School found that prerecorded nature sounds can prompt relaxation by helping listeners adopt a more outward-directed focus of attention—and the more stressed out someone is, the better they seem to work.[26]

As we learned from Alex Smalley earlier, we seem to have the most positive reactions to soundscapes that we enjoy and can attach a memory to. So if you're a beach fan, the next time you're stuck inside and feeling overwhelmed, try popping on one of the 183,000,000-plus recordings of ocean sounds on Google, closing your eyes, and taking a break in the mental seaside of your choosing. While extractions of nature can never quite live up to the real deal[27]—I love how Frances Kuo, whose research was introduced in the parks chapter, has described this: "Nature seems to be like a multivitamin. You can get different benefits from different kinds of exposure. . . . But to get all of them, you kind of have to be there"[28]—they're certainly better than nothing.

Take an Epsom salt bath.

Sitting in a bath while listening to your soundscape can add another sensory element to your immersion. Throw in some Epsom salts to further re-create the experience of being in the sea. As you settle in, close your eyes and let the sounds transport you out of your bathroom and onto a beach you may not have thought about for a while.

Make a rain date.

According to Alex Smalley's research, people also tend to consider sound-scapes that include audible wildlife, like birdsong, more therapeutic than those without it. Abiotic sounds of the landscape are enriched by the sounds of animals—as long as we perceive them as nonthreatening. So, the next time you're bummed out by a rainy beach day, remember that the sound of the raindrops hitting the water, the waves lapping on the shore, and the squawk of the seagulls signaling a change in pressure can combine into one incredibly soothing soundtrack. Be sure to open up your windows and take it all in.

Reframe your reminders of the beach.

I, like so many others, am a sucker for shells. Looking at them used to re-mind me of the beaches they came from and the people I enjoyed them with. But since reading Anne Morrow Lindbergh's account of a snail's shell she found during a solo vacation at the seashore in her book *Gift from the Sea*, I have a new perspective on these mementos.

> "His shell: It is simple; it is bare; it is beautiful. Small, only the size of my thumb, its architecture is perfect, down to the finest detail. . . . My shell is not like this, I think," she writes, using the shell as a metaphor for her own life as a busy mom. "How untidy it has become! Blurred with moss, knobby with barnacles, its shape is hardly recognizable any more. Surely, it had a shape once. It has a shape still in my mind. What is the shape of my life?"

She eventually moves beyond shells and marvels at the simplicity of ocean life in general: the landscape is not one of distractions or frivolities; it's the elements in their purest form. The beach is where we go to shed layers instead of don them, to reconnect with simpler pleasures. Now, when I look at my shells, I'm a little envious of their modesty and simplicity and wonder how I can streamline my own life in pursuit of the same.

Journal on the ocean's themes.

The human-ocean relationship is a case study in trust, control, and surrender. You can reflect on how these themes play out in your own life with ocean-inspired journaling prompts. Set aside some time (perhaps with wave sounds playing in the background and a photo of your favorite beach nearby?) to free-write on the following questions.

- What were you doing the last time you felt totally focused on the present moment?

- When's the last time you did something brand-new? What was it? How did you feel afterward?

- What's one challenge you are currently facing? How can you surrender some control over the situation?

- Write a detailed description of a natural landscape that makes you feel totally at ease. Keep this place in mind to return to the next time you're stressed or overwhelmed.

The Action

Perhaps unsurprisingly, we innately prefer clean, abundant aquatic environments to dirty, overharvested ones. Litter seems to negate some of the coast's psychological restorative benefits,[29] and people report greater reductions in heart rate and increases in self-reported mood when looking at species-rich aquatic tanks versus partially full or empty ones in aquarium settings.[30] So in addition to being a nice way to thank Mother Ocean, living a more sustainable seaside life could eventually come back to boost your own health too. Once you've taken to the water to be held by its waves or get lost in its soundtrack, it's time to pay back the favor. Here are three of the most pressing threats to ocean health today, and what we can do about them.

Plastic Waste

It's hard to say with certainty how much plastic from land ends up in the ocean each year, but one of the most-cited research models pegged it as between 4.8 and 12.7 million metric tons.[31] For some context, the midpoint of that estimate—8 million metric tons—would cover an area thirty-four times the size of Manhattan ankle-deep in plastic waste.[32] (And I thought New York was dirty already.) Ocean-bound plastic starts as things like litter on the street, micro-fibers in clothing, or polymers in rubber tires before being washed away in rainfall or flushed down sewer systems into the sea. In developing countries with poor waste management systems, much of it comes directly from landfills.

Some of plastic waste's impacts on the ocean are visible: by this point, we've all cringed at pictures of turtles trapped in six-pack rings or fish with bellies full of plastic straws. But there's another plastic threat that remains largely unseen and unknown. Over time, as everlasting plastics degrade into tinier and tinier pieces, they eventually hit microplastic status, when they are five millimeters long or smaller. We can't always see these microplastics with the naked eye, but we can go ahead and assume that they're everywhere: in the air, in our food, on land, and, yes, all across our oceans. As much as 99 percent of the plastic in our ocean is invisible.[33] Emily Penn, the cofounder of eXXpedition, a series of all-women sailing voyages studying the impact of plastic pollution on the ocean, tells me that when her teams looks at samples of ocean water using a microscope, it's basically impossible to tell the difference between plastic microparticles and plankton, both equally abundant under a lens. "It makes you really start to understand the problem," Penn tells me. "Actually, there's not one big island of plastic in the middle of the ocean. It's these tiny pieces that are so hard to see that we can't even distinguish them, let alone the fish."

It's too soon to tell how these microplastics will go on to affect human and aquatic health in the long term (since plastic is, in the grand scheme of things, a relatively recent invention). Still, the fact that they have become so ubiquitous is reason enough for concern.

The Mindset Shift:
"I know that there is no such thing as 'away.'"

This phrase "no such thing as away" gets used a lot in the zero-waste community. It's a reminder that something doesn't just disappear when you throw it in the trash or recycling bin. When I hear it, my mind usually travels to the ocean; I imagine a patch of beach that's so covered in layers and layers of the plastics that I've used over the years that the sand no longer peeks through. This is an incredibly dark way to think about plastic waste—and if I've just pushed you to picture the same thing, I apologize—but it's effective!

Whenever I have this vision, it does nudge me to consider whether I really need to buy that new thing that's packaged in plastic, since I know there's no way of truly getting rid of it. Some forms of single-use plastic that I find easier to avoid are the produce baggies at the supermarket (throw loose produce in the cart and wash it when you get home, or bring your own cloth bags to the store); plastic wraps (store food in jars, reuse aluminum foil, or invest in some reusable silicone baggies or beeswax food wraps instead); coffee and beverage bottles (pack your own drinks!); and some cleaning and personal care packaging (buy cleaners in refillable bottles, opt for paper-wrapped bar soaps and shampoos). Scouring bulk bin aisles and shopping farmers markets can also help you find unpackaged food, and some services now deliver home staples like cleaning wipes, hand soaps, and shampoos in reusable, returnable containers.

Cutting down on our personal plastic waste is important, but ultimately the plastic pollution problem (like almost every other environmental issue) will not be solved by individual action alone. Governments and larger corporations need to get involved so that the responsibility doesn't fall on consumers to find a way to dispose of something that they didn't even want in the first place. (When you're buying toothpaste, you're buying the toothpaste; the annoying tube it comes in is just a vehicle to get that toothpaste to you.) Eventually, companies will need to take the same responsibility for their packaging as they do for the products inside it.

Overfishing

Around a third of the world's marine fisheries are now considered overfished by the United Nations, meaning they're being depleted faster than they can naturally rebound and are at a higher risk of stock depletion or collapse.[34] The human impacts of this overfishing have been swift: when I spoke with Julia Lucas, an elder of the Hesquiaht First Nation on the west coast of Vancouver Island in Canada, she told me she remembers that while she was growing up, fish were in abundance in her community. Now, she gets about six quarts of seafood a year. If current fishing practices continue, some estimate that 88 percent of stocks will be overfished by 2050.[35]

The ocean is a notoriously difficult entity to regulate. Coastal countries all have their own rules and regulations about how strictly to protect their nautical miles from overfishing, the pursuit of endangered species, and destructive fishing practices like trawling (casting a wide net that catches and kills many different species, not just the one you intend to sell) and blast fishing (using dynamite or other explosives to kill all the fish in one area quickly).

But the ocean exists in a delicate balance, and all its creatures play a role in maintaining that balance. Dips in certain fish populations, therefore, are felt by the ecosystem as a whole. Lucas remembers the day an elder told her that salmon, a main source of food in her community, had been all but lost because of the overfishing of its prey, the herring.

The Mindset Shift:
"I want to know where all of my food comes from."

In America at least, it's fair to say that most meat eaters are less curious about the origins of their fish dinner than their burger. Part of it probably has to do with the fact that sustainably raised seafood is more difficult to identify than sustainably raised meat. Unlike beef or pork, you can't slap an organic, pasture-raised label on wild-caught fish. Unless your fish was farm raised, you really have no way of knowing where it comes from, what it ate, or where it spent the majority of its life. Some things you can ask about, though, are what species it is and where and how it was caught.

Emi Koch, whose community-based research studies the impacts of low fish availability as a consequence of overexploitation, habitat degradation, and climate change on small-scale fisheries, is from a coastal town in California where fish tacos and craft beer are on every menu. She's noticed that while diners are always asking waiters and bartenders about the origins of their beer, they hardly ever question where their fish comes from. What if we could build more of a craft movement around seafood in this country? What if more of us took pride in knowing about nearby fisheries and how they operated? I'd wager that it would put pressure on the fishing industry to more thoughtfully consider how to take from the oceans in a more respectful and sustainable way in the long term.

So the next time you visit a restaurant, question where and how your fish was caught. Doing so might be a little awkward, and the person you ask might not know the answer. But at the very least, your curiosity could make them—and any of your dining companions—a little more inclined to ask around in the future too.

Acidification

The ocean is a massive carbon sink (meaning it accumulates and stores more atmospheric carbon than it emits), but I like to think of it as more of

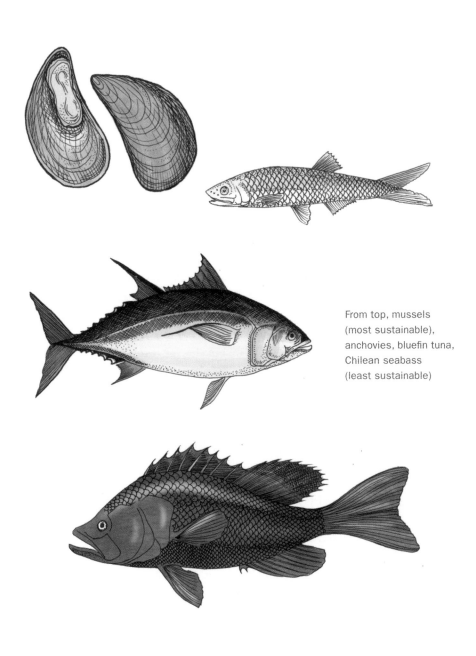

From top, mussels
(most sustainable),
anchovies, bluefin tuna,
Chilean seabass
(least sustainable)

a garbage disposal. This sink is fueled in part by phytoplankton, micro-scopic algae that drift near the water's sunny surface and help absorb CO_2 from the atmosphere through photosynthesis. Through natural processes, like when these phytoplankton are eaten by larger predators and then re-leased as waste, some of this surface CO_2 sinks to deeper depths (see where the disposal analogy is coming in?), eventually settling on the ocean floor, where it can remain safely stored out of the atmosphere. There are parallels between the ocean's carbon cycles and the ones you'll find on land, and the trailblazing marine biologist, explorer, and founder of Mission Blue Sylvia Earle has likened the damage to the ocean to the clear-cutting of a forest.

Instead of chopping down the ocean, though, we're choking it. As global emissions of CO_2 rise, this CO_2 builds up in surface waters and makes them more acidic (water plus carbon dioxide equals acid). Ocean acidification hinders the ability of marine organisms, especially sensitive structures like coral reefs, to thrive and regenerate. The irony is that the ocean is one of our biggest buffers against climate change (it can absorb about 30 percent of the carbon dioxide released by humans[36]), but by overtaxing it, we're harm-ing its ability to do its job. "The air we breathe, the regulation of tempera-ture, everything that provides a hospitable planet goes back to the existence of the ocean," Earle tells *Atmos* magazine.[37] "The more we discover about life on Earth, the more interconnected we find that everything is."

The Mindset Shift:
"I recognize the interconnectedness of all things."

Nothing in nature exists in a vacuum, and the ocean is no exception. When I asked Easkey Britton about her advice for being a better environmental-ist, she said that it starts by simply recognizing the ocean's link with literally everything else: "When we talk about climate change and the climate cri-sis, we're really also talking about the ocean." This means that anything you can do to reduce your CO_2 emissions and role in global warming will also help the big blue sea, and all that it holds.

CHAPTER THREE

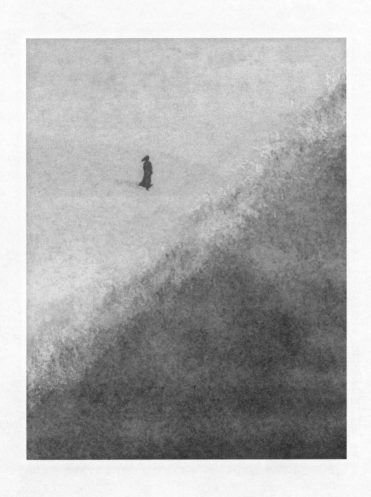

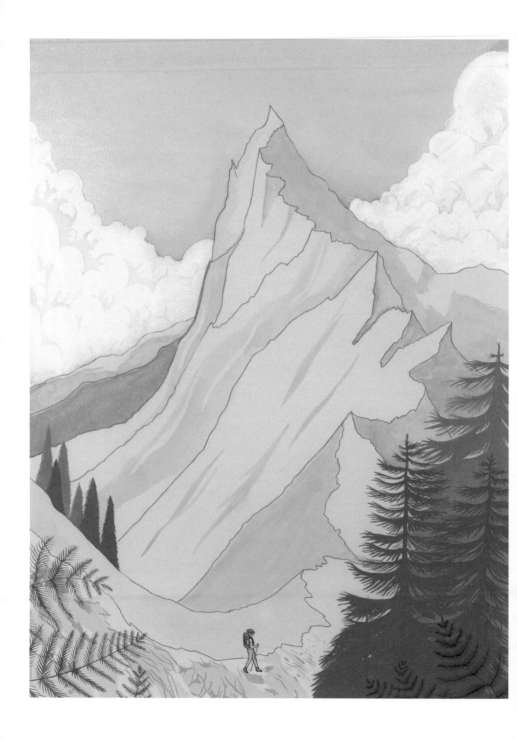

MOUNTAINS & HIGHLANDS

perspective, awe, breakthrough

After two hours (or was it three?) of ascent, we're on level ground again. From an elevation of fifteen hundred feet, the world below takes on a softer quality: the slippery forest floor that gave us so much trouble on the way up is now gently tucked under the cover of green. The steep rocks we struggled to climb are now just another piece of the expansive view. The stress I was feeling on the ride here even feels a little duller, as if my worries at ground level shrank in proportion to the height gained. My friends and I aren't the only group of hikers at the peak of Acadia National Park today, and I imagine everyone on the mountaintop is experiencing something similar: the refreshingly wide perspective that a climb can bring.

The Remedy

Mountains are where the sky first meets the ground, and they account for nearly a quarter of our planet. As the tallest landmasses on Earth, they provide valuable ecosystem services for the world below, like collecting water and stifling wind. The mountains also represent retreat and evoke reverence in visitors and the approximately 915 million people who dwell in their shadows.[1]

As for the health benefits of this landscape, you'll think of some obvious ones quickly: walking up a mountain's incline is a difficult, sweat-inducing physical activity. But as I learned hiking in Acadia that day, this landscape's impact on mental well-being also builds steadily over the course of a climb. By piecing together emerging research on green exercise, biodiversity, and awe, we can get a sense of how mountains widen our frame of view in more ways than one. Let's trace how the landscape does so, starting at the bottom and working our way up to the peak.

Starting from the Bottom: Setting the Stage for Green Exercise

Relatively few scientific studies have sent people to the mountains and tracked how their bodies and minds responded. This limited pool of mountainous exercise research is partly logistical: it's much easier to set up a controlled study at ground level than it is at elevation, and mountains are far away from most of the college campuses where the majority of environment and human health studies are conducted. Plus, research on the health benefits of more accessible greenery lends itself to policy change and can be used to support the creation of a new park or patch of trees. A new mountain? Not so much. This means that to explore what makes mountains healthy, we need to look to studies from other landscapes and extrapolate the findings.

To start, we can dig into the literature on green exercise (GE)—any exercise done in natural green space. Existing GE literature suggests that doing an exercise outdoors can be more beneficial than doing that same exercise inside. Researchers have found that the physical benefits of movement and the mental benefits of being outside seem to work synergistically, and the whole becomes greater than the sum of its parts. GE's potential psychological advantages include improved self-esteem, more positive mood,[2] and recovery from short-term stressors.[3] Physically, people seem to feel less exertion during GE,[4] and their postexercise blood pressure returns to normal more quickly after an outdoor workout than an indoor one.[5]

We don't yet know what exactly it is about green exercise that provides these added benefits, but Jo Barton, a GE researcher and reader at the University of Essex, thinks it's a confluence of many factors—including the way that outdoor exercise engages all the senses and just tends to be more fun. "We've shown that green exercise is more enjoyable [than indoor exercise] and there is a greater intention to repeat the activity," she tells me. "It also facilitates social interaction more effectively, which probably feeds into the enjoyment."

Thanks to their elevation gain and steep slopes, mountains are among the most dramatic places to undergo green exercise, solo or with a friend. Of the many mountain exercises, hiking in particular tends to be an enjoyable, popular way to work up a sweat. One 2016 literature review says that hiking can be a significant health intervention because it's an opportunity to sightsee, explore, and often connect with other people, as well as to exercise.[6] In other words, people are typically more inclined to want to spend time on a hike than in a gym, making hiking a form of exercise that could have an outsized impact on physical and mental health, according to the GE hypothesis.

Navigating the Trail: How Biodiversity Restores the Body and Mind

Another clue about the health benefits of the mountains comes from Stanford in a widely cited series of studies testing the mood and cognition of healthy participants after a ninety-minute walk in either nature or an urban street.[7] Those in the group who took the nature walk returned saying that they felt less burdened by negative rumination—repetitive thought loops that are markers of depression and anxiety—while the urban walkers did not. A run through an MRI scanner confirmed that nature walkers had less neural activity in the subgenual prefrontal cortex, activated during periods of sadness and negative self-reflection, than the urban walkers did. Those who walked through nature also scored better on a working memory test, suggesting that since they were less focused on rumination, their minds were free to focus on other mental tasks. Finally, they reported a more positive mood overall than urban walkers did, potentially because of that decreased rumination.

ART provides one explanation for how extended walks in nature might pull us out of such negative thought loops. If you'll remember from the introduction, ART suggests that nature gives our brains an opportunity to recharge from the mental fatigue of daily life and focus on gentler, less cognitively demanding stimuli—the pattern of a leaf, the striation of rocks, or the color of the sky.

Mountains provide the hallmark qualities of restorative natural spaces as the Kaplans described them: a complex environment interesting enough to coax our attention outward and keep our brains occupied. "A restorative environment must be of sufficient scope to engage the mind," Stephen Kaplan wrote of his theory.[8] "It must provide enough to see, experience, and think about so that it takes up a substantial portion of the available room in one's head."

Multifaceted mountains fit Kaplan's description to a tee. The temperature, lighting, and cloud cover at the bottom of a mountain is rarely the same as it is at the top. The vegetation and animal species you'll find at the base also tend to be different from those at the summit. Mountains are so biodiverse that, sometimes, they stump even experts. "Mountains are simply too rich in species," the director of the Center for Macroecology, Evolution and Climate at the University of Copenhagen, Carsten Rahbek, reflected after one of his review papers, "and we are falling short of explaining global hotspots of biodiversity."[9] Nearly half of the world's thirty-six biodiversity hotspots he's referring to are in mountainous regions.[10]

This species richness is partly due to the unique topography of mountain ranges. Air temperature and weather patterns change as you go up a mountain, and large mountains tend to be more dry and barren on one side and lush and green on the other, depending on how the wind moves as it's pushed up and down peaks. This creates the conditions for many types of plants and animals to thrive not far from one another. Also, mountains tend to be less fragmented by roads and human industry, meaning that they have larger swaths of habitable area (though, as I show later in this chapter, this is changing). Whereas isolated areas tend to be dominated by a few species,[11] connectivity fosters greater diversity.

This biodiversity might further increase mountains' capacity for mental restoration. In 2007, Richard Fuller, the conservation biologist we first met in the parks chapter, published a study finding that people's positive emotions and cognitive restoration increased in urban green space with more species richness.[12] This appreciation for biodiversity was innate. People could more or less predict the degree of species richness around them, and they didn't need to know the surrounding plant and animal species by name to benefit from them.

When I caught up with Fuller to ask how more plants, butterflies, and birds could lead to psychological benefits, he said that it could be because of the way this biodiversity invites us away from our normal thought processes, in keeping with Kaplan's theory. "A more complex environment theoretically should lead to more restoration because that environment requires your attention to a greater extent. There's more mystery in a more complex, biodiverse place," he tells me, adding that the more biodiversity a place has, the more dynamic and ephemeral it becomes—further separating it from the static and predictable built environments we inhabit.

Mountains are a through line where different species can meet and mingle over a relatively short distance, giving us plenty to engage with during a hike to higher ground.

Gaining Elevation:
How Awe Opens Us Up to New Perspectives

As we ascend a lush mountain trail, traversing its physically demanding terrain and taking in its mentally gripping layers, we open ourselves up to the best kind of distraction. (It doesn't hurt that cell service in the mountains is often lacking.) We can step away from a stressful and repetitive inner dialogue and into something more freeing. All the while, the most mentally engaging part of a mountain still waits for us at the peak.

Once people reach the top of a scenic lookout, their eyes tend to widen, their jaw goes slack, a gasp escapes their lips, and goose bumps might peek through their skin. These are telltale signs of awe at work.

Awe is the emotion we get when faced with "perceptually vast stimuli that overwhelm current mental structures, yet facilitate attempts at accommodation."[13] In other words, it's what we feel in the presence of something that exceeds expectation and makes us question our current understanding of the world and our place within it. It's an emotion that fascinates psychology researchers because of the unique way it seems to promote learning, creativity, and prosocial behavior.[14]

While music, art, animals, and inspiring human achievements can all lead to positive awe, vast nature scenes, like the one you see from a mountaintop, are especially effective at evoking the feeling.[15] While the capacity of specific landscapes to provoke awe has not been extensively researched, one study found that those polled considered mountains more likely to evoke awe than forests, rivers, oceans, or beaches.[16]

Melanie Rudd, an associate professor at the University of Houston, is one researcher who associates awe with the mountains. "I've always had [a] connection to mountains," Rudd, who grew up in Washington State looking at awe-inspiring Mount Rainier every day, told *Psychology Today* in 2019, "so when I started doing research on awe, one of the obvious stimuli to use was mountains."[17]

One thing Rudd has explored with her research is how awe can shift our perception of time: "Awe can make you feel like time is more expensive because it really sucks you into the present moment," Rudd tells me. "Your mind isn't floating around to the future or the past. It's really absorbing everything in the moment. This greater sense of time can influence your decision-making." Indeed, after tracking how people said they wanted to spend their time after feeling different emotions, Rudd found that subjects were more willing to volunteer their time to help other people after experiencing awe, likely because they felt like they had more of it to give.[18] They also expressed a stronger desire to seek experiences over material things, again, possibly because they felt as if they suddenly had more time to spend on them.

Awe experiences like the ones we have in the mountains may also open us up to more critical thinking. Most positive emotions (e.g., happiness, pride) don't tend to change anything about the way we see the world; feeling them often reinforces our existing ideas about right and wrong, good and bad. Michelle Shiota, a prominent awe researcher, has said that in this way, many positive emotions tend to leave us cognitively sloppy.[19] When we have them, we are quick to jump to conclusions about what caused them, without questioning the validity of our assumptions. Awe, however, seems to do something different. Since it so closely connects us to the present and challenges our immediate understanding, it causes us to make fewer assumptions about our surroundings and adopt a more curious attitude.

"Awe makes you want to alter the mental schema in your brain, which is very unique. Most people are terrified of changing how they see things or revising their knowledge," Rudd explains to me. "But awe surrounds that cognitive component in a positive feeling, a positive experience, and thus it is one of the few states in which altering the way you see things is not threatening."

While it's unclear how long this expansive, malleable worldview lasts, one investigation on healing awe experiences outdoors suggests it's longer than you might think.[20] This research monitored two groups of people with high rates of PTSD—military veterans and young people from underserved communities—as they came face-to-face with awe over multiday whitewater rafting voyages in California. Participants reported their emotions and stress levels before, during, and one week after the trip. GoPro cameras also filmed the journey, allowing researchers to compare self-reported well-being with footage of facial expressions and body language.

"When we looked at those emotions, put them into our regression models, awe was the only emotion that we measured that significantly predicted whether or not people's wellbeing would improve at that follow-up one week later," Craig Anderson, a researcher on the study, told *Outside Podcast* of the findings.[21] The experience and the lasting sense of awe it elicited reduced both groups' PTSD symptoms.

Though not conducted in the mountains, these findings show that the awe we feel outside can reverberate, even after the initial rush of it fades. Largely invisible save for the tangible mark it leaves, awe may not last forever, but the fact that we felt it at one point is what's significant.

Approaching the Summit:
A Peak Experience That Borders on Spiritual

My first exposure to the power of awe in nature was Florence Williams's seminal book, *The Nature Fix: Why Nature Makes Us Happier, Healthier, and More Creative*.[22] In it, Williams writes about how *awe*—like the type she felt hiking the mountains of Colorado—is derived from an Old English word for the sensation one gets in the presence of a divine being: equal parts reverence and disbelief, and a healthy dash of fear. It's no wonder that the mountains, with their awe-inducing views and grand scale, are often considered home to higher powers. The Greek gods settled on Mount Olympus to watch over the mortal world below; Mount Fuji is dedicated to Shinto gods and goddesses; and Mount Sinai was where Moses received the Ten Commandments. In Bible scripture, mountains and hills are mentioned hundreds of times, and some of the world's most breathtaking churches were built on mountaintops to be closer to God.

In his book *These Mountains Are Our Sacred Places*,[23] Chief John Snow describes how the Rocky Mountains serve as "a place of hope, a place of vision, a place of refuge" for his Stoney people of western Canada. Mountains are also the stage for their vision quests, a sacred Indigenous rite of passage that involves fasting in order to enter a state of openness to divine

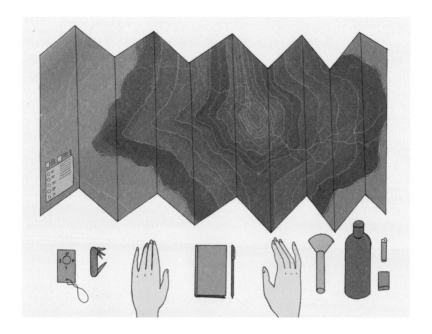

guidance. "Upon these lofty heights," Snow writes, "the Great Spirit revealed many things to us."

The psychiatrist and founder of analytical psychology Carl Jung considered the mountains an archetype, a universal symbol, for personal growth, discovery, and transcendence. "The mountain stands for the goal of the pilgrimage and ascent, hence it often has the psychological meaning of the Self," Jung wrote in *The Archetypes and the Collective Unconscious*.[24] This could help explain why so many cultures, though separated by time, space, and ideology, have felt a similar pull to the peaks.

When speaking to modern-day mountaineers, you get a sense that they, too, have felt a veil lift on their climbs, like they hiked straight into a more divine realm. A few years ago, Wasfia Nazreen, the world's first Bangladeshi to climb the highest mountain of every continent, described the feeling on top of Everest to me: "I really felt like there was something higher than me that took over. . . . My life flashed before me, and I felt this overwhelming sense of gratitude, for being alive, for being where I was." More recently, the climber Tashi Sherpa, who has summited Everest a remarkable ten times, told me that "the excitement level is extraordinary" every time he reaches a peak. The reward for discipline, focus, and patience can evoke an ecstasy that borders on religious.

Like the deepest trenches of the ocean, the highest peaks of mountains are not places most humans are physically equipped to be—yet people pursue them anyway, surely pulled along part of the way by something relentless but unseen.

"After most available peaks have been conquered," the mountaineer and author Ned Morgan writes in his book, *In the Mountains: The Health and Wellbeing Benefits of Spending Time at Altitude*, "spiritual and ethical self-examination may be the new object of mountaineering."[25]

The Descent: Integrating Lessons Learned at Great Heights

It's not uncommon to hear of people who begin a hike with a problem and return with the solution in mind, as if it had been dropped off while they were away.

In *The Nature Fix*, Williams describes her experience walking mountain trails: "When my feet were moving, I would think about whatever I needed to think about and the farther I went, the more I would space out. Sometimes I could by accident compose some writerly sentences in my head, or some insight might waft up, unbidden."[26] Famed writers, thinkers, and creators through history like William Wordsworth and Henry David Thoreau similarly credit mountains with some of their brightest ideas.

Then there are the physical creations that the landscape pulls out of us. When forester Benton MacKaye was perched in the Green Mountains of Vermont in the early nineteenth century, he was struck with a "planetary feeling" looking at the world below.[27] The emotion—awe, surely—left him with the itch to create, and years later he broke ground on his vision: the Appalachian Trail, now the longest hiking-only footpath in the world.

These unplanned but welcome ideas that strike in the high country correspond with what science now knows about nature, rumination, and creativity: when we return to our thoughts after some time outdoors, we might find their sharp edges slightly less sinister, having been dulled by the beauty around us. Any landscape can free up our minds to perspective change, but mountains, for all the reasons described, seem to be especially good at it.

As we walk back down them, surrounded by tall trees, age-old rocks, or ice if we are at altitude (which all come with their own special forces that I cover in later sections), the grounded lives that get closer with each step remain largely the same. But we might find that it's us who have, in some way, changed.

The Practice

Whether you're heading out on a backpacking trip, going on a day hike, or taking in a mountain view from ground level, here are some ideas for enhancing the journey.

IF YOU HAVE 5–10 MINUTES:

Walk a trail slowly, without a destination in mind.

Even if you don't have time to gain much elevation, you can still have a memorable experience on a mountain trail. Denise Mitten, sustainability and adventure education professor and nature health researcher at Prescott College, tells me that even mundane moments can be transformative so long as we approach them with an open mind. "It seems like people in general have transformative experiences when they're open to what's going on, when they don't have an agenda of how they think things should be," Mitten tells me. This happens when we see the land around us as a space to leisurely traverse rather than quickly get through.

"Pace makes a huge difference," she adds. "So stop and smell the roses—seriously." In this meandering state, you might find yourself noticing more of what landscape has to offer.

Expand the breath to eleven counts in the presence of mountains.

Melanie Rudd, the awe researcher we heard from earlier, has found that slow and controlled breathing can ground us in the present moment (and subsequently expand our sense of time) in a similar way that awe tends to.[28]

Apply this research by following a slow, mindful breath pattern of a five-second inhale and a six-second exhale as you gaze at a mountain view in order to open yourself up to, as Rudd puts it, be awed by something you might not have noticed or fully appreciated otherwise.

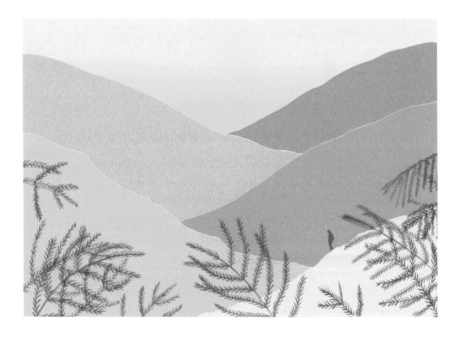

Consider a problem at the start of your hike, and write about it at the end.

Before you start your climb, consider one problem you're facing or one area of your life where you could use some clarity. At the end of the hike, free-write on it and see if you've stumbled across any new insights during the journey.

This ritual is inspired by Bonnie Smith Whitehouse, an English professor at Belmont University in Nashville, Tennessee, who lectures on the creative inspiration that lies in nature using some unique methods: when I interviewed Whitehouse for an article in 2019,[29] she told me how one class a semester, she'll have her students journal on a question before starting a hard hike and then come back to it every time they needed to take a break on the way to a summit. She encourages them to "focus on your footsteps and your breathing" along the way, and then use their journals to extract any insights that came up during the experience. "When you combine walking and journaling," she said, "it can really pack a punch for your well-being."

Revisit the same route season after season.

In most parts of the world, a trail will look different in winter than in summer. The seasonal shift is a reminder that time changes everything, and it's why the Good Grief walking program in Calgary brings participants who are mourning the loss of a loved one on the same walk on the same trail multiple times throughout the year. Sonya Jakubec, a mental health nurse and associate professor at Mount Royal University who works with the program, tells me this revisiting can cause people to consider how their inner landscapes have gone through a transformation since the last time they walked through that area: how their grief and loss look different in the new surroundings.

Whether you're grieving or not, going on a hike with the intention of using nature's cycles as a cue to tune in to your own cycle is always valuable practice.

Let awe find you.

You don't need to climb to the top of Everest or take up backpacking to experience awe in the outdoors. In fact, during that whitewater rafting study introduced earlier in this chapter, the researchers found that participants felt the most awestruck not in the frothy rapids but in the calmer waters where they had a chance to relax and take it all in. So go ahead and set a goal to hike to an overlook that you've never been to before—one with the expansive and unobstructed views that awe loves so much—but don't fret if life gets in the way and you aren't able to make it there. Oftentimes, awe takes less coaxing than you think; the key is just to set the scene for it by continuing to expose yourself to new stimuli.

The next time you do begin to sense awe coming on, Rudd says the only thing left to do is be present with the emotion. "When I do start to feel awe," she shares, "I really savor that experience and enhance it as much as possible. I focus and suck everything in—sights, sounds, smells—and try to form a strong memory." Doing so, she says, makes the feeling of awe easier to mentally revisit later during tense, narrow-minded moments.

Open your heart to the view.

This heart opener practice is helpful for slowing down and becoming more receptive to your surroundings. I've found that doing an exercise like this can evoke the presence Rudd suggests settling into in the face of awe. While it would be epic to do this sitting on top of a scenic overlook after a long hike, doing it at ground level while looking at the mountains (or any landscape you have access to that day) is powerful in itself.

- Press play on a song that you love—preferably one that builds steadily and has a strong beat. My favorites for this practice include "We Will Run," by Jens Kuross, and "Hold Me Like a Fire," by Reuben and the Dark.

- In a seated position, close your eyes. Open your arms out to either side, like you're going in for a hug, and bend the elbows at ninety-degree angles. The shape you make will resemble a cactus with two branches.

- Move your hands back and forth to touch, keeping the arms bent. It will feel a little funny at first, but keep pumping the arms to the beat of the music and keep the eyes closed. Try to keep going, moving the arms back and forth across your body, until the song is complete. (This doubles as an arm and back workout.)

- Once the song is up, open your eyes and take in the view around you. Since this movement is meant to engage the heart, you might find yourself feeling more attuned to the landscape, more present. Again, make the conscious effort to soak in the feeling for future reference.

Wander somewhere that feels untouched by humans.

During his career as a superintendent with the National Park Service, Dan Wenk watched as most visitors hurriedly drove Yellowstone's main roads, stopping at attraction after attraction to tick boxes off a bucket list, without indulging in the over one thousand miles of backcountry trail the park had to offer. Keenan Adams, a federal public land manager based in Puerto Rico, has noticed something similar in his neck of the woods: "People experience a fraction of public land because they stay on the beaten path. To get a different public land experience, you need to get off the beaten path," he tells me.

Most people never stray farther than a quarter to a half mile away from the main road when they go to a national park. Yellowstone is a prime example: well over 95 percent of the people who visit the park never get more than a half mile from the main road, most of them a quarter mile. . . . They don't allow time within their day to explore or to dive deeper into the experience. They don't allow themselves to take advantage of opportunities that present themselves because of a schedule.

—DAN WENK,
former superintendent of Yellowstone National Park

Many of the gifts of the mountains reveal themselves slowly: settling in a species-rich area, stumbling on an awe-inspiring view, and walking until ruminative loops are broken all take time. Only when we loosen our grip on our schedules and let the landscape take us where it will do we open ourselves up to the "emotional renewal," as Wenk describes it to me, that comes when we are totally alone with nature, our thoughts, and our experience.

CONNECTING FROM AFAR:
Look at photos or videos.

It turns out that there's something to those preset desktop backgrounds that show the granite walls of El Capitan and sunsets over the Sierras: photos and videos can elicit a bit of awe in us too[30]—the more immersive, the better. To tap into the feeling of the mountains from afar, Rudd recommends keeping a folder of awe-inspiring nature images on rotation on your phone or computer. There's a point at which the same photo will stop delivering an awe response, so swap them out every so often to keep things fresh.

Stargaze.

Even if you're nowhere near the mountains, looking up at a starry sky can also lead you to that "nothing and everything" sensation that they deliver so well, according to this memory from Roz Savage, whom we met in the oceans chapter.

> Suddenly, I had this sort of cosmic moment of feeling so tiny and insignificant in the scale of the whole cosmos, but also feeling so at one with it all. Like I was nothing and everything at the same time.
>
> —ROZ SAVAGE,
> ocean rower, on stargazing over the Pacific

Leave space in life for the unknown.

When we put ourselves in new situations, awe has a way of meeting us there. It's less inclined to show up when we repeat the same behaviors day after day. Any creature of habit might find this a tough pill to swallow, but remember that awe-inspiring moments don't need to be spent in a place as grand as a mountaintop to be significant: you carve a little space for awe every time you take a different route home, visit another area of your neighborhood, or shake up your schedule for the day. When seeking everyday adventures, prioritize ones that might expose you to something new and send your brain into curiosity mode.

Nature is really good at this, since it tends to be dynamic and ever-changing. So even if you've walked the same park path a million times, you still might be able to find something new and awe-inspiring about it by slowing down and giving the area your full attention.

Take on an outdoor challenge.

Walking through nature for extended periods takes perseverance. As Elsye Walker, known as Chardonnay on the trails, the first Black woman to thru-hike the Triple Crown (the Pacific Crest Trail, the Appalachian Trail, and the Continental Divide Trail), reminds me, it's called thru-hiking for a reason: it requires moving through challenges, not skirting them. In doing so, you learn what you're capable of, and that feeling of accomplishment can be addicting. It's why Chardonnay and many other thru-hikers return home from months-long trips thinking, "I want to have that feeling again. You want to push yourself to see how far you can go."

We can feel the pride and glory that comes with overcoming nature's obstacles in any landscape we have access to—whether it's a long run through a forest, a kayaking voyage in a river, or an extended bike trip through grassland.

Journal on the mountain's themes.

The mountains give us perspective, expose us to awe, spotlight how we approach challenges, and open us up to spirit. The following questions and prompts touch on similar themes and can help lead to the type of breakthroughs you might get on the trail:

- What metaphorical mountains are you climbing these days? What in your life feels like an uphill battle every step of the way? What would it look like to zoom out on that problem and put it into perspective?

- Where in your life are you following trails laid out for you? Are you taking the time to look up from them, or are you too focused on the path ahead to notice your surroundings?

- When was the last time that you felt in awe of your surroundings?

- Reflect on an experience that changed your view of the world. Write down what you thought before the experience, how your perspective changed, and what you think it was about the experience that was so powerful.

The Action

Besides scenic beauty, mountains also provide important ecosystem services: they carry rivers that deliver fresh water, and as we continue to exhaust agricultural resources in the lowlands, they could become more essential for food production too. Mountains represent a space of escape and reprieve from the world below, but they, too, are in danger of falling victim to human influence, industrialization, and climate change. Here's how to help protect the landscape from three key threats.

Human Impact

Thanks to their altitude, mountains are retreats from the world below— places where fewer people tread and the touch of industry is less apparent. Once hikers visit them, though, there's always a chance that they bring with them disruptive habits from ground level.

In the Hindu Kush Himalayan (HKH) region, home to some of the world's highest mountains, including Mount Everest and K2, litter has become a huge problem. In 2019, the Nepalese government removed 24,200 pounds of trash from Everest,[31] but many more tons of food wrappers, cans, oxygen bottles, and discarded climbing gear still sit on the way up the peak. These mountains are reserves of ice and snow (the HKH is known as the world's "third pole" because of its large volume of fresh water), and more trash continues to be unearthed with the snowmelt. "The beauty of nature is harming itself," Tashi Dorji, an ecosystem specialist who works at the International Centre for Integrated Mountain Development based in Nepal, tells me of what's going on in his native mountain region.

The same goes for some mountainous national parks in the US, where increased foot traffic is damaging local ecosystems. "There's an old saying I've heard that goes something like 'No single raindrop thinks it's the cause of the flood'—no single visitor thinks it's the cause of the damage or the erosion or the wear and tear you see over time," Dan Wenk, of Yellowstone, explains. But in the mountains, as in the rest of nature, tiny disruptions do add up.

The Mindset Shift:
"I pledge to leave nature just as I found it."

This isn't to say that we should stop visiting this landscape altogether, since many mountain communities around the world are financially dependent on tourism dollars. But when we do head to the hills, we should do so without leaving a trace.

The seven Leave No Trace principles, a series of stewardship rules first introduced in the US backcountry in the 1980s, give us a good sense of how to act outdoors—where there are no waste management systems to clean up litter or cameras to see who is disrupting animals or heading off-trail. Here's a brief introduction on how to honor each one on your next hike:

- **Plan ahead and prepare.** This one's as much for your sake as the mountain's: do your homework and know what your hike entails before you go so that you don't put yourself or others at risk.

- **Travel and camp on durable surfaces.** Trails and campsites are strategically placed to cause minimal destruction to the land and keep human impact contained. As tempting as it can be to veer far off them, trust that they're there for a reason.

- **Dispose of waste properly.** Never leave trash or debris behind on a hike; put it back in your pack if needed.

- **Leave what you find.** Just like you shouldn't add anything new to a mountain environment, you shouldn't take anything away from it.

- **Minimize campfire impacts.** Always stay conscious of your surroundings when starting a fire, and be sure to clean up and restore the land to its previous condition afterward.

- **Respect wildlife.** As mentioned before, mountains are often hotbeds for many different species. Read up on local wildlife before your journey so that you have an idea of what to expect on the trail. When you do spot an animal, resist the urge to get closer or yell about it to friends up ahead: give it some space and silence.

- **Be considerate of other visitors.** Give other hikers a smile and a wave as you pass by. We all play a role in making the trail an inclusive and welcoming space for everyone.

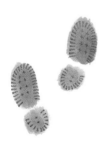

In addition to these rules, respecting the land we're traversing means recognizing its history and culture. Before you head out on a new hike, read up on who that land currently belongs to, who it might have historically been taken from, and what communities currently depend on it for their livelihoods. Ask yourself how your visit helps or harms these people, and consider how you could make a more direct contribution to them.

Industrial Development & Resource Extraction

Though a mountain's harsh terrain makes it harder to exploit to a certain extent, industrial development is still a threat at altitude. According to a recent report, nearly 60 percent of the world's mountainous area is under human pressure.[32] The construction of tunnels and roads for tourism and mountaintop removal for mining and energy production significantly alter mountain landscapes and threaten the people who call them home. As more mountains are industrialized, impacts like water contamination, habitat loss, and landslides and floods spurred by erosion will become more common.

The majority of this development is happening at the base of mountains, but we can assume that it will continue to creep farther and farther up peaks as time goes on and lowland resources are exhausted, unless regulations are put in place to stop it.

The Mindset Shift:
"I support conservation efforts near and far."

In the US, the federal government owns and oversees 640 million acres of land, including national parks (most of which are in mountainous areas), national forests, and national wildlife refuges.[33] On the local level, state and community governments are always acquiring new public lands too, thanks in part to the work of land trust agencies.

Keenan Adams, whom we heard from earlier, has extensive experience working on land acquisition and management and says that these land trusts are where individuals looking to make a difference in conservation will want to turn. You can make a monetary donation to your nearest trust (most states have one) to help it acquire new public lands and protect existing ones from development, or volunteer your time to lend a hand to the trust's fundraising and conservation projects. "It all boils down to local politics," he tells me of the decision to set aside new land for conservation.

"If the local communities want it, it can happen if the money is there." If you happen to own land, you can also partner with your local trust on a conservation easement. In doing so, you'll still own and be able to use your property as normal, but the land trust will monitor it to ensure that it is properly conserved into the future.

Donating time, money, or land to land trusts is one way to step beyond Leave No Trace principles and actually improve on and expand the natural areas near you—mountainous or otherwise.

Diversity Loss Due to Climate Change

Mountains are incredibly diverse reservoirs that can support rivers and glaciers, grasslands and forests, plants and animals with wildly different needs, and people from a variety of cultures, over a relatively short expanse. (The term mountain *range* never made so much sense.) This means that mountains are feeling the impacts of climate change in more ways than one.

The first notable impact is directly on plants and animals. As a mountain's climate warms, its plants and animals need to take refuge at higher elevations—and not all of them survive the journey. Considering that habitable mountain land becomes smaller the higher up you go, and new habitats also mean new predators, scientists have named this type of vertical migration "the escalator to extinction."[34] Climate change could also make the areas higher up on a mountain more hospitable to humans, further opening them up to development.

A second climate impact threatens people living in the mountains: when global warming melts mountain ice caps and throws off precipitation and weather patterns, it predisposes the landscape to flash floods, landslides, and wildfires. In the HKH region alone, Tashi Dorji tells me that many younger people whose families have lived in the mountains for generations are packing up and heading to the cities due to increasingly erratic weather patterns and diminishing resources. With them, the heritage and culture of this part of the world is leaving too.

Biodiversity is like an insurance policy that makes mountain landscapes more resilient to change: the more species an area has, and the more variation that exists within these species, the less likely that area is to completely disintegrate when challenges arise. Every time an area loses some biodiversity, the less equipped it is to rebound from future threats, setting off a dangerous chain reaction. You could say that the same risk exists for people: the less cultural diversity that exists within a human system, the less likely that system is to successfully adapt to change. By protecting the diverse array of plants, animals, *and* humans that call a mountain—and any landscape, really—home, we are buffering ourselves from the very real danger that comes with becoming monolithic.

The Mindset Shift:
"The awe in my life inspires action."

There's no one solution that will save mountain biodiversity from climate change (but wouldn't that be nice?). Such a diverse region will require an equally diverse set of solutions and demand participation across governments, academe, and industry. Surely, mountains could use some help from us individuals too. To find out what you can give to them, why not use awe—and the expanded worldview it inspires—as your guide?

The research tells us that awe should at least temporarily give us a wider, less selfish frame of view. This is a perspective that the conservation movement undoubtedly needs. So the next time you are taken aback by an awesome view, use the moment as an opportunity to consider how you can use your unique skills to forge a healthier planet that supports diversity of all kinds. Who knows, the answer you get in that moment could set you on the path to a new project in conservation or beyond. I can think of no better way to honor the mountains than to hold on to the expansive worldview they inspire in you, long after you make your hike back down.

CHAPTER FOUR

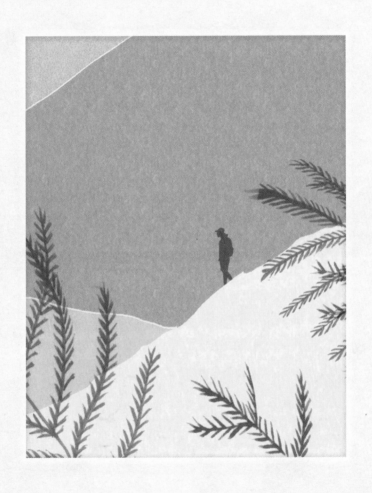

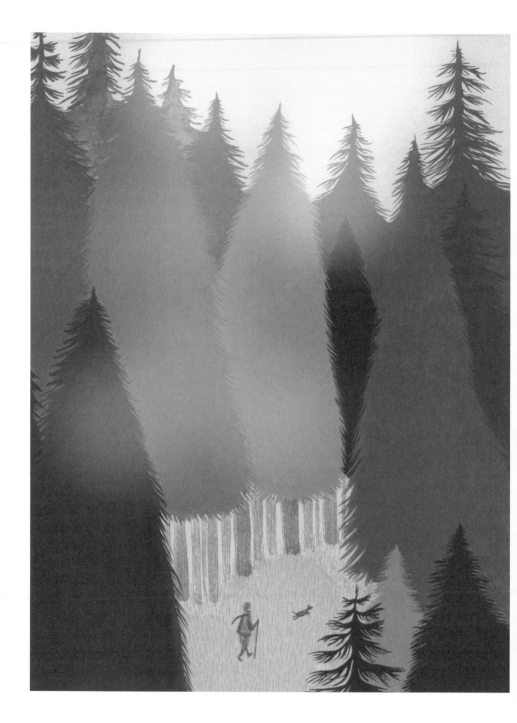

FORESTS & TREES

vitality, patience, wisdom

I walk into the forest, and the first thing that meets me is the silent stillness. The canopy forms a fortress where chaos and distraction from the outside world is not welcome. In the shadow of trees, I'm hit with a strange urge to get quiet myself. Their size and presence demands my immediate attention.

Looking up, I can imagine the first yellowing leaves of the season dropping in the months ahead, eventually disappearing under a blanket of Vermont winter snow. Looking down, I can see patches of exposed dirt, the imprints of previous visitors sitting on the craggy ground. I smile, thinking about how the forest is a rare place where the past and future can meet, introduced under the cover of canopy.

The Remedy

The Forest Resources Assessment describes a forest as any land over 0.5 hectares (about 1.2 acres) that's at least 10 percent covered by tree canopy.[1] By this definition, a little over 30 percent of land worldwide is forested,[2] but the landscape is home to an outsized 80 percent of terrestrial species.[3] Like mountains, well-maintained forests can be chock-full of biodiversity and the climate change insurance it provides. And like oceans, healthy forests are carbon sinks, storing emissions in the trunks and roots of their trees. In the process of sucking up CO_2 and other pollutants, trees send fresh stores of oxygen back into the environment. It's why forest air feels so fresh on the inhale, like it somehow seeps farther into the lungs. Beyond this respiratory boost, a walk in the woods comes with myriad health benefits, as well as lessons in reciprocity, exchange, patience, and the value of listening with all of one's senses.

How Forest Bathing Became the Focus of Researchers Worldwide

Relative to other landscapes, we actually know a fair amount about how forests affect human health, largely thanks to the *shinrin-yoku* movement that sprouted in Japan about forty years ago. In English, *shinrin-yoku* is referred to as "forest bathing," though the name is slightly misleading: the practice is more of a sensory immersion than a literal one, and you don't need to drag a clawfoot tub into the woods to try it.

Instead, forest bathing began in Japan as a way to test whether the country's expansive forest system could help stressed-out city dwellers find some calm. Sure enough, from the first experiment in the Akasawa forest in 1982,[4] researchers and physicians have since found that forest bathing could deliver powerful psychological benefits—and some surprising physical ones too.

In the years since, the country has funneled millions of dollars into forest bathing research and designated dozens of trails to walking in the name of science. In his book *Forest Bathing: How Trees Can Help You Find Health and Happiness*, Qing Li, a leading scholar on forest bathing, writes that "shinrin-yoku has become standard practice, a way in which Japanese people manage their stress and look after their health."[5]

They're onto something: since that early research, studies have shown that forest bathing can reduce blood pressure, sympathetic nervous system (a.k.a. fight-or-flight) activity, and stress hormones[6] while improving sleep quality,[7] immunity, and attention—and these benefits can last up to thirty days, according to Li's book.

However, many of the forest bathing trials in Japan have been small, and it's difficult to know which perks came from the forest and which ones were the natural result of stepping away from screens and everyday stressors. So researchers across Asia and Europe are now taking to their own forests to validate the findings and see exactly what it is that makes this landscape so life-affirming. They, too, are finding many healthy qualities concealed in the canopy.

Though the term is new, the practice of forest bathing is a return to a simpler and more intuitive way of interacting with the woods. And an accessible one at that: it requires a "safe and beautiful forest" environment, though there are no rules about how much tree cover or vegetation that environment needs to have, Yoshifumi Miyazaki, another prominent nature therapy researcher, tells me. The hallmark of forest bathing, and something that separates it from a typical forest walk, is its emphasis on going slow and engaging your senses.

A typical session begins by smelling the clean air, looking at the trees, listening to the activity of the canopy, tasting the breeze, and feeling the ground beneath one's feet. Beyond increasing mindfulness, these invitations connect us to the smells, sights, tastes, sounds, and textures of the woods—all of which have healing qualities of their own.

The Smells:
Why Trees' Fragrant Armor Protects Us

Most of a forest's health benefits can be traced back to its trees: nature's mighty pillars that appear separate on the surface but are actually connected through intricate underground webs. It's through this soil network that trees engage in a type of conversation. In human terms, they whisper words of incoming threats, sound the alarm when they're stressed, and share food and water as needed. The fairytale-esque process is made possible by mycelium, a fungus that latches onto tree roots and extends them so far and so wide that, underground, it can be impossible to tell where one tree ends and another begins.

Suzanne Simard, a professor of forest ecology at the University of British Columbia, discovered this "wood wide web" in Canada, when she observed a birch tree sharing life-giving carbon with an obstructed fir tree that had been cut off from its energy source, the sun. In later experiments, the fir tree returned the favor and lent some carbon to the birch when it had started to lose its leaves.

This finding was published in 1997,[8] and in the years since, Simard has found that some older trees even exhibit maternal instincts when they share resources with forest youngsters. While these elder "mother trees" link up with many others in the forest, they are more inclined to protect their kin.

Science still hasn't uncovered all the ways that trees are sharing and communicating underneath our feet (maybe they're all gossiping about us?), but we do know that once a tree is attacked by an insect, fungus, or other predator, it sends a chemical signal to alert other trees in its underground network to stand guard. Neighboring trees can then emit more phytoncides, oils that are nature's bug spray, to ward off predators. These phytoncides are what gives a forest its distinct woodsy scent. And while trees give off more of them when they're under threat, most species always emit at least some phytoncides as a type of insurance policy. The phytoncide count in the air varies constantly, and seems to be affected by variables like temperature, sunlight, and humidity.[9] Evergreens like pines and cedars are more fragrant, since they don't lose their leaves in winter and thus wear their phytoncide armor at all times.

Miraculously, this fragrant substance that protects plants seems to help out us humans too. To study the health outcomes of phytoncides in forest air, researchers in Asia have isolated their active compounds, called terpenes, and had subjects inhale them in a lab. A handful of different ter-

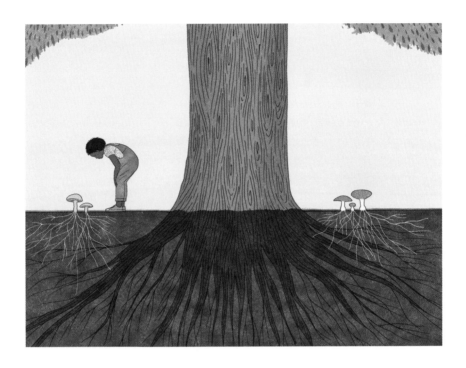

penes have been tested, such as D-limonene (a citrusy aroma given off by the pine family and citrus trees),[10] α-pinene (an earthy scent, also emitted from pines),[11] and cedrol (a herbaceous smell found in cedar trees).[12]

In these studies, smelling terpenes for as little as ninety seconds was enough to evoke a relaxation response in participants. Compared to lab air without terpenes, the forest-scented air increased heart-rate variability (the measure of the variation in time between each heartbeat), a sign that the parasympathetic nervous system was activated, and improved self-reported mood.

When walking through a forest—especially an older one, with lots of tree varieties connected by thick underground networks—we reap the benefits of these terpenes working in tandem. In addition to having a relaxing effect on the mind, this smorgasbord of smells could protect the body in a spectacular way. Qing Li discovered this when he took a small group of people on a multiday trip to the forest, measuring their NK cell activity before and after the excursion.

NK cells are white blood cells that form the body's first line of defense against pathogens. They attack and kill foreign, suspicious-looking entrants, including viruses and cancerous cells, meaning that people with higher NK activity will typically have a lower incidence of disease. Over a three-day forest bathing trip,[13] Li found that the number and activity of participants' NK cells significantly increased, by around 50 percent each, compared with baseline levels. Even more impressive, these numbers were still higher than baseline levels after participants were tested thirty days after the trip was over. A follow-up study found that those who live in forest environments year-round tend to have higher NK cell activity than those who live in urban environments, based on a small sample group.[14]

This immune support might be a direct benefit of phytoncides, or it might be a result of phytoncides' stress-relieving properties (stress, after all, tends to hamper our ability to fight disease). Either way, Li suggests getting out and taking a whiff of forest air at least once a month for the sake of your mental and physical health.

The Sights:
Why the Patterns of Trees Look So Familiar— and Feel So Comforting

As discussed in previous chapters, many people feel calmer just looking at certain natural landscapes, and forests are definitely one of them.

One 2020 study out of Asia found that a cohort of women felt more relaxed, as evidenced by brain activity, when looking at a forest for fifteen minutes compared with an urban environment.[15] An older study in a suburban hospital in Pennsylvania found that patients whose recovery room windows overlooked deciduous trees were released from the hospital faster and required fewer painkillers than those whose rooms looked out on brick walls.[16] Led by professor of architecture at Chalmers University of Technology in Sweden Roger Ulrich in 1984, this finding was considered groundbreaking at the time and is still widely referenced in literature on the links between nature and human health. For our purposes, it's interesting because it suggests that the restorative impact of forests could be due partly to the sight of its individual trees.

But what is it about the look of trees that we find so therapeutic? One fascinating possibility lies in their shape. When you look at a tree, you'll notice that its branches form a repeating pattern that gets smaller and smaller as they extend outward. In mathematics, this is called a fractal pattern—one that can be repeated an infinite number of times, each offshoot a condensed version of the one that came before it. This pattern is useful for the tree, as it allows it to cram more surface area into a small space and soak up more energy from the sun.

The pattern also seems to appeal to humans on some level. In one study, when people observed stripped-down, computer-generated outlines of fractals found in nature[17]—those that are not exact replicas of a pattern but contain some variation—in a lab setting, their brain waves changed. Their minds entered a more relaxed yet activated state, signaling that the images were holding their attention. "I think it's rather amazing that these very simple black-and-white pictures get these kinds of results," Caroline Hägerhäll, an author on the study (whom we met in the parks and gardens chapter), tells me. "They're not really fascinating or fantastic to look at."

Other research has also found that looking at intricate fractal arrangements (like those in a dense forest) might somehow free up the mind for other cognitive pursuits: in a study that asked university students to complete a difficult puzzle after looking at high-fractal or low-fractal stimuli,[18] the students reported that the puzzles felt easier to complete after they looked at the high-fractal stimuli, even though they were more complex.

This innate attraction to even bare-bones fractal patterns could be due to our physiology. After all, the human body is full of fractals, with blood vessels spread through our system like branches from a tree. And how's this for meta: when we look out onto expansive scenery like a forest, our eyes naturally move in a fractal pattern as they attempt to take everything in.[19] A prominent fractal researcher, Richard P. Taylor, head of the physics department at the University of Oregon, has hypothesized that this equips humans with a certain "fractal fluency,"[20] a tendency to find fractal patterns in nature comforting in their familiarity. We like looking at trees because we recognize ourselves in them.

Beyond their complex fractals, the size and scale of trees are also significant. Tall trees provide some of the awe factor we explored in the mountain section, while forcing the gaze up to heights it doesn't usually go. "Generally you're looking straight ahead to see where you are and orient yourself and not trip," Hägerhäll tells me. "But if you're a person walking on the ground, the trees will fill a lot of your visual space."

By inviting the gaze upward, trees force us to take in more of our surroundings and be struck by even more of their soothing visuals: the soft, dappled light through the canopy, the dynamic movement of the leaves in the wind, and—as we now know to look out for—the familiar fractal patterns of the branches.

The Tastes:
Why the Forest's Fresh Air Is So Healthy

The average wood wanderer can engage the element of taste simply by taking in the air of a forest, so clean and crisp that it goes down like a glass of cold water.

Part of the freshness of the air is due to its high oxygen count: "Every walk in the forest is like taking a shower in oxygen," the forester Peter Wohlleben writes in *The Hidden Life of Trees: What They Feel, How They*

Communicate,[21] a fun read for anyone interested in forest dynamics. At the same time, trees also act as nature's air filters. In the process of sucking up carbon dioxide from the atmosphere and converting it into all that oxygen, they trap soot, dust, and other pollutants in their leaves. When it rains, these particles wash downward and get absorbed by soil,[22] where they can stay out of our lungs (though, of course, trees emit their own irritants too, as anyone with seasonal allergies will know).

Beyond going down easy, a clean supply of filtered oxygen supports respiratory health, and one report by the US Forest Service found that trees and forests in the US prevented 670,000 incidences of acute respiratory symptoms like asthma in 2010—mostly through the retrieval of ozone gas and NO_2.[23]

Tree terpenes can also help with air quality and temperature regulation. When these fragrances are released by trees, moisture condenses around them, which has a slight cooling effect. The shade of the canopy, of course, also makes forests cooler, more comfortable places to be.

This landscape's clean, temperate air is good for the brain, seeing as air pollution[24] and excess heat[25] can contribute to stress, depression, and other mental health conditions over time. It makes sense: when we feel physically comfortable in our surroundings, it's a whole lot easier to be in a better mood. So the next time you take a deep breath of forest air, notice its fresh, clear taste and pay attention to how it feels going down.

The Sounds:
Why Forest Sounds Register as Restorative

Another defining characteristic of a forest ecosystem is its sound: the rustling leaves, whispering brooks, and chatty critters.

To test how people react to this rich soundscape, researchers in Japan took a one-minute recording from a forest environment and another from the crowded streets of downtown Tokyo.[26] Twenty-nine female university students listened to both recordings in a lab while their heart rate was monitored. After listening to the forest soundscape, participants logged lower heart rates and decreased sympathetic nervous system activity, signaling that they felt calmer in the presence of those sounds, as compared with the urban noise. A similar study,[27] also out of Japan, found that the forest sounds relaxed a cohort of twelve men who had a gambling disorder, easing stress and reducing negative emotions.

These studies were very small, and it's unclear what sorts of associations their participants had with forests going into them. (As we now know, history, memory, and personal preference all play a role in how we react to nature sounds.) However, separate, more robust studies have found time and time again that most people prefer natural sounds to anthropogenic (human-made) ones. And with their thick walls of trees and vegetation, forests tend to stifle out such anthropogenic noise pretty well.

When an area is less afflicted by human-made noises, the native wildlife is also more likely to share soothing sounds unabated. If cities are one-note, forests are symphonies. The harmonies of animals, trees, wind, and the land create an audio track that's rich and interesting.

While other naturally quiet places like remote deserts and empty fields just after snowfall also tend to be low in human-made noise, they might actually register as *too* silent to the point of being uncomfortable—especially for urbanites who have built up a tolerance for commotion. While quiet places are predictable and nonthreatening to a certain extent, they can also feel isolating and eerie. One test of people's reactions to a virtual reality forest that had some natural sounds compared with one that was totally silent found that the sound added to the virtual landscape's potential for stress recovery—possibly because explorers of the silent landscape worried that a predator was about to pop out and surprise them.[28] We'll dig deeper into humanity's complex relationship with silence in the ice and snow chapter, but for now, we can say that forests provide just the right amount of it.

While the soundtrack of every forest is different—and a tropical jungle will sound more heavy metal than soft folk—on average, this landscape tends to be a tune that's pleasant enough to make us drop our shoulders, quiet our inner dialogues, and enjoy the experience of just listening.

The Feelings:
Why Playing in the Dirt
Can Be Nourishing

Finally, the physical feeling of forests can help bolster well-being. In one study, a plate of uncoated white oak wood induced relaxation more than marble, tile, or steel.[29] Just touching the bark seemed to calm brain activity and increase parasympathetic activity, which is heightened during relaxation.

After gently running your hand along some trees of any temperature, bending down and picking up a handful of forest soil can also prove enriching. Woodland floors are abundant in microbes—creatures too small to be seen with the naked eye[30]—thanks to how trees support healthy, diverse soil. Every time deciduous trees shed their nutrient-rich leaves for the winter, they feed the ground below. Tree roots also help out soil by improving aeration, increasing capacity to hold water, and forming mutually beneficial partnerships with soil fungi like the mycelium we touched on earlier. (In return for sending a tree's messages, the mycelia receive a lifetime supply of sugars that they can't create on their own.) As a result, forest soil communities tend to be a lot richer than those on grasslands or farms.[31]

One soil bacterium of particular interest is *Mycobacterium vaccae*,[32] which scientists believe can help increase serotonin levels in the brain and regulate mood. Early research on *Mycobacterium vaccae* has been so promising that physiologists at the University of Colorado Boulder are now attempting to turn it into a "stress vaccine" for humans after successful trials feeding it into mice to increase resilience and fend off anxiety.[33]

How's that for proof that playing in the dirt shouldn't just be for kids? Making physical contact with a wide variety of beneficial soil microbes is a healthy habit to get into, especially in today's increasingly sterilized world.

Beyond the Senses:
How the Understory Puts the
Human Journey into Perspective

A forest's fragrant phytoncides, intricate fractal patterns, fresh air, inviting soundscapes, and varied textures come together to create a rich landscape that can be either invigorating or relaxing, depending on what it is you need. And talking with forest bathing guides around the world, I get the sense that the forest can be medicinal in more ways than one. Through those conversations, I've heard how the woods can shift to become a source of wonder for uninspired times, a force of clarity on difficult decisions, a respite from chaotic days. To anthropomorphize the landscape for a moment: forests are like seasoned therapists, pulling from deep wells of knowledge that come with years—many, many years—of lived experience.

Some tree species can, after all, outlive humans hundreds of times: Wohlleben writes that a two-hundred-year-old tree is about the equivalent of a forty-year-old human being. Trees' longevity is made possible by their slow and controlled growth. They go through endless transition, but they do it with such patience that they appear stagnant to our human gaze. Their periods of loss—of leaves in the winter, of sap in the spring—and regrowth follow each other in loops eternal. They shed and pick up, die and become reborn, all the while exuding some of nature's most vibrant colors.

In a world riddled with anxiety for the future, this steady assuredness and grace through change is something to learn from. As Julia Plevin, founder of the Forest Bathing Club and the author of *The Healing Magic of Forest Bathing: Finding Calm, Creativity, and Connection in the Natural World*, puts it to me, "Trees live their lives in meditation. You can feel that energy when you're around them."[34]

We feel drawn to trees because, in them, we see more ideal versions of ourselves. Every walk in the forest is an opportunity to imagine ourselves anew, to learn from the insights gleaned over hundreds of years of patient listening.

These lessons don't always come easily. While individual trees are often positively portrayed (the wise and all-knowing stump of *The Giving Tree*, the Grandmother Willow of *Pocahontas*), expansive forests have historically been places to fear. Dark, enclosed, and mysterious, the woods have spooked characters in religion, myth, and fable through time (Snow White had her fight with bats and clingy flesh-eating twigs in the haunted forest; Little Red Riding Hood was tricked by the wolf when she veered off the wooded path).

While lingering at the forest's edge is safe, to wade deeper into the woods is to invite danger in your life. Coming out the other side, though, is a triumph.

In this sense, trudging through the woods can be a metaphor for facing the darker parts of the human psyche. Confronting negative thoughts and emotions is threatening, it's uncomfortable, but oftentimes it's necessary, and we emerge better for it. That's certainly what Judith Sadora, a wilderness therapist who works mostly with teens grappling with trauma, depression, and racial identity, has seen in her work. In addition to helping her clients become physically and mentally stronger, Sadora says that the wilderness has fueled her own journey toward self-analysis and, ultimately, self-acceptance. "Wilderness to me means a level of enlightenment, a level of growth," she tells me. "I grew up Christian, and for a long time I thought wilderness was something that was a sin, a place that people go to mess up. I'm still a Christian, but I've deconstructed that for myself: wilderness is not someplace that I go to get rid of myself or to condemn myself. . . . It's a place where I go to find myself and be okay with it."

The Practice

Most of the research on the healing capacity of the woods was done in extreme conditions: sterile labs or lush, remote woods. If you don't feel comfortable in dense, unmanaged forests (a lot of people don't![35]), visiting

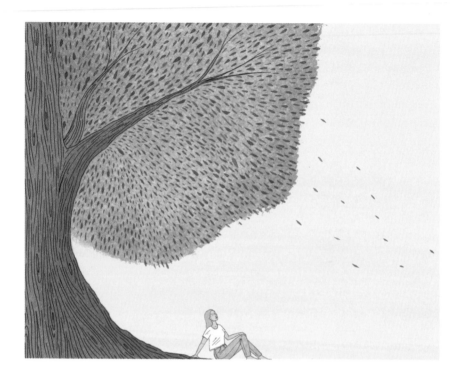

them may cause more stress and fear than restoration. Instead, look for a
middle ground: an urban forest, a popular wooded trail, or even a path of
street trees can all be fertile ground for the following exercises.

IF YOU HAVE 5–10 MINUTES:

Look at the tree communities in your area.

Those short on time can still have a meaningful few moments with the canopy around them. On your next outing, simply look at the patterns and
colors of one particular tree, then notice how they play with others in their
cluster. Even if the other senses can't be fully engaged, this intentional ob-

servation has a relaxing effect. In research out of Asia, forest views[36] have repeatedly[37] made participants feel more "comfortable," "natural," and "soothed" and less stressed than urban ones.

Take your lunch break under the canopy.

When he's not leading forest baths for research, Qing Li finds a similar peace by spending his midday work breaks in a small city park near his office. While eating lunch, he sits under a tree and engages with his surroundings using all the senses. He isn't the only one who finds the canopy a comforting eating companion: when I wrote to the legendary Jane Goodall for an interview during COVID-19's lockdown,[38] she told me that she, too, had been spending a sensory lunch break outside, in the yard of the home where she was quarantined. She sat under a favorite beech tree, listened to the daily robin song, and softly sang back between bites.

Get to know one tree.

Chances are, you pass hundreds of trees every day without paying much attention to what they're up to. This "tree blindness," as it's been dubbed by botanists,[39] can quickly be cured.

Start small, by choosing one tree that sticks out to you and is easy to visit and revisit. Look up what type of tree it is if you're not sure, and whether it's native to your area. Every time you pass it, make a point to slow down and see what you notice about it. Has it lost a branch? Are its leaves changing color at all? If you're so inclined, you can take regular pictures of the tree over a period of months or years. Let the album be a reminder that although the tree may have always looked stagnant to you, it was really growing up before your eyes the whole time.

Richard Powers, the author of *The Overstory*,[40] a stunning novel told from the perspective of trees, describes the process of overcoming his own tree blindness through observation as a "religious conversion" that made him feel like he was "being bound back into a system of meaning that doesn't begin and end with humans."[41]

Feel into the five senses.

Seek out the quietest patch of trees you can find for this mini moment of mindfulness. Once you've found a spot to stand on, close your eyes if you feel comfortable. Take a few deep breaths and place your attention on the smells around you. Then, imagining that you're standing in the middle of a snow globe, identify the sound that is farthest away from you, the one that would be vibrating off the glass. Move on to the sensation of your feet on the ground as you rock back and forth slightly. Open your mouth and take a deep breath in, noticing the flavor and texture of the air. Finally, open your eyes and let them land on the trees in front of you, taking in their patterns big and small. Head back into your life with a slightly greener awareness.

IF YOU HAVE AN HOUR:

Be a tree hugger.

In the forests of India in the 1970s, a group of villagers started hugging large trees to keep loggers from cutting them down, all the while chanting "This forest is our mother's home; we will protect it with all our might." Their bravery inspired the Chipko, (a Hindi word for embracing), which popularized the term *tree hugger*. There's a disconnect between this history and the often-derogatory way we talk of tree huggers today. But based on what we now know of forests, there are lots of reasons to hug trees.

If physically hugging a tree feels a little too woo-woo for you, sit near one instead. Observe its expansive ecosystem and tune in to its small details, starting at the base of its trunk and working upward to its leaves. Get to know it, and then let it get to know you: consider a problem you have or a question you're grappling with and listen for any insights that might come through the forest. Stay open and receptive to the knowledge wedged in the canopy: it might surprise you.

Leave behind an offering.

In the name of reciprocity, Julia Plevin likes to cap off her forest bathing sessions by asking the group to make an offering to the land. "We get so much from the Earth, but what do we give?" she'll ask them. (Blank stares and murmurs of "climate change?" sometimes follow.) Leaving behind a prayer, a song, or even just some water from your water bottle is a simple way to thank the forest after your next wooded walk.

One of the key points in forest bathing is to be really slow. It's less about getting there than about just being here. There's some kind of emotional and mental clarity that comes along with the slowness.

—YOUMIN YAP,
forest therapy guide in Singapore

IF YOU HAVE LONGER:

Take a forest bath.

The typical forest bath lasts about two to three hours, but it doesn't need to cover more than half a mile of ground. A guide in your area can lead you through these mindful walks, or you can follow your own curiosity and go on a self-directed forest tour.

There are very few rules here—but a slow pace is essential, Manuela Siegfried, a forest bathing guide outside San José, Costa Rica, explains to me. "Awaken the senses and slow down so you can really connect to the forest in this sensory and more personal way," she suggests. As you're walking slowly to the point of exaggeration, stay open to the details around you and let your mind settle where it will. This framework can help direct you:

STEP 1. For the setting of your walk, choose a forest or patch of trees that feels safe and comfortable. It can be secluded or more public, but ideally should be relatively free of human noise and have plenty of natural sights and sounds to tune into. Details like running water, mossy stones, and birdsongs can all engage the senses in a big way. Qing Li adds that the taller and more dense the trees in the area, the better.

STEP 2. Take note of how you feel, mind and body, before heading into the woods.

STEP 3. Once you step into the forest, start with the five-minute, five-senses meditation shared earlier. Feel free to come back to it at any point.

STEP 4. Walk slowly through the forest, with no real plan or goal in mind. Notice the novelties the trees and the soil and the plants share with you that day, remembering that they're constantly changing. Here are some cues to help you tune in:

- Gaze up at the patterns of the branches and leaves, looking out for *komorebi*,[42] the Japanese word for light filtering through the canopy of a tree.

- In addition to the sounds your ears immediately pick up, try to listen to the layers of noise that are more subtle. "As people, we just tend to put our attention on the loudest and the most obvious," Youmin Yap, a forest therapy guide in Singapore, tells me. "The practice helps to bring people's perspective to the other side, and pay attention to the softness that is present in the background."

- Lightly touch the bark of tree trunks, the moss on rocks, or any other aspect of the "sensory extravaganza," as Yap calls it, of the forest that appeals to you. (Just watch out for anything poisonous.)

STEP 5. Take a few moments to reflect on the forest's character that day. What energy did you pick up on during your mosey through the woods? How do you feel now, compared with before your walk? Write down your thoughts so that you can refer to them the next time you give this practice a try to see how the experience differs.

CONNECTING FROM AFAR:
Diffuse woodsy essential oils.

Using essential oils, we can literally bottle up the fragrant phytoncides of the forest and reap some of their health benefits on demand. In one of Li and Miyazaki's studies led by Nippon Medical School, participants spent three nights in a hotel room that smelled of hinoki cypress (a common woodsy scent in Japan) essential oils.[43] After their stay, guests' NK (white blood cell) activity was up across the board, while their stress levels had decreased.

Stock up on spruce, fir, cedarwood, and hinoki essential oils and smell or diffuse them any time you're inside but really want to be outside. While researchers opted for a longer diffusion time in this experiment, capping yours at around three hours will be plenty—oils start to lose their smell and potency after that.

Listen to your ideal forest soundscape.

The exaggerated sounds of birds, running water, and singing cicadas can instantly transport us to busy tropical jungles, while the subtler quality of leaves swaying and dirt crunching can take us to serene evergreen woods. That's the beauty of this landscape; it takes on many forms. Choose a forest recording that corresponds to what you're craving on any given day, close your eyes, and fade into the tonal embrace.

Journal on the forest's themes.

The following questions are based on the very foresty themes of trust, community, and hard-earned wisdom:

- What or whom do you depend on for support? What do you give to that person or thing back in return?

- How does seasonality play a role in your life? Do you slow down and start to shed in winter, or do you expect yourself to run on constant summer mode?

- When was the last time you needed to stay patient and how did it go?

- When you get outside, what's your favorite of the five senses to engage? We tend to be highly visual creatures, but how could you more actively engage your other senses every day?

The Action

Beyond being nice to look at and relaxing to walk through, forests are guardians against global warming. They're busy carbon sinks that absorb CO_2 from the atmosphere and store it in the leaves, trunk, and roots of trees (dry wood is about 50 percent carbon by weight) as well as in soil and other vegetation.

To the slow pace of forests, climate change must feel especially rapid—and especially disruptive. Here are three ways to support forests so they can continue to support us.

Clear-Cutting & Burning for Agriculture

As trees age and grow, their capacity to sequester carbon increases. This makes intact old-growth forests (around 150 years or older) some of our most powerful allies in the fight against climate change. Nestled in their developed underground root systems, thick leaf canopies, and layered branches, you'll find three hundred billion tons of carbon,[44] roughly the amount that humans have emitted into the atmosphere over the last 150 years.

It isn't locked in there forever, though, and every time we chop down a section of forest, the carbon it holds is released into the air once again. This makes mass deforestation events all the more disturbing—and dangerous. Since humans began clearing forests, we've cut down 46 percent of the trees on Earth,[45] releasing greenhouse gases, disrupting the intricate balance of the surrounding forest, destroying wildlife habitat, and threatening the people who depend on trees for their livelihood with the felling of each one.

The Mindset Shift:
"Every time I buy food, I vote for the future I want to see."

Needless to say, protecting the few remaining old-growth forests we have from destruction is essential. But widespread, apocalyptic fires in developing countries, like the one that engulfed the Amazon rainforest in 2019, illustrate how socioeconomic factors can derail forest conservation. Unlike many of the wildfires we're seeing here in the US, the Amazon fires were no accident. They were the amalgamation of hundreds of smaller fires set by farmers clearing forest land. They were clearing the land to make way for farms, and they were making farms to earn a living wage. This type of intentional forest clearing is still happening in the Amazon and throughout other poor nations, such as the Congo Basin region in Africa and the rainforests of Borneo.

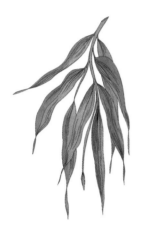

It's too simplistic to write off the individuals clearcutting these places as corrupt and immoral and call it a day. In many cases, they do so because they're more concerned with using this land to get food on the table in the short term than protecting the rest of the planet from the devastating impact of greenhouse gas emissions (which, by the way, they usually contribute very little to otherwise) in the long term. Instead, we need to question the systems that make them have to choose between saving a forest and making a living in the first place.

"Protected areas are safe from exploitation only when their collective resources as intact systems are valued above and beyond their immediate economic value," the forest ecologist Robin Chazdon wrote in a letter to the editor in response to a paper in *Nature*.[46] Preserving mature forests, then, will likely require breaking up with the capitalist, supply-and-demand models that now fuel the global economy, or at least majorly reimagining them to better protect nature.

This won't happen overnight. Agriculture (specifically, beef production) is the leading driver of deforestation worldwide, so if you're looking for a more immediate way to help reduce your role in deforestation, look to your food first.

In an increasingly globalized food system, it can be difficult to trace what we're eating back to its roots and know that it wasn't grown on deforested land. Buying local won't fix the systems driving mass deforestation, but it will ease some of the pressure on them.

So the next time you walk through a grocery store for your weekly haul, pay attention to how many countries are represented in your cart. Then, question which ingredients you can find grown closer to home, from producers who are transparent about their land management. If you have the means and the access, support them by buying from local food systems in your area, whether it's a farmers market or community supported agriculture (CSA) program. Deforestation may seem like a faraway problem, but it's something we have more of a stake in than we might think.

Poorly Executed Reforestation & Afforestation Projects

In addition to protecting existing forests from destruction, planting new ones can help draw carbon out of the atmosphere and back into the ground. And these days, tree planting is big business: tons of organizations and frameworks aim to plant what adds up to trillions of trees around the world through a mix of afforestation (planting trees in previously treeless areas) and reforestation (planting trees on land that was previously forested) projects.

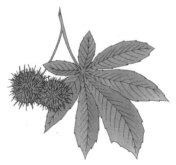

Donating money to their efforts has become a popular way for businesses and individuals to support the environmental movement and offset their own carbon emissions. While this reforestation model is a good deal on paper, it's not without its flaws. It's very possible—and quite common—to botch the job of planting trees, especially when attempting to do so on a large scale.

For one, without an understanding of the land you're planting on, you could choose the wrong tree for that environment. Pick one that doesn't do well in that soil or climate, and it'll end up dying off. Introduce a nonnative tree species, and you run the risk of it disrupting existing plant and animal life.

Planting a whole forest using one or two tree species is equally short-sighted. The resulting ecosystem will be suitable for only a limited range of plants and animals, not to mention vulnerable to rising temperatures and pests. (As we learned in the mountains section, biodiversity acts as insurance against the worst impacts of climate change.) Overly uniform forests also tend to burn much faster than diverse, mature forests, making them vulnerable to destructive fires.

Any kind of climate change initiative really needs to look at building the resilience of local communities. . . . Adaptation is ultimately going to happen at the local level.

—SUSAN CHOMBA,
project lead, Regreening Africa

The Mindset Shift:
"I don't take environmental projects at face value."

The best reforestation programs plant trees that naturally thrive in their given area. These programs don't plant trees in isolation and overly manage them; they plant the building blocks of entire woodlands and then let nature take its course, until the trees start to look and act like older growth. This approach often takes more time and money, but it pays off in the long run in healthy, resilient forests that have a higher chance of storing carbon well into the future.

When I spoke with Robin Chazdon, she said that in the search for a more ecologically savvy reforestation project, it's wise to look for companies that are transparent about what kinds of trees they plant and how they tend to them; what kind of land they plant on and how they chose it; and how much of your donation will go to transaction costs versus be used on the ground. Plan Vivo, Ecosia, and Socio Bosque are a few that she thinks are doing good work from an ecological perspective. Notice that she didn't say to go with the project that is planting the most trees or covering the most ground. As far as tree planting goes, quantity doesn't necessarily signal quality.

The nuances of tree planting remind us that not all restoration projects are created equal. Just because an organization claims to be helping the environment doesn't mean it deserves your time or money. When donating to any pro-environment group, it's still essential to do your research and ask questions.

Mismanaged Tree Cover

When outside organizations come into poor areas and add trees without consulting community members, chances of long-term success are low. "Anybody can go into a community area and just cut trees for fuelwood," Susan Chomba, a social scientist and forest governance expert in sub-Saharan Africa, tells me. When you focus on the needs and interests of the local people, she tells me, the dynamics of restoration change. To ensure that a tree stays standing, she says locals need to be informed about *and involved in* the planting process.

"When you focus on the needs of the people, things are different," Chazdon tells me. "Now they're invested. They view it as a livelihood activity, and they're able to make some money from it, not just because they're being paid by the government. It changes the whole dynamics of it."

For an example, we can look at Chomba's Regreening Africa project,[47] which is regenerating forest land in eight African countries through collaborations with local landowners. For the vulnerable communities she works with, trees are more than carbon sequesters; they are a source of livelihood. Chomba's team presents locals with a suite of trees that are adapted to their areas, and then gives them the final say about what is planted—whether it's fruit-bearing trees that can give them food to sell at the market or varieties that will produce enough timber to build a house.

Engaging communities creates a sense of ownership, Chomba explains. That ownership helps ensure that the vegetation will stay in the ground and stay well managed into the future, so it can do its job of reinvigorating degraded land—a win for that environment and its people.

The Mindset Shift: "I know environmental restoration doesn't need to come at the expense of human livelihood."

The next time you participate in or donate to a tree planting, make sure it considers both the ecological and cultural context of the land. Don't just ask what kinds of trees will go into the ground; ask about the people who will be putting them there and taking care of them too.

Chomba and Chazdon both recommend looking for decentralized plantings that involve local environmental committees (this might mean working with them directly, or going through an intermediary institution or NGO), since they're the ones who will know about the laws and local government structures that will protect the trees into the future, long after they take root. Supporting a community model for any environmental initiative—not just reforestation—will make your dollars and time go further.

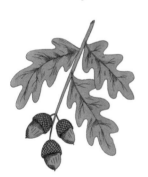

Finally, remember that like trees in a forest, environmental solutions glean strength in numbers. While tree protection and restoration has the potential to preserve land and livelihoods, it is not a solution to climate change in itself. Forests alone can't absorb all of the CO_2 we are releasing into the environment (and, in fact, trees lose some ability to store carbon as the world warms[48]), so these actions always need to be paired with emissions reductions.

CHAPTER FIVE

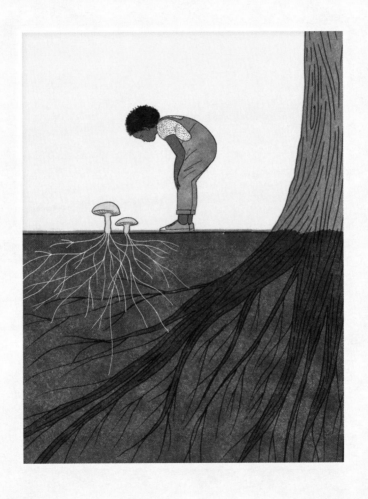

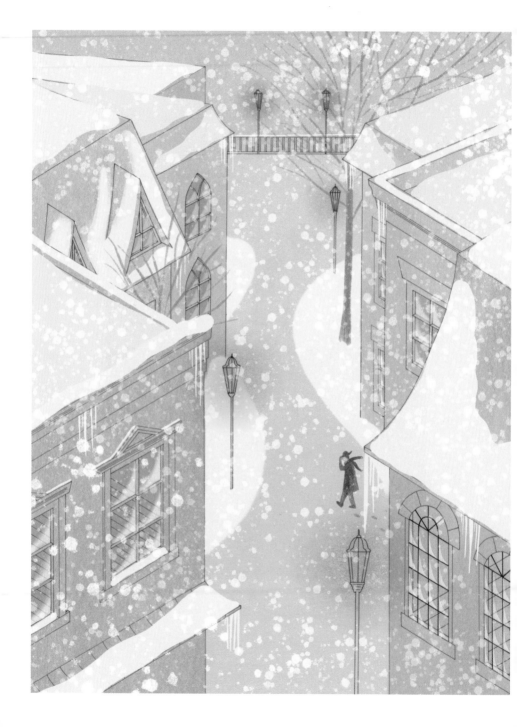

ICE & SNOW

silence, resilience, reward

The snowy weather slaps a filter on my usual view. Under the coat of white, details soften and merge. It's hard to distinguish between much of anything: the sidewalk and the grass, the tree branches and the shrubs are all covered in the same reflective veil. Land and sky blend as sunlight peeks through to cast a million crystal chandeliers as it hits Earth. I want to wrap myself in it all. But then, I open the window—or, rather, it blows open on me—and the chill hits. Cold is a polarizing thing, and I am usually not one to embrace it. But today is one of those days when, as I watch the blanket of snow thicken, Brooklyn sleeping warm underneath, I just need to get out and feel it for myself. As always, I'm so glad I do.

The Remedy

While not a landscape in itself, snow and its relatives—ice, sleet, and so forth—can turn any natural scene into a new place entirely. In higher latitudes, dipping temperatures, darker days, and icy conditions make outdoor excursions, save for the occasional snow sport, much less appealing in winter. Of all the weather patterns, ice and snow are two of the most likely to keep Americans (myself very much included) huddled inside.[1]

Like animals, we hibernate for much of the snowy season—but some initial investigations on white space conclude that we'd be better off getting out in it more.

The Psychological Case for Getting Outside in the Snow

Nature doesn't become any less restorative once it's blanketed in white. Far from it. While a walk through the cold snow may not lead to the same positive emotions (depending on the person) as one on a sunny, temperate day, it still seems to restore the mind in a similar way.

One of the best indicators we have of this is a winter 2008 study on the very chilly University of Michigan campus.[2] In it, participants were instructed to walk through urban areas and the school's tree-clad arboretum—in subfreezing temperatures. Their short-term memory and attention improved by 20 percent on average after the cold nature walk, but saw no change after the cold city walk.

"We found the same benefits when it was 80 degrees and sunny over the summer as when the temperatures dropped to 25 degrees in January," Marc Berman, an associate professor of psychology and cognitive neuroscience, said in a write-up of the study. "The only difference was that participants enjoyed the walks more in the spring and summer than in the dead of winter." This suggests that an outdoor experience can be cognitively beneficial even if it doesn't lead to particularly positive emotions. Like so many things in life, we don't need to love it—or even particularly like it—to be changed by it.

When I asked a handful of other environmental psychology researchers based in colder climates about the snow, the theme of preparation came up again and again.

If you go out for a winter walk expecting it to be frosty and wet, they said, the experience will likely align with those assumptions. This compatibility is a prerequisite of attention restoration theory. The most restorative experiences, Jason Duvall, the University of Michigan lecturer we met in the parks chapter, explains, are the ones where there is a match between expectation and reality. "If you have the right kind of mindset, the right kind of expectations about going out in winter, you prepare yourself, you wear a coat, you put your thick socks on, you can have a really enjoyable restorative experience," he tells me, with the caveat that there is, of course, a limit to how much discomfort we can take, even when prepared: "I'm doubtful we would see a restorative benefit if you're walking through a gale-force wind with your eyes closed and sleet is hitting you in the face."

Snow is nature reminding us who's in charge. And if getting outdoors is painful to the point of being dangerous, it won't make you feel much in the way of restoration. So maybe skip the blizzard walk, but by all means head out for the light dusting.

By continuing to get out in the snow when it's safe to do so, you'll also create opportunities for favorable cold-weather memories to collect and crystallize. You might be thinking: Wait a minute, I thought enjoying an experience doesn't matter as far as restoration is concerned. Well, while a neutral or negative feeling may not impede your outdoor experience, a positive one can only add to it.

The Mysterious Ways That the Cold Affects the Body

Once you're prepared for them, cold landscapes can prove uniquely invigorating. Cold therapy in all its forms (ice bath or cold morning shower, anyone?) has long been used by extreme athletes to speed up muscle recovery. Recently, it's received a new wave of interest as one of Wim Hof's three pillars. Hof, an extreme ice athlete, rose to fame by setting world records that sound like something out of a Marvel movie: he's climbed Mount Kilimanjaro in shorts, run a half marathon above the Arctic Circle barefoot, and stood in containers filled with ice (again, in shorts) for hours at a time.[3]

Though he's earned the nickname "The Iceman," Hof says that there's nothing superhuman about him. He's simply trained himself to withstand extreme cold and reaped the benefits—which he says include better sleep quality, sharper focus, and a stronger immune response—in the process.

In a TEDx talk,[4] Hof stands in a clear box as ice is dumped on top of him bucket by bucket. After a few minutes, snow up to his neck, the human snowman stands still, without so much as a shiver escaping him. Somehow, he's managed to keep his heart rate and blood pressure down in the freezing cold when it should be speeding up—making him an active participant in human processes that were previously thought to be automatic. Researchers are now investigating how this enigmatic figure is able to do the seemingly impossible. Meanwhile, Hof is teaching the masses to befriend the freeze through books, retreats, and video courses. Hof's story is a prime example of the complex human-cold relationship and all that we have yet to learn about it.

Cold exposure on a far safer and more comfortable scale can also be beneficial, good news for those of us not ready to go full Iceman. Exercising outside on a cold winter day, for example, can help your body move more efficiently because your heart won't have to work as hard, you'll sweat less, and you'll expend less energy, Adam Tenforde, an assistant professor of sports medicine, tells Harvard Health Publishing.[5] Brief exposure to chilly temperatures can also prompt the brain to release mood-supporting endorphins, and cold therapy has been investigated as a potential treatment for anxiety and depression.[6] So while it may be uncomfortable at times, safely continuing your nature exploration in the snow can still be great for the mind and body.

The Dusting:
How Snow Teaches Us to Hear Silence

Once the cold snow starts to settle into blankets and freeze, its healing potential further solidifies. That's when the silence sets in.

Silence, as Gordon Hempton, an acoustic ecologist and founder of One

Square Inch of Silence,[7] defines it, isn't the absence of sound but the absence of noise. *Noise* is relatively loud, simple auditory information that denies us access to complex, often more valuable natural *sounds*. A street ablaze with chatter, sirens, and cars passing is, undoubtedly, noisy. But from Hempton's perspective, a snowy scene that is equally alive with wind, swaying leaves, and social critters can still be considered silent.

He has spent decades traversing the world's most remote places to relish in and record these sounds of wilderness absent of man or machine. They are becoming harder to find. One chilly winter morning, on a Face-Time call from his truck, Hempton laments that noise now pervades almost every ecosystem. Natural quiet, he fears, could be yet another resource to go extinct within the next ten years if we don't act to protect it.

These days, he says, the groans of fighter jets shock the surface of the land and ocean below,[8] and the whir of car engines ricochets off nearby trees and shrubbery. And cities? Forget it. The noise in cities has become so omnipresent, so normalized, that we forget it is, in fact, a pollutant— and a dangerous one at that. After sifting through data on how prolonged exposure to noise can increase one's risk factors for heart disease, insomnia, and cognitive impairment, the World Health Organization estimated that one million healthy life years are lost to traffic-related noise annually in the western part of Europe alone.[9]

The silence after snowfall offers respite from such costly commotion. With fewer people out and about, fewer cars on the road, and a coating of snow to dull any leftover hubbub, what remains is a rare quiet that is important to pay attention to.

Humans through time have used still moments like these to tune in to themselves and, in some cases, a higher power. Timothy Gallati, one of the few scholars to receive an advanced degree in capital S Silence (from Harvard, no less), pointed me to one article in the constitution of Cistercians, a monastic order in the Catholic tradition, that phrases its power perfectly. This constitutional clause directs brothers to be "zealous for silence, which is the guardian both of speech and of thought." This was written in *1119*.[10] Over nine hundred years later, the whir of machines and ping of notifications have made quiet and all it espouses even more holy, even more worthy of our ears.

A naturally quiet space, after all, presents the opportunity for honesty, for thoughtful consideration of both speech and thought. It's a gentle invitation to shovel our internal landscape, work around the sticks and rocks of the mind, and clear a path forward. As Gallati tells me, "It's where expectations end and real discovery and wonder starts."

Committing to such discovery is not easy work, and Gallati adds that silence and its "immediate relatives"—stillness, solitude—can be destabilizing in the information age.

Indeed, in a sobering 2012 survey of how Americans spend their time,[11] only 17 percent of respondents reported "relaxing/thinking" in the previous twenty-four hours, while 95 percent reported doing some other, more active leisure pursuit (mostly, watching TV). In another series of studies on college students, those polled found being alone with their thoughts for just fifteen minutes so uncomfortable, so "aversive," that "it drove many participants to self-administer an electric shock that they had earlier said they would pay to avoid."[12]

This is likely one reason that many people find quiet landscapes like a snow-covered field or city street unsettling at first. Like a pause in a conversation, these spaces present a silence that we long to fill. It's only through working past this initial discomfort that we find the gift waiting on the other side of silence.

Research is emerging to support this quiet utility. Somewhat by accident, a physician and professor of internal medicine at the University of Pavia in Italy named Luciano Bernardi found that the most relaxing part of music, the part that lowers heart rate and blood pressure, is not the bridge or the chorus but the moments of pause between verses.[13] Silence, it seems, is even more valuable following periods of sound, in the same way a blanket of snow feels ever more inviting following the cacophony of a storm.

So the next time you find yourself in a silent winter's moment, linger in it. Instead of trying to fill the silence, let it fill you.

The Powder:
How Snow Challenges Us to Stay Present

As snow sits, it becomes less ethereal and more dirty. It slickens into ice. Its weight can overtake a tree or home, or collapse on itself and fall downhill as an avalanche. These changes don't happen over the course of seasons but seconds. Snow wears transformation on its sleeve, and for many people, this volatility is off-putting. But ask any outdoor adventurer who calls snow their stage, and they'll reframe that unpredictability as an opportunity.

Take Chris Fagan, who, in her late forties, chose to ski for forty-eight days across Antarctica with her husband, a 220-pound sled, and the goal of reaching the South Pole before they ran out of food. She left behind a comfortable life—a preteen son, a stable career—to traverse one of the harshest terrains on the planet, complete with subzero temperatures and biting winds that she remembers being "ever-present."

Then there's backcountry snowboarder Dani Reyes-Acosta, who tells me, laughing, "A lot of the things I choose to do are straight-up suffering." And outdoor and high-alpine figure skater Laura Kottlowski, who has ditched the rink in favor of open-air frozen lakes. She sets out before sunrise, climbs for hours, sometimes up to altitudes of 11,000 to 15,500 feet, in frigid temperatures for the mere chance of finding ideal weather windows where she can use her skates to carve intricate patterns into the ice.

These women choose to take the path of most resistance, to embrace chilly landscapes because of their harsh unknowns and not in spite of them. As a self-proclaimed winter wimp, it's hard for me to understand why. Are they built differently? Does the stripping slap of heavy wind, the unrelenting sourness of cold, just not affect them the same way?

The answer is, of course, no—the cold's downsides are just as unpleasant for them as they are for me. The difference is that in snow and ice, they've found opportunities that outweigh temporary dangers and discomforts.

The opportunity for presence is a big one. Listening to their stories, I get the sense that stark white can evoke a meditative state unlike any other,

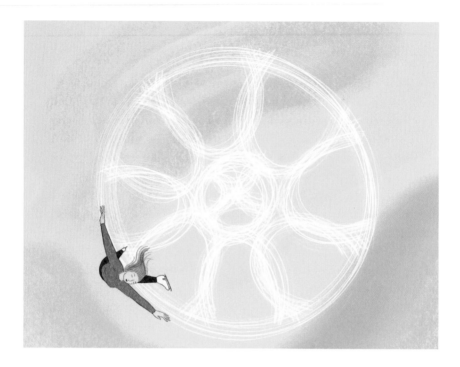

one that is centering and limitless all at once. All landscapes lead to this presence to a certain extent, but the more forceful ones like ocean, snow, and desert seem to turn it up a notch.

Fagan tells me that at one point in her journey, when the wind died down enough that she could hear herself think, "there was this profound silence and it kind of washed over me in this moment of connection to everything in the world. . . . You're in the most alone place you can ever be, and all that you see is the white nothingness around you, and my body started to go away—it merged with what was happening around me."

Reyes-Acosta feels similarly smudged into the landscape every time she takes to her board. From there, she says, snow becomes a metaphor for some of life's greater lessons. The constantly shifting conditions on ice-capped mountains are humbling hints that even with proper preparation, so much is out of her control; anything can happen at any moment. As she puts it to me, "There are a million different ways that land can be unstable."

With that in mind, she rides down and makes her mark in the snow—knowing nothing for sure except that the imprint of her board will eventually disappear. "There's a sense of impermanence," she says of the feeling she has snowboarding. "The impermanence of life, the impermanence of what we leave behind." Kottlowski's figures, Fagan's footsteps, too, have inevitably all long faded to ice. But that doesn't keep them from continuing to carve.

The way these women describe the winter makes me think of a blank page: it can either be terrifying or empowering, depending on how you look at it. And ultimately, when we choose to see the opportunity in snow, ice, and cold, we can walk away having experienced a freeing surrender—one that will serve us long after we find warmth once again.

The Deep Freeze:
How Ice Reminds Us of Our Place in Time

Finally, with enough cold and pressure, once-ephemeral and fragile snow freezes and compacts, transforming into one of the world's most persistent and persuasive of landmarks: glaciers that shape entire countries and continents with the weight that they carry.

In regions where glaciers dominate, minutes become mind-bending. Frozen edges of the world like the Arctic and Antarctic have everlasting days in the summer and unrelenting nights in winter, creating what the writer Barry Lopez deemed "hourless moments."[14] The glaciologist, geographer, and National Geographic Explorer M Jackson feels a similar time warp when she steps onto the ice: "It's hard to get distance. It's hard to get scale. It's hard to get smell. It's hard to get color. It's hard to get time out there." Ultimately, she tells me, it's a boundlessness that's inspiring. "Your whole world never shrinks; instead, your whole world cracks open much, much bigger when you're with ice."

Since glaciers hold Earth's history in their depths, they have a way of making us feel small, short-lived, and delightfully insignificant. Like gazing out onto an expansive vista or watching a river stretch toward the horizon, looking at a glacier (in real life or, more realistically, in a travel magazine or on TV) is a humbling feeling, and a strangely freeing one at that. In its depths lies the vastness of geologic time, or "deep time," as John McPhee first wrote of it in the 1980s.[15] McPhee coined *deep time* as a way for geologists to describe "time in quantities no mind had yet conceived." Considering it is a way to stretch the limits on time as we experience it, and put our lives into perspective in the process. In today's world where news cycles by the minute and requests for our attention come by the second (and are only getting faster), widening our clocks outward can offer a much-needed reprieve.

Most of us will never get to see glaciers or learn their dizzying lessons on time up close, especially considering the rate at which we're losing them. But every snowflake can serve as a similarly humbling reminder of the larger forces at play in our universe: the way in which beauty and power, strength and fragility, the immediate and the eternal, can coexist in our world.

Winter is full of ambiguities like this. The season provides opportunities for quiet reflection as well as intense peak exertion—neither of which is comfortable. Snow and ice, after all, give nothing away easily.

The Practice

These activities can help you forge your own path in the snow. Inspired by those who know winter best, they offer doable, meaningful ways to get outdoors all year round. If you live in an area that doesn't get much snowfall, feel free to modify them into rituals for rainfall or otherwise inclement weather.

Consider what you're leaving behind.

Once the final dust of snow falls, a single blanket of white emerges, reshaping the land into a place to be explored for the first time. Fresh snow is a canvas, and to walk across it is to leave your own unique mark. The next time you head out, be a bit more mindful of the path you're leaving behind. Consider taking a cue from Laura Kottlowski and offering up some art along the way; drag your feet into a shape, outline your name, make a snow angel, play around. Let what you create remind you of the one-of-a-kind beauty that comes when you and nature meet.

> Quiet is not a thing to do. Quiet is a way of being. . . . Quiet is a feeling, and it's a path, and it will lead you to where you need to go.
>
> —GORDON HEMPTON,
> acoustic ecologist

Turn up the volume on silence.

Sound and silence experts Gordon Hempton and Timothy Gallati both say that to fully engage with quiet spaces, you need to enter them with an open and curious mind—and a willingness to listen. (*Silent* and *listen* share the same letters, after all.) "If you're thinking about what you're doing, what you're hearing, then you aren't listening," Hempton explains to me.

Try out his routine for tuning in to the space around you on your next snow outing. First, choose a spot to stand (or walk around, if it's really cold) for a moment. Then, listen and pinpoint the sound that's the farthest away from you, at the edge of your auditory horizon. Next, tune in to the faintest sound you can hear. Then, to a sound you can hear but can't see, like the wind. Then, simply notice how you feel.

Once you stretch your awareness in this first spot, move to another one and repeat the listening exercise again, letting the soundscape reveal itself to you and taking note of how it makes you feel. Repeat this silence tour for as long as you like, or as long as your bare ears can take.

IF YOU HAVE AN HOUR:

Go outside after preparing for the snow, physically and mentally.

To borrow from the Norwegian phrase, there really is no bad weather, only bad clothes. Even if you are someone who loves the winter and has fond memories of the snow, heading out into a storm ill-equipped will only lead to suffering. "It's not going to be a restorative experience because you'll have to remain vigilant," Rich Mitchell, an epidemiologist, geographer, and professor at the University of Glasgow, tells me.

> Instead of getting stressed about the cold or the wind or the whiteout or the terrain, I realized it's futile. It's using up my limited resources, my limited energy, and it's taking me from a positive mindset to a negative mindset.
>
> —CHRIS FAGAN,
> endurance athlete, speaker, consultant,
> reflecting on her time in Antarctica

In addition to the proper base layers, as Chris Fagan's experience shows, donning the right mindset can help make your winter experience more positive. Before you head out, flex those visualization muscles and spend a moment mentally preparing for—and surrendering to—the weather. Picture the first slap of wind, the burn of frosty air on your skin, the dampness of snowfall. Remember that your outing can still be a treat for the mind through it all.

Go on a walk with a winter awareness plan.

We learned in the parks chapter that going out into nature with the aim of spotting something (birds, other critters) or adopting a certain perspective (an artist looking for beauty in nature, a botanist on the hunt for a unique plant species) can help make the experience richer and more positive.

While winter scenes may look flat on the surface, they're actually teeming with life and opportunities to engage, explore, and discover. In many areas, winter is a great time to observe animals you can't in other months, like birds that have flocked to your area from out of town. Your winter awareness plan could include looking out for them, watching how snow collects in different trees, listening to how the sound of your footsteps has changed with the season, or observing other ways that life keeps chirping on through the freeze.

Take it all in from inside.

For days when getting outside really isn't an option, taking in a snowy winter scene from indoors can be the next best thing. To set yourself up for mental restoration, crack open a window and engage all the senses: track one flake with your eye as it floats down to the ground, sticking your hand out to feel its imprint. Smell the crisp air; open your mouth to its taste. Listen to the way the world outside your home has calmed down, letting it be permission for you to do the same.

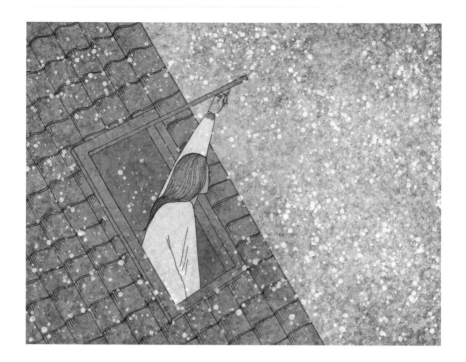

Scout out the silence in your home.

If your area doesn't have much in the way of snow, Timothy Gallati says that you can still take a "sound walk" through your home to discover the quiet that winter weather brings.

"Not all areas of your home are the same," he explains to me. "As you walk through, say, a doorway, notice the transition from one room to another . . . What are the differences between these spaces?" Slowly, through a process of discovery, Gallati says this activity can help you pinpoint a special spot in your home that feels inviting, quiet, and peaceful. Designate that area a meditative or reflective silence practice, like the one Hempton shared earlier in this chapter.

Let cycles remind you of all your relations.

Snow, and weather in general, is cyclical. At the end of the day, a snow-storm is just a collection of elements falling to the ground before eventu-ally evaporating into our atmosphere yet again. Our bodies are governed by the same cycles: the air we breathe, the water we drink, the food we eat all travel through the environment in shape-shifting forevers.

For Connor Ryan, a skier and member of the Lakota tribe, there is great solace in these cycles. When he goes outside—be it on a snowy mountain or a dry sunny day—they are what he looks to for peace and reassurance.

"In Lakota, we say, *Mitakuye-Oyasin*, which means 'all my relations,'" Ryan tells me. This teaching says that all beings—human and nonhuman—are connected on a web of life, related in the sense that they share the same foundation. "We're in this constant balance of relations. And to me, it's one of the most comforting feelings to consider."

In moments of stress or overwhelm, he remembers that with every in-hale, he is borrowing from the planet's pool of oxygen, with every exhale he is returning carbon to the atmosphere. Eventually, that carbon will make its way to a tree, which will then turn it back into oxygen. Amid moments of chaos, this mindful breath taking can remind us that we always exist in larger cycles of life.

Take a random snow day and start fresh.

Is there anything better than a snow day when you're a kid? It's an excuse to devote an entire day to fun and relaxation—and you never really know when one's coming. The anticipation—the "will they or won't they close schools?" of it all—is probably the most exciting part (for kids, at least; I can imagine it's a different story for parents).

There isn't really an adult equivalent. But don't we all deserve a day of completely unplanned celebration—whether it's snowing outside or not? While responsibilities might get in the way of taking an entire day all to yourself, maybe you can take a few "snow hours" instead. Leave this time completely open to allow yourself to do whatever feels right in the moment.

After your snow day, reflect on what it taught you and where in your life you could use a fresh start. Imagine that a blanket of snow has just fallen on that part of you. Whether it melts to reveal the same landscape, or something totally new, is up to you.

Journal on the snow's themes.

Use these questions and prompts to consider how snow's themes of silence, resilience, and reward show up in your life.

- When was the last time you did something that felt uncomfortable? What was it and what was the result?

- What opinions or feelings have you held on to for so long that they've "frozen" over the years and become hardened, fixed, and solid?

- Where in your life do you feel stillness? Do you perceive this stillness as constructive or destructive?

- Consider how the weather affects your mood. What is your favorite type of weather? What's your least favorite type, and what about it bothers you? If that weather keeps you inside, journal on what it would look like to befriend it a bit more.

The Action

In a changing climate, snow and ice are some of the first things to go. Those who spend time in polar regions know this all too well. It's why Chris Fagan didn't wait until her son had grown up to travel to the South Pole, and why Dani Reyes-Acosta doesn't hesitate to follow the snowpack wherever it leads her. They aren't sure how much longer these frozen places will stay frozen, how long they will remain solid enough to explore on two feet.

To understand some of the biggest threats to snow and ice around the world, we're going to zoom in on specific regions. The Arctic and Antarctic are case studies for how all of Earth's frozen realms are under fire, and what we can do to save winters near and far.

Global Warming

You knew this would be number one! With nineteen of the twenty hottest years on record happening since 2000,[16] the planet is quite literally melting before our eyes. And the frozen Arctic region of the north is feeling the burn more than most—warming at more than twice the rate of any other place on Earth.[17]

To freeze is to immortalize. Something as ancient as a glacier feels like it should be impenetrable, but as we now know, humans have found a way to make the eternal temporary. Glaciers may take thousands of years to form, but they are disappearing in our lifetimes. Climate change and its impact on polar regions show that even the deepest of time can end in alarm bells.

Scientists have only been surveying Arctic sea ice since 1979, but in that short time, the summer ice cap has shrunk by more than 40 percent, and the average thickness of the ice has been cut by more than half, according to a Carbon Brief report.[18] It seems that the Arctic is particularly susceptible to high temperatures and glacial melting because of something called the albedo effect: when the Arctic's ice is intact, it's bright enough to reflect a lot of sunlight back into the atmosphere. But as it melts, it exposes a darker underbelly of land or water, which absorbs more of the sun's rays and further fuels warming.

That isn't the only problem with exposing the layer of soil and rock that sits beneath Arctic ice. Also known as permafrost, this previously covered land, also known as permafrost, is like the planet's freezer drawer—a place

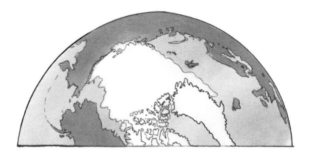

Arctic sea ice 1979

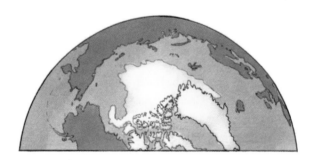

Arctic sea ice 2020

where our "leftovers" (think: carbon dioxide, decomposing animals, microbes, etc.) can remain frosty and undisturbed. When glaciers melt, exposing the permafrost below, all those leftovers are warmed back to life once again, and from there they can cause serious problems. Beyond bringing potentially dangerous pathogens back to the surface, thawing permafrost frees up carbon that was previously locked in place.

Of course, as the journalist Dahr Jamail writes in his book *The End of Ice: Bearing Witness and Finding Meaning in the Path of Climate Disruption*, "what happens in the Arctic does not stay in the Arctic."[19] By the National Oceanic and Atmospheric Administration's estimate,[20] there's twice as much carbon present in northern permafrost region soils than in our atmosphere. It's a dangerous match that, if struck, would fuel warming to new extremes across the globe and could turn worst-case temperature projections into a horrifying reality.

This ice loss would leave an indelible mark on the human landscape too. As M Jackson reminds me, "Where there are glaciers, there are people."

Atop one patch of now-bare land in Iceland where the Okjökull glacier once sat, a memorial plaque reads, "In the next 200 years all our main glaciers are expected to follow the same path. This monument is to acknowledge that we know what is happening and what needs to be done. Only you know if we did it."[21]

The Mindset Shift: "I keep things cool at home."

Getting global emissions levels in check and preventing ice melt will undoubtedly require a stacking of strategies—one of which starts in the icy domains in our very own homes. I'm talking fridges.

Project Drawdown, a climate organization that ranks strategies on their potential to reduce emissions, lists refrigerant management as the number one climate solution.[22] Yep, it beat out plant-based diets, transitioning to solar power, phasing out plastics, and all the other salves we hear so much about.

It turns out that hydrofluorocarbons (HFCs), a class of chemicals that keep our fridges and air-conditioning units cool, are actually extreme sources of heat when they leach into the environment. Depending on their chemical makeup, these refrigerants have one thousand to nine thousand times greater capacity to warm the atmosphere than carbon dioxide, according to Project Drawdown.

"Refrigerants currently cause emissions throughout their life cycles—in production, filling, service, and when they leak," Project Drawdown's book *Drawdown* reads. "But their damage is greatest at the point of disposal." That's when these chemicals are released into the environment 90 percent of the time. So if you're a fridge owner looking to make a difference, the most important thing you can do is ensure that your machine is properly disposed of when the time comes, by a company that's been certified Responsible Appliance Disposal (RAD) by the Environmental Protection Agency. It's a radically simple solution that has an outsized impact.

Globally, hundreds of countries have committed to phasing out HFCs in the coming decades, so at least we don't have to worry about more refrigerants being created. While this won't single-handedly solve global warming, it's a good reminder that with the right legislation in place, we can cut certain sources of warming relatively easily and protect some of the world's most fragile ecosystems in the process.

Resource Extraction

Extreme polar regions like Antarctica are more lively than they look on the surface. Even though parts of the continent are inhabited by vast expanses of snow, sky, and not much else, others are rich in biodiversity.

Cassandra Brooks, a marine scientist and assistant professor in environmental studies at the University of Colorado Boulder with a special focus on Antarctica, describes the ocean surrounding the continent as a last frontier—a place where thousands of species exist and new ones are discovered with each expedition. "The waters are absolutely teeming with life," Brooks tells me, "and we're talking about waters that are below the point of freezing."

In such cold, isolated conditions, the web of life is relatively simple: phytoplankton convert carbon in the atmosphere and are eaten by Antarctic krill, prehistoric-looking, cork-sized critters that fuel the rest of the food chain. The universal cuisine of the region, they keep penguins, seals, and a variety of fantastical fish full and satisfied. To survive in these unforgiving waters, many of these fish also depend on proteins in their blood that act like antifreeze. One species, the icefish, actually ditches red blood cells altogether and absorbs oxygen directly through their transparent skin instead.[23] Farther down on the ocean floor, sea stars, jellyfish, urchins, and sea spiders form communities so colorful that they could be mistaken for a tropical reef.

On land, the biodiversity continues—albeit on a smaller scale. Microscopic life abounds below the snow and ice, forming vibrant underground webs. We can see them up close in areas shielded from ice by mountain ranges, like the McMurdo Dry Valleys, where the land is so impossibly parched that it looks like the set of a Star Wars movie. The landscape is so similar to that of Mars that scientists are now studying it for clues about what microscopic life could exist on other planets.

To learn about these systems is to be amazed by them. And any place that's home to such unique life and landscape is bound to draw interest from human industry. While Antarctica is protected from drilling and mining thanks to the Antarctic Treaty of 1959 (the same can't be said for the Arctic, where drilling is now a real concern), other extractive practices have found their way to the region. The supplement industry is now harvesting krill for their omega-3-rich oils, for example, while high-end fisheries are catching local toothfish (better known as Chilean sea bass) to sell at a premium to diners around the world.

Brooks sees industrial fishing as a major threat to the future of this special region—one that could keep getting worse. "When the ice melts, vessels can get into places they never could before," she says. Overfishing in

Antarctica could throw off the perfectly tailored food chain and lead to nutrient imbalances in the water. The impacts of this would be felt elsewhere, since Antarctica contains the strongest current system in the world and affects water quality, weather patterns, and air temperatures globally.

The Mindset Shift: "I have a stake in places that I'll never visit."

While Brooks is quick to acknowledge that it's difficult for individual action to reach places like Antarctica, she does say that avoiding fish caught in the region can keep it intact into the future. Beyond that, she says the best way to invest in Antarctica and polar regions in general is just to learn about them. Reading stories, flipping through photos, and watching documentaries about these faraway places can help make their conservation feel more urgent.

Disconnection

The foreign beauty in places like Antarctica and the Arctic is both a blessing and a curse. On the one hand, such unique areas are worth protecting. On the other, they are so different from what so many of us are used to that they almost don't seem real. Home to unfamiliar plants and animals, sights and sounds, bitingly cold and dark for half of the year, maddeningly bright for the other, they are places that many of us are curious about but few ever dream of visiting. The same can be said for any winter landscape, really. The snow is synonymous with getting cozy by the fire, staying inside, shutting the doors and windows—any way to shield oneself from the cold world "out there."

This becomes a problem when you consider that climate change is, above all, a crisis of disconnection. So many environmental issues start the minute we separate ourselves from nature. These days, we frame the outdoors as a place beyond our homes, nature as a place outside our bodies.

Distinctions like this can be dangerous. When we don't feel connected to something, it becomes really easy to neglect.

But, if you'll allow me to get meta for a second, there really is no such thing as separation. Everything in nature is connected, and every time we shut out a place, we're casting off part of ourselves.

The Mindset Shift:
"I'm willing to make sacrifices in the present to ensure a sustainable future for all."

I have long known instinctively that, yes, sure, humans *are* nature, so by polluting the planet, we are also polluting ourselves. It's an idea that I have been exploring in my writing for a while, albeit subtly. It wasn't until I spoke with Connor Ryan, the skier we met earlier, that these connections really hit me in the face. He, more eloquently than anyone I'd heard before, framed a warming climate, disappearing winters, melting snow not as an environmental issue but as a matter of human survival.

In his Lakota culture, winter is called *Waniyetu*, which translates to "snow time." A number of winter months also are named for the snow—there's the month of snow blindness, followed by the month of the big snows. Snow plays such a central role in Lakota culture because it gives way to life. The majority of fresh water on Earth, after all, is stored in ice caps and glaciers.

"The experience of Indigenous understanding often gets over-spiritualized," Ryan tells me. "What does sacred really mean? In my inter-pretation, I've come to realize that sacred means it's vital to life. And for that reason, all the land, all the water is sacred."

Being an environmentalist is often considered a selfless act that requires sacrificing something—be it red meat, plastic, or international flights. From this more elemental perspective, though, being an environmentalist is not selfless. It's just a new way of putting yourself and your community first.

"The thing I'm really protecting is my own ability to live and the ability of people after me to live," Ryan says of his own activism—though he's hesitant to call it that. "There's a lot of people who have said, 'I'm not an activist, I'm Lakota.' That's how I feel about it: I didn't wake up one day like 'I want to become an environmental activist because I saw *An Inconvenient Truth*.' I didn't need Al Gore or CNN or Greta Thunberg to convince me. Because of the cultural understanding that I have, water is going to be my highest priority. To me, that's the most sensible thing. I'm a human being. I'm water, so I'm going to protect the water."

Valuing natural elements like air and water like we do manufactured ones like money and material possessions is, of course, easier said than done in our current society. It's an issue of immediacy: the day that the coastline rises feels far, maybe even lifetimes, away. The day that bills need to be paid is never more than a month away.

But in tracing this value system to its logical end, I can't help but keep coming back to a prophecy from the Cree Indians: "When the last tree is cut down, the last fish eaten, and the last stream poisoned, you will realize that you cannot eat money."

Disconnection is the threat, and it's reinforced by manufactured urgency. Maybe, then, saving ourselves is a matter of slowing down to a more glacial pace—one that isn't concerned with the wealth collected over decades but eons.

CHAPTER SIX

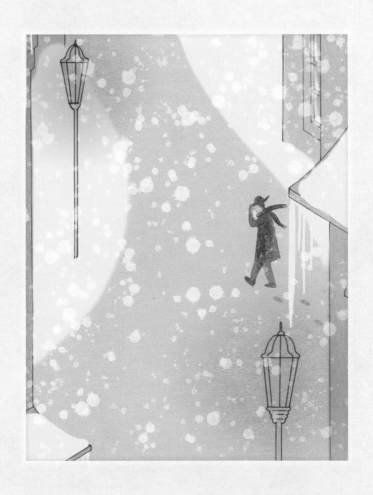

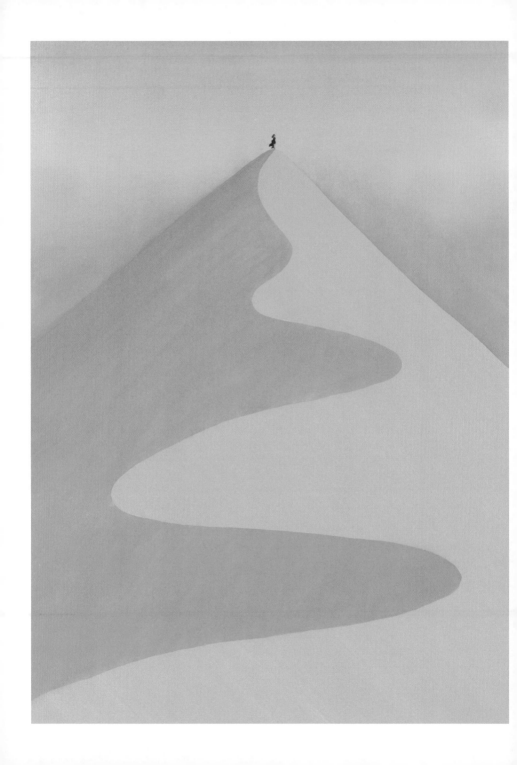

DESERTS & DRYLANDS

erosion, reinvention, reveal

Some people light incense for the smell; I light it for the smoke, for the contained explosion of match to wood that sends plumes dancing through the air until their edges fade to nothing. Going, going, gone. Watching the ribbons of smoke at once settles me into my immediate surroundings and takes me somewhere far away—to the desert where the elements are always in performance with one another, where concerts of air and fire have been playing all day and all night, since the beginning of time.

Like many who didn't grow up in the desert, I assumed the landscape would be an unwelcoming one. But my first time stepping foot into the Sonoran Desert of the American West, I found myself pulled in and not turned away—enchanted by the honesty of desert lands and the quality in the air that I can only describe as mystical. It's a place I happily return to, if only in my mind.

The Remedy

Deserts are what most people would consider "hard" landscapes. They are, as you know, dry. By definition, they get less than ten inches of rain a year and are suitable only for highly adapted plants, animals, and people who have hardened to do without fresh water. The result is a more exposed landscape, one that wears weathering and decay on its sleeve. Deserts are also massive: they occupy about a fifth of Earth's land area and touch every continent (most of Antarctica is considered a polar desert, since so little of its water comes in the form of rain)—and as we'll learn later, they're only getting larger.

While the desert's breakneck heat and dry sun are dangerous in large doses, they can be therapeutic in smaller sips. Here's what research has shown about how to find balance in this land of extremes.

The Daylight Effect: How the Sun Can Contribute to a Steady, Positive Mood

Like frozen landscapes, deserts can quickly go from restorative to risky. Sunburns and dehydration have a way of ruining the whole "relaxing nature outing" thing and keeping our brains focused on pain instead of environmental pleasures. But when we are prepared for time out in the desert, many of its elements can be invigorating for mind and spirit.

Take the sunshine: when we step out into a desert environment on a sunny day, we give the body the natural light it needs to produce vitamin D. In addition to strengthening bones and supporting immunity, the sunshine vitamin seems to build mental strength.

Researchers have identified a link between vitamin D deficiency and depression on multiple occasions, but they don't totally understand how vitamin D affects mood.[1] It could have more to do with the mental benefits of nature more generally, seeing as people who get more vitamin D (from the sun, at least) also tend to spend more time outside, a healthy practice on its own. Or there might be a more direct explanation, tied up in the way vitamin D helps regulate certain neurotransmitters.

In addition to telling our body to create vitamin D, the uninterrupted desert sun keeps our internal clock ticking along. A quick recap on how this timepiece works: exposure to morning sun signals that it's time to start the day, while darkness before bed cues the body to prepare for sleep. When we keep a consistent sleep-wake time with the help of natural light, it regulates our mood and deepens our sleep (which then goes on to improve mood some more), hence why sun-mimicking lighting is popular during the long days of winter in cloudy, dreary places—but not as necessary in sunny spots like the desert, where daylight tends to be brighter and darkness darker.

All that sun and little rain also means that those who live in the desert have opportunities to get outside year round and reap the mental health benefits of doing so. In sum, sunshine is mentally restorative, and the desert has it in droves.

Beyond this initial perk, so far only one study has set out to directly measure the health benefits of deserts—or "brown space"—compared with those of green space. (Remember, most of the existing environmental psychology research is done in lush parks or on green college campuses, not cacti-clad scenes.) It was a small trial at the University of Nevada, Las Vegas (UNLV), in which ten of the school's students took a thirty-minute walk in five environments—indoors, in an outdoor urban center, in greenery, and in two scenic desert settings: Red Rock Canyon outside Las Vegas and Death Valley National Park in California.[2]

Walking through these last two areas yielded the same high comfort and calm scores and low stress rates as walking through green space for the students, who lived in the desert and were accustomed to its risks. "Taken together, these data provide evidence that exercise in a desert environment is just as beneficial as the exercise performed in a green environment," the study concludes. These results imply that, as James W. Navalta, the lead researcher and an associate professor of kinesiology at UNLV, explains to me, an environment doesn't necessarily need the fragrant phytoncides of trees or the lush patterns of green leaves to be mentally restorative. Pared-down landscapes of sand, sky, and sun, when navigated safely and with care, hold a similar potential.

Bring On the Heat:
The Cleansing Capacity of
the Desert's High Temps

In most deserts, with sun comes warmth. And love it or hate it, heat has long had a place in healing too: Finnish home saunas, Russian banyas, Turkish baths, Native American sweat lodges, and Korean jjimjilbang have all long used high temperatures to spiritually cleanse.

These purification techniques also seem to pay off physically: a longitudinal study that followed more than two thousand Finnish men over nearly twenty years found that those who took four to seven sauna bathing sessions per week (yes, they really like saunas) were less likely to develop memory diseases than those who only took one sauna session weekly.[3] After adjusting for factors like age, alcohol consumption, and heart disease, the authors concluded that "in this male population, moderate to high frequency of sauna bathing was associated with lowered risks of dementia and Alzheimer's disease."

In Japan, the occasional sauna bath has been correlated with improved mood and decreased anxiety.[4] Rates of cardiovascular disease, hypertension, and respiratory illness also seem to be lower among those who soak.[5]

Though it may not have the steam of a sauna, the desert's trademark heat (when navigated with caution) has been known to have multiple benefits, which include reduced stiffness and swelling and increased flexibility.[6] Perhaps it's no wonder that the five global blue zones where people live the longest—Okinawa, Japan; Sardinia, Italy; Nicoya Peninsula, Costa Rica; Ikaria, Greece; and Loma Linda, California—all sit in warmer climes.

Of course, even the hottest deserts (thankfully) don't reach sauna-level temperatures, but as the UNLV research demonstrated, being active outside on a warm, dry day can also be clarifying.

An Expansive View: How the Desert Horizon Inspires Creative Problem Solving

Desert skies, thanks to their lack of tall trees or heavy vegetation, are the picture of expansiveness—and research suggests that they might give way to equally spacious ideas.

Neuroscientists have noticed through research that when people attempt to solve problems or come up with creative ideas, their eyes naturally gravitate to blank spaces.[7] (Think back to the last time you noticed someone gaze at a blank spot on the wall when asked a tough question.) This visual tick minimizes outward distraction so that we can stay focused on the internal issue at hand. The cognitive neuroscientist and study author Carola Salvi tells me that, interestingly enough, we tend to blink more when problem solving for the same reason. It's another way of blocking information from entering the brain.

If vast emptiness is a natural resting place for the working mind, this would make the open, unobstructed views of the desert (and other expansive vistas like fields) ideal for thinking through problems. More enclosed landscapes like forests can, of course, promote deeper thinking too, due to their ability to reduce stress (which also pays dividends for creativity). They are also capable of evoking awe, which, as we learned in the mountain chapter, leads to new perspective.

But maybe, when it comes to creative ideas, at least—which Salvi says tend to be the ones that make novel connections between seemingly unrelated concepts in the brain—there's no comparison to the desert horizon. This would explain why many great artists through time, from Georgia O'Keeffe to Paul Bowles to Salvador Dalí, have called this landscape a muse. Its blank spaces provide ample room for us to fill in with the widest breadth of ideas, words, and brushstrokes.

The Mighty Medicines
That Grow in Desert Lands

The desert is a difficult place for life to thrive, so everything that exists in this landscape has persevered to be there. Take the blue agave native to the southern US and Central America, with thick leaves covered in spikes to protect precious stores of water within. Or the saguaro cactus, native to the Sonoran Desert of the American Southwest, which, like many desert cacti, conserves water by opening its "pores" to feed on carbon dioxide at night instead of during the evaporative heat of the day. Amazingly, some researchers now believe that many members of this species germinated at the same time, 1884, a year that was uniquely cold and wet due to a volcanic eruption in Indonesia that altered weather patterns.[8] Born of catastrophe and challenge, these desert species flower rarely (blue agave, once a decade; saguaros, once they reach the age of seventy), but when they do, it's a sight for sore eyes. Desert blooms are the ultimate show of the beauty that comes from restraint.

Some of these adaptations that help modest desert plants withstand the heat can be refreshing for us too. Aridity-adapted aloe can be used for soothing and softening the skin, wild licorice for calming coughs. In some Native American traditions, sage is burned to cleanse and purify, and juniper, referred to as the "desert's elder," is thought to pass on resilience and strength in its smoke.

The desert, in all its friction, is also where many gems first come to form. Colorful quartz, opulent garnet, delicate turquoise: they can all be shaped by centuries of pressure in inhospitable desert conditions. Desert rose selenite, created by water, wind, and sand, is perhaps the most spectacular of all: it forms in a flowerlike pattern and can grow to be an elemental bouquet that weighs over one hundred pounds. When considering these plants and gems, I can't help but think of the desert landscape itself as an artist and creative, an alchemist that can conjure beauty out of thin air.

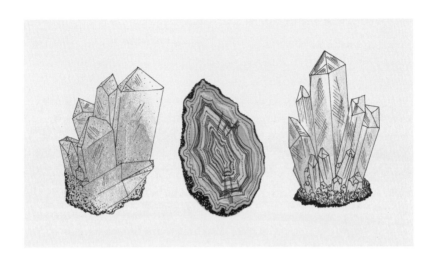

A Wild Journey:
How Deserts Break People Down
to Build Them Back Up

Human resolve, too, has a way of becoming crystallized in this landscape. In sacred texts and secular stories throughout history, the desert has set the stage for the archetypal hero's journey.

When a protagonist enters the desert, you can bet that they will be stripped down to their most foundational self along the way. Inevitably, one of the landscape's hazards—a sandstorm, a water shortage, an enticing mirage—always shaves down the passerby's resolve, layer by rough layer. These legends make many outsiders wary of entering the desert in the first place. Why expose oneself to a land of erosion, of dry earth and bare rock, rife with the stinging sharp edges of weathering?

It's worth remembering that when a piece of land erodes, it doesn't just vanish. It gets carried somewhere else—the bottom of a valley, the bed of a river—to lay a new foundation. Perhaps the desert allows us to do the same.

Douglas E. Christie, a theology professor at Loyola Marymount University who has a special interest in contemplative traditions, ultimately sees this landscape as one of transformation. "I'm quite aware that the desert is not everyone's landscape. This sense of fear or foreboding is part of it," he tells me. "I think it's an instinct that many of us feel: 'It's just too exposed. I'm too exposed.' Because of that, however, [the desert] becomes a symbol of not only struggle but renewal."

The phoenix rising from the ashes, the sudden burst of creativity after a period of drought; these breakthrough moments prove that collapse can precede growth. After old habits are drained by the heat, resolves tested by the sun, desert goers can begin the process of rebuilding from what's left. "If you stay with it," says Christie, "you find yourself becoming more vulnerable, more tender, less guarded."

The Alchemist is the story of a young shepherd named Santiago who sets out for the Egyptian desert in search of treasure. Along the way, a merchant forewarns that a higher power, the Soul of the World, will inevitably test him on his quest. "It does this not because it is evil," the merchant says, "but so that we can, in addition to realizing our dreams, master the lessons we've learned as we've moved toward that dream. That's the point at which most people give up. It's the point at which, as we say in the language of the desert, one 'dies of thirst just when the palm trees have appeared on the horizon.'"

To go through a desert is to trust that after periods of drought, the palms are just a few steps away. Every time we keep on pushing through constraints, moving toward some grander vision, some oasis on the horizon, we embody this lesson. We internalize the desert and are better for it.

The Practice

"Deserts may be the only landscapes in the world defined by most cultures in terms of *what they lack* rather than the uniqueness of *what they have*," the ecologist Gary Paul Nabhan writes in his book *The Nature of Desert*

Nature.[9] The following practices can help attune you to the underappreciated abundance of this multilayered landscape, from up close or afar.

Find creativity on the horizon.

Put Salvi's research into practice and let your gaze rest on the open desert sky the next time you're trying to think creatively. Studies have shown that we actually tend to come to "aha" moments of realization when we step away from a problem at hand, so there's value in building these horizon breaks into your workflow.

"When you're stuck in a problem and can't solve it, continuing to think about it is not going to lead to a solution," Salvi explains. "The best thing to do is just stop thinking of it and go on a walk if it's nice out, and come back and try to reinterpret it."

Learn a thing or two from plants.

Desert plants are the picture of resilience. Arid succulents absorb water through a wide, shallow root system and quickly store it in their leaves and stems as a reserve. (It's why their leaves are so bloated and fleshy compared with more tropical varieties.) This measured way of being allows them to live in a dry landscape that's not suited for most life. This root system also ensures there is plenty of room between neighboring plants. You'll notice that cacti are hardly ever crowded one on top of the other, making it easier to home in on the detail of each one. On your next desert stroll, do so. Consider how each plant you see has managed to survive after being dealt a seemingly unfavorable hand. Let them show you what can come from restraint, diligence, and a little space. As environmentalist Edward Abbey wrote of the plants of Arches National Park in *Desert Solitaire,* "Love flowers best in openness and freedom."[10]

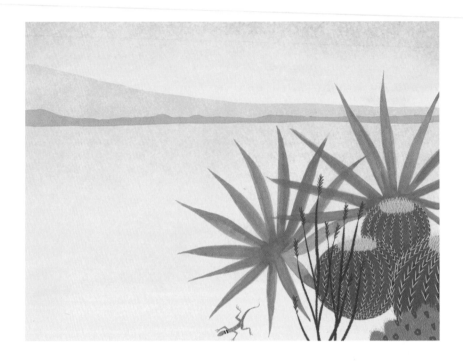

Look out for life where you least expect it.

Though he would ultimately go on to spend years studying it, the desert wasn't always a landscape that felt welcoming, or particularly interesting, to Douglas Christie. He remembers driving through the Mojave Desert on his way to the Sierra Nevada mountains as a teenager and seeing it as a means to an end—a desolate place to pass through before the *real nature* could begin. "It was completely lost on me," he recalls. "It was just emptiness and barrenness." This is a common feeling: since the desert lacks the usual signs of human productivity, we (mistakenly) assume that it's also infertile by nature's standards.

It wasn't until Christie was invited back to the Mojave with a group of biologists that he began to recognize the landscape for what it was: vibrant, varied, enticingly moody. "Their eyes and ears and senses were so finely attuned to the subtle nuances of place," he says. Following their slow, observant lead gave him the chance to get to see not just the desert but the world in a new and more contemplative way.

On your next desert outing, channel your inner biologist and discover the life that has been there all along. Keep a steady eye out for the unfurling of a new leaf or a colorful bud emerging from a cacti. Consider how a place can go from desolate to vibrant with a simple shift in perspective.

CONNECTING FROM AFAR:
Let off some steam.

Those who are far from the desert sun (or a personal sauna) can still make their own warmth. One of my favorite ways to bring on the heat is by taking a facial steam: pour boiling water in a large bowl and drop in a smell-good element (essential oils, loose leaf-tea, herbs) of your choice. Close your eyes and hover your face over the bowl, being careful not to touch the water, and drape a towel over the back of your head to contain the heat.

Stay in the hot, fragrant steam for five minutes or so (I'll usually time it to the length of one song), focusing your attention on your inhales and exhales, which will be amplified in the tight cocoon. The heat of the steam, the sound of the breath, and the smell of the oils or herbs converge into an experience that mimics a desert voyage: slightly uncomfortable but wildly cleansing. My complexion always appreciates the journey too.

Get outside during a new time of day.

People (and animals) who live in hot desert environments often need to build their schedules around the temperature. This means exploring the outdoors during the early morning hours, before the sun has reached its peak, or in the evenings once the air cools. You can take a cue from them by going on a walk outside during a time you wouldn't usually do so. The natural environment takes on many forms throughout the day, shifting in the sun and shadow, so this practice can show you a new side of your land, wherever it may be.

Light incense.

As I shared earlier, incense sticks have become my gateway to a desert state of mind. When I'm tucked inside on a snowy winter's day or during a rainstorm, I'll light them to beckon the qualities of the desert that I most crave: its smells, its heat, its artful haze.

Bring this landscape home by lighting incense of your own (a candle would work too) and observing it for a moment, letting your attention rest on its smoke. You can then use the stick as a fragrant timekeeper for the ritual of your choosing: be it a meditation, journaling session, visualization, or yoga flow, continuing the practice until the last of the stick burns and you can open a window to clear the smoke and reenter your own landscape once again.

> There are few places in the world where you can experience both the silence and the space that you can in the desert. It's quite extraordinary to rest your eyes on that vast, distant horizon and not feel it interrupted. . . . I think what many people experience in that silence and space is that it starts to open up something in us.
>
> —DOUGLAS E. CHRISTIE,
> professor of theology,
> Loyola Marymount University

List your fears to disarm them.

Walking through the open desert can feel like traveling back in time. Maybe it's all the myths that have taken place in deserts through history. Or it could be the fact that the savannahs in which humans evolved likely had some degree of desertlike expansiveness to them. The vast openness is familiar. Its barren heat is written somewhere in our history.

As a primal landscape, the desert also evokes the most basic of human instincts: love, loyalty, but also fear. Fear is a natural, valuable response when our baseline needs aren't being met (say, when we don't have water), but it's something that we also feel during times of relative safety (say, when a deadline is coming up at work). One way to connect to the desert from afar is to face some of these more manufactured fears head-on.

Make a laundry list of your fears from the tangible (for me: airplane takeoffs, public speaking, possums) to the more formless (loneliness, regret, death). Write until you can't come up with anything else, then keep going for a few more. When you're done, look at your list and consider how these fears shape the actions you're taking or not taking, how it's leading to an unfulfillment, a drought. No need to judge; just consider. Acknowledging fear is the first step to dismantling it.

Journal on the desert's themes.

All the words I've used to describe the desert—heat, harshness, opportunity—can easily apply to any one of life's obstacles. When you're in a challenging, uncomfortable period, this is the landscape to journal on. Here are some questions to get you started:

- What do you tell yourself when you're feeling afraid? Fear, while there for a reason, is not always truth. Write down a snippet of your inner dialogue and look back on it to see what part of your fear voice is true and what is exaggerated.

- Consider a part of your future that is uncertain: How does that uncertainty feel to you? Expansive, like a clear horizon? Scary, like being stuck in a desert without water?

- What's your "mirage"? What vices do you cling to for comfort through hard times that might not actually be so helpful in the long run?

- What's your "oasis" at the end of your current period of discomfort? How will you know that you've worked through the worst of it and arrived at some kind of other side?

The Action

Existing deserts need to be protected, but also contained. In recent decades, we've lost millions of acres of land to erosion and degradation—a disturbing trend that could prove disastrous. According to UN data,[11] human populations in dry desert lands are growing at a faster rate than any other ecological zone, and, by 2030, nearly half the people on Earth could be living in areas of high water stress. Here are some of the major reasons that land around the world is drying out and what can be done about it.

Industrial Agriculture

America's large-scale farming operations are in a tight spot. On the one hand, there are more mouths to feed than ever, and farms need to rev up production to keep pace with a growing population. On the other, the methods that they've always used to do so could soon be their own undoing.

Farming in the industrial age is highly formulaic. If you walk onto a typical commercial crop farm in the US, you'll see neat rows upon rows of the same crop, a practice called monoculturing. When the time comes, they'll all be harvested, and a tiller (one of those big lawn-mower-looking contraptions) will roll through to shake up the soil to get it ready for the next round of seed. Rinse and repeat, season after season. Ranches are similar: lots of cattle are packed on the same plot of land to maximize yield. These rigidly efficient systems are predictable, consistent, and reliable in their repetition. In other words, they go against basically every law of nature there is.

While controlling for the variability of nature is good for a farmer's bottom line, it's often damaging to the land. When the ground is left uncovered in between harvests or herds, more of the rain that falls on it gets lost to evaporation. The less rainfall the soil can soak up, the drier it will become over time. When tillers come through, the land gets poked and prodded even more, until all that's left is a system that's been tampered with so much that it loses its beneficial microbe colonies. Like the microbial communities that dwell in our guts, these networks of tiny critters digest nutrients, making them more readily available to plants. As they're stripped away, crops suffer and eventually become water-starved, nutrient-poor, and more prone to pests and diseases.

Once agricultural land is arid and lifeless enough, it becomes nearly impossible to grow anything. Its owners will need to either give up or move to another plot of land to cultivate using the same methods. If we continue this cycle, eventually there won't be much viable land left. There is, however, another option.

The Mindset Shift: "I mimic the regeneration I see in nature."

Regenerative agriculture more closely mimics the way things grow in nature—slowly, gently, and in constant collaboration. It's a return to an Indigenous, preindustrial system that replaces machine tilling with a human (or animal) touch, monocultures with a variety of different crops, and synthetic fertilizers with compost. The result is soil that's rich in beneficial microbes that provide crops with more nutrients, absorb more water, and provide protection against pests.

> The foundational principles of regeneration are biophysical and chemical. And within that perspective, a farmer really isn't the producer of anything. As farmers, we are truly engaged in the stewardship of energy and its transformation, from nonedible into edible forms. And the foundational principle of how that happens is mostly microbiological—both in the intestinal gut of animals and the intestinal gut of the Earth, which is the soil.
>
> —REGINALDO HASLETT-MARROQUÍN,
> president and CEO,
> Regenerative Agriculture Alliance

By restoring soil health, regenerative techniques can also help pull more carbon out of the atmosphere. More healthy soil means more healthy plants. Healthy plants absorb CO_2 from the atmosphere through photosynthesis and convert it to energy: the CO_2 that they don't use is sent back into the soil, where it's converted into humus, which gives soil its rich, deep brown color. In this form, carbon is more stable; it happily sits underground and out of the atmosphere, where it can contribute to warming.

Mollie Engelhart is one farmer who has seen the potential of regenerative practices to reverse desertification and restore land firsthand: when she bought her seventeen-acre Southern California property from a conventional farmer in 2018, she remembers it was "a hot mess"; layers of dry soil had blown away to expose fields of rock.

Over the first few seasons, "the soil got better and got better and got better," Engelhart tells me on a call from her farm, Sow a Heart.[12] She's proud to report that the latest soil test showed the farm is now absorbing water at a rate five times faster than when she bought it, setting grounds that are more conducive to growth. When she gave me a peek at the farm outside her window, to my sore Brooklynite eyes it looked like Eden. Mountains set the backdrop to lush, green grass and crops that winked under the California sun.

So why isn't every farmer in the world adopting these seemingly win-win practices? No surprise here: it's largely a matter of funding and incentives.

Financial constraints keep longtime growers locked into the old way of doing things. Changing over to a more regenerative system takes time, new equipment, and a new mindset. In the transition period, there's always the risk of losing crops (and, by extension, money) before you gain them, and most farmers just can't afford to risk this hit. (Engelhart, who is also the chef and owner of Sage Plant Based Bistro, a chain of restaurants, says that she was only able to go regenerative because she had money coming in from her other successful business.) Another complicating factor is that in the US, there's actually a cash incentive for many farmers to carry on with monocropping. Government subsidies are reserved for farmers to grow massive amounts of staple crops like corn, wheat, and soy. These subsidies are meant to provide a steady source of income in the case of extreme weather events and droughts, but ultimately they encourage practices that make these catastrophes more likely.

The government distributed $240.5 billion in farming subsidies between 1995 and 2020.[13] Twenty-six percent of the funds went to just 1 percent of farms.[14] Those large-scale operations are the

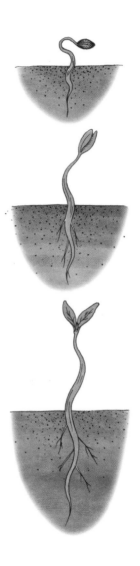

ones we need to target for ecological transition. If they changed their ways (say, if they were subsidized based on their carbon sequestrations instead?), the impact on the land and climate would be enormous.

At the same time that we readjust rewards for the 1 percent, we need to start relocating funds to those who have been historically disadvantaged. For starters, the young and first-generation farmers who Engelhart says could benefit from a reduction in the down-payment rates currently charged for farm property. As it stands now, they are prohibitively high to prospective farmers who are just starting out and don't come from the old guard.

Then, there's the need to support BIPOC and Indigenous farmers, who created this holistic management practice in the first place but have historically been disenfranchised from owning land in this country (95 percent of farmers in America are white[15]). Through his organization, the Regenerative Agriculture Alliance,[16] Reginaldo Haslett-Marroquín builds regenerative food supply chains, with a focus on regenerative poultry systems deployment, primarily in the US Midwest. And he tells me that intentionally seeking out a wide diversity of farmers, businesses, and public service institutions is the only way to build them. Regeneration is, after all, fueled by diversity: on a micro(be) level, it requires a wide array of organisms working together to strengthen soil. On a human scale, it requires a range of opinions, backgrounds, and perspectives.

This total reimagination of agriculture won't happen overnight. The most impactful way we can support this systemic shift is to buy from local farmers growing regeneratively and stay vocal. Ask your supermarket or farm stand how their food is grown and if regenerative is on their radar. Write to larger food and textile companies to ask if they are buying from regenerative farmers or financially supporting them through their transition period. Contact your policymakers to encourage them to support bills that treat agriculture like what it is: a land restoration tactic and a potential climate solution.

Salinization

Dry environments, where the rate of evaporation exceeds the rate of precipitation, are more prone to soil nutrient imbalances. If drylands are irrigated using mineral-rich water or improperly drained, once that water evaporates, it leaves salt residues behind. Without steady fresh rainwater to wash them away, these salts can build up in soil over time. Anyone who has watered their houseplants with hard tap water may have seen this process play out on a small scale: as your plant absorbs the water, some of its minerals are left behind to form a white coating on your soil or pot.

While easily fixed in a single houseplant, this salinization can prove harmful to large ecosystems. In an increasingly water-starved world, according to a report by the UN,[17] around sixty-two million hectares have been affected by salinization. The report estimates that each week, the world loses an area larger than Manhattan to salt degradation, rendering country-sized swaths of land unsuitable for plant growth.

This salt buildup is just another example of why fresh water is such an essential resource for life on Earth—and why we need to treat it as such.

The Mindset Shift:
"I know that water isn't a renewable resource."

California's Central Valley is one area where wells repeatedly run dry and soil salinity is increasingly becoming an issue. I did some reporting on the water crisis in the agricultural hotspot in 2018, and an interview I had with Christiana Zenner, an associate professor of theology, science, and water ethics at Fordham University, has stayed with me ever since. Zenner has spent her career fighting against the commonly held idea that fresh water is a renewable resource. It's not. And if we continue to treat it like it is, millions more people will know what it feels like to turn on their tap and have nothing come out, and millions more acres of farmland will go bust.

There are many ways to cut down on your water use. Sure, taking a shorter shower and turning off the tap when you brush your teeth helps, but being a more mindful shopper makes more of a dent in your water footprint. Everything we consume, from food to clothing to electronics, necessitates a ton of water to create, so being picky about what you buy is key. As always, lasting water reductions will require government buy-in through programs like mandated water-efficient farming and high tariffs on excessive water use. In the meantime, we can all get used to the idea that water is not a renewable resource by being grateful for the water we do have and using it wisely.

Desert Expansion

Our deserts are far from fixed. Their borders are as fluid as the sea's, and they're rising even more quickly.

Forces like weather patterns, climate change, and human degradation are causing some deserts around the world to expand before our eyes. The Gobi, for example, continues to creep closer to Beijing and send sand into the city when the wind is strong enough, causing traffic to stand still and windows and doors to lock shut in a city whose air is smothered in plumes. Further inland, the Ningxia region of China has had 57 percent of its land affected by desertification, as three surrounding deserts creep on it from all sides.[18] In the Sahara, where Sumant Nigam, a climate dynamacist and chair of the Department of Atmospheric and Oceanic Science at the University of Maryland, has conducted research, a shifting climate is leading to a desert in flux. "The Sahara waxes and wanes with the seasons," he says, but on average its southern border is advancing south by about a kilometer every year. The Sahara as a whole has grown by 10 percent since 1920.[19]

To those who live nearby, the advancing desert is a real threat. In China, hundreds of thousands of people have been displaced by the Gobi and relocated to planned communities, their homes marked with their status as "ecological migrants."[20] Deserts don't just harm those in their immediate path: their sand can travel great distances, and dust kicked up in the Gobi has traveled all the way across the Pacific Ocean, to California, Oregon, and Washington State. In Rome, dust from the Sahara now reaches the city nearly every one day in three,[21] and with it come higher death rates from cardiovascular illness.

The Mindset Shift: "I don't treat land like dirt."

Faced with encroaching deserts, some communities have begun to physically shield themselves. China is over forty years into a "Great Green Wall" project that seeks to plant a line of trees around the growing Gobi. The idea is that this natural border will act as a buffer zone by fixing nutrients into the arid soil below. So far, sixty-six billion trees have been planted to contain the Gobi, which has been nicknamed the yellow dragon for its power, unpredictability, and breath of fire.

Reading about this project, I can't help but think of the more politically motivated walls humans have constructed over the centuries—the ones that create artificial divides to separate an area from a perceived other. Don't get me wrong, I'm a tree evangelist and am heartened to know that China is reporting early success in their massive planting. But I have a hard time believing that a blockade of any kind, even a green one, is the answer to this problem. After all, as the expansive travels of desert dust prove, the natural world knows no borders.

Taming this proverbial dragon on a global scale will surely take more than a single shield. It will also require cooperation, not division.

I usually don't like to entertain the whole "human civilization is doomed" climate dialogue, as I don't think that dread necessarily leads to action, but ever-expanding deserts are one of the few trends that do send me into catastrophe mode. This is, after all, a landscape that stokes our most primitive fears of disruption, decay, and ultimately death.

In his book *Sand Talk: How Indigenous Thinking Can Save the World*, Tyson Yunkaporta, a senior lecturer in Indigenous Knowledges at Deakin

University in Australia, writes that "a city tells itself it is a closed system that must decay in order for time to run straight, while simultaneously demanding eternal growth."[22] He theorizes that this thirst for growth is why humanity's oldest civilizations—from Sumer in Mesopotamia to ancient Egypt—eventually ran dry. They are all blanketed in sand, dulled by desert. They stripped their surroundings bare and now lie in ruin.

"Why do we misuse and treat land like dirt?" asks the United Nations Convention to Combat Desertification.[23] It's a fair question. Protecting the world's land from further degradation requires a change of perspective— from seeing the soil as something to own to treating it as something to work alongside. We must factor soil health into all our decisions as a species moving forward, or the ground will disappear beneath our feet.

CHAPTER SEVEN

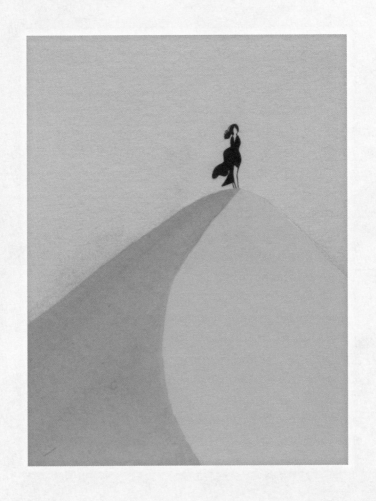

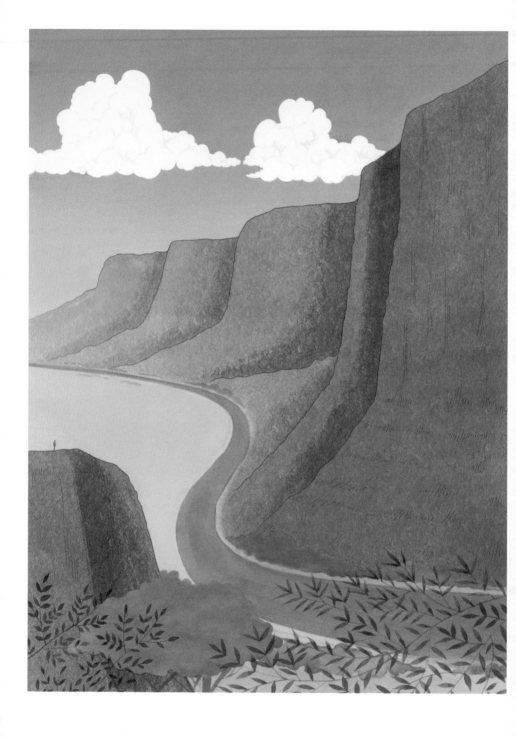

RIVERS & STREAMS

cycles, direction, transcendence

I hear the river before I see it. The faint whir of static tells me that I'm getting close. After a few more wrong turns, I spot its water glistening in the early summer sun: a return to a familiar scene and the younger self who occupied it. I'm reminded of where I was when I first met this river, and where I've been since.

It's been years since I ran along Rock Creek, a tributary of the Potomac River that winds through Washington, DC, before emptying into the Atlantic by way of the Chesapeake Bay. And I mean physically run—the path next to the meandering creek is where I first started to see running less as a means of torture and more as a mind-clearing exercise. It was a discovery that changed my health and life for the better. I credit running with helping me break free from a period of crippling anxiety, and I feel indebted to the river, my initial cheerleader, for making that possible. I watch its waters clear rocks, so steady in their movement, so forceful in their flow, and wonder what they have seen since I was here last. I take it all in for a moment, then keep on running downstream.

The Remedy

Rivers are nature's dutiful messengers. They are constantly carrying the world's fresh water to its next destination, confidently twisting and turning through landscapes of all kinds as they go. They're connectors, and their banks have long been conduits for life.

Human civilization still lives and dies by their flows; we depend on rivers for fresh water and fertile land for growing food. Though they cover less than 1 percent of the planet's surface, rivers make it possible to live on this Earth— and in some cases, to transcend it. Rivers and smaller streams and creeks are flooded with mystery and symbolism, and their currents can carry us to new parts of ourselves. To trace what makes this landscape so special, let's start at its beginning, the headwaters, and make our way downstream.

The Headwaters:
The Science Behind Why Winding Rivers
Can Put Us at Ease

Stand at the start of an unfamiliar river and its path will appear to go on forever, into places unknown. This sense of secrecy is part of what gives rivers their charm, according to Stephen Kaplan and Rachel Kaplan of ART fame. The Kaplans suggest that we're hardwired to prefer landscapes that we can understand (and therefore feel safe in), but still explore (they have some element of surprise or novelty). Rivers fit the bill: whitewater aside, they are relatively safe and stable, yet also mysterious, with meandering bends, varying current speeds, and obscured depths. The Kaplans claim that our preference for a landscape rises with its coherence (whether its elements make sense together), complexity (whether it has enough going on to keep us engaged), legibility (whether it's possible for us to navigate it or picture ourselves navigating it), and mystery (whether it promises to provide more if we walk deeper into it).[1] It makes sense, then, that rivers, with their winding paths and rich array of plant and animal life, play a prominent role in the psychologists' early writing on landscape preference.

The Experience of Nature: A Psychological Perspective,[2] a 1989 Kaplan text that spells out why certain parts of nature hold psychological appeal, mentions rivers more than fifty times. It explains that a river winding out of sight is a prime example of a mysterious landscape that is impossible to fully perceive and therefore offers visitors the opportunity to fill in the blanks "according to the play of his own fancy."

Olivia Laing writes of the visceral appeal of winding waters in her book *To the River: A Journey Beneath the Surface*: "There is a mystery about rivers that draws us to them, for they rise from hidden places and travel by routes that are not always tomorrow where they might be today. Unlike a lake or sea, a river has a destination and there is something about the certainty with which it travels that makes it very soothing, particularly for those who've lost faith with where they're headed."[3]

There is some research to support this ease that Laing feels in the presence of rivers. Preference has been correlated with restoration potential, meaning we consider aesthetically pleasing places to be more relaxing too. And as we explored in the oceans chapter, landscapes with water can prompt positive thinking and mood, and ones that have a mix of blue and green seem to make us feel happiest of all.

Cognitively speaking, then, rivers have all the elements of a restorative landscape, and a mysterious one at that. Walking along (or rowing down) them is an exercise in embracing the unknown, in decoupling comfort from control. We may not know what lies ahead of us, but that doesn't mean we can't rest, restore, and daydream by the riverside.

The Waterfall: Why Rivers Can Be Paths to Transcendence

After rivers clear the mind, they can fill it up again with new and potentially transcendent experiences, in which one transcends the earthly plane to connect to God or a higher power, transcends the body to experience a oneness with the environment, or transcends the ego to come closer to self-actualization.

In search of the cognitive root of a spiritually transcendent experience, a team of researchers from Yale and Columbia asked a small pool of healthy participants to recall a situation in which they felt a connection to a higher power or a spiritual presence—be it God, the universe, or a natural landscape.[4] This situation was relayed to them during an fMRI scan as researchers monitored their brain activity. Activity in their inferior parietal lobule seemed to quiet down. This lobe has been linked to spatial awareness, reading other people's intentions, body image, and orienting ourselves in the world around us. It also processes sensory information like smell, touch, and temperature. The fact that its activity slows when we place ourselves in spiritual experiences suggests that this lobe plays a role in our self-other representations.

Researchers are increasingly interested in how these transcendent moments happen—and why they seem to happen more when we're outside. Rivers offer two potential pathways to these mental breakthroughs: waterfalls and rapids that can provoke awe, and slower trickles that offer opportunities for reflection. Let's start by parsing the more dramatic pathway.

When I caught up with Kathryn Williams, a professor of environmental psychology at the University of Melbourne who studied transcendence in nature for her PhD,[5] she recalled that participants tended to report moments of awe, wonder, and amazement in nature that was large in scale and novel in scope. "It was about the scale of the environment," she tells me. "Things that were big made the person experiencing them feel small in the context of a much larger world." Waterfalls were one natural feature that Williams says evoked those hefty awe experiences in participants—as did tall trees.

These dramatic views can steal our breath but give us some kind of new perspective in return, leading to what the twentieth-century psychologist Abraham Maslow named "peak experiences," in which we feel "disorientation in space and time, ego transcendence, and self-forgetfulness; a perception that the world is good, beautiful, and desirable."[6] Maslow, who is best known for his hierarchy of human needs, said that these peak experiences were a route to self-actualization, which he considered the highest form of humanity.

Wild river scenes also fall under the category of sublime environments, as the philosopher Immanuel Kant described them. Kant theorized that sublime landscapes, distinct from beautiful scenery, were innately threatening to their observers. They either possessed the capacity to harm (rushing whitewater, sharp rocks) or were so vast as to make onlookers consider the infinite universe, in all its unsettling mystery (water continuing on, past the horizon).

When we observe such a sublime landscape from a place of relative safety, Kant thought that we grapple with its interplay of beauty and danger, the wonderful now and the great beyond. "You've got this kind of admiration of this external landscape that relates to internal reflection on who we are as subjects," Nicole A. Hall, a postdoctoral researcher at Texas A&M University, tells me of sublime experience. According to the theory, as we consider our own lives during these moments of sublimity, we brush up against our own duality, our own humanness, in ways that are powerful and difficult to fully comprehend. "We can conceptualize that we're having an experience of something that we can't fully form," says Hall. Like subliminal messaging that is impossible to grasp, these sublime nature scenes are beyond our scope of understanding. After all, political philosopher Edmund Burke called sublime "the strongest emotion which the mind is capable of feeling."[7]

Returning to Calm Waters:
How Rivers Make Way for Personal Reflection

In contrast to its sublime whitewater, a river's gentler ripples can provide another gateway to spiritual discovery. In a study on spiritual experiences in American wilderness,[8] a small group of women went on a weeklong canoeing trip in northern Minnesota, keeping journals along the way. One participant wrote, "What often happens is that as I become familiar with a particular place, I also become re-familiarized with myself and how I fit with the rest of the world. . . . For me to experience 'that which is spiritual,' it has to be nature, with water, with trees." Another writes, "The water and trees became more beautiful when I was able to go off by myself and just sit, perched on a rock away from the rest of the group. . . . It made me feel like I had a home again, like I really belonged."

These entries speak to another type of transcendent experience, one that stems from quieter, familiar moments that make way for personal reflection. "Nature is a place that allows you to reflect on things that might be difficult to reflect on. That's a pathway through which spiritual well-being can occur," Katherine Irvine, a senior researcher of conservation behavior and environmental psychology at the James Hutton Institute in Scotland, explains to me. Irvine is interested in the ways that biodiverse outdoor environments can lead to spiritual health—of which there seem to be quite a few. She theorizes that peacefulness, tranquility, and awe are a few potential pathways to a spiritual experience, as are feelings of attachment to or a sense of belonging to a place.[9]

Belonging and attachment are feelings that rivers seem uniquely poised to bring out of us. There's something about this landscape that keeps people coming back to it over and over again, like I recently did with Rock Creek. And when we return to these rivers of our past, they can prompt us to take a moment and reflect on how we've changed since we last sat on their banks. It's in that return that special places can become sacred places.

One question that continues to stump environmental psychologists is how long the health benefits of a nature experience stick around. Does the reduction in stress we feel after a walk in the park have a time limit? Do we have to use up the creativity that an expansive view inspires right away, before it fades with the sun? When it comes to everyday encounters, we're not entirely sure (though researchers have floated 120 minutes outdoors a

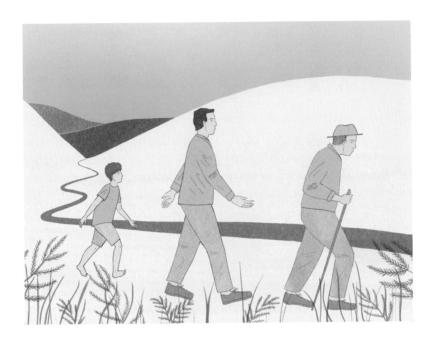

week as a baseline to aim for if you want to reap nature's well-being benefits[10]). But when you factor in transformative experience, you realize that some outdoor moments never really leave us. They can shape the direction of our lives, and in that sense, they transcend time and live in perpetuity, like a river flows.

The Middle Run:
How Our Relationship with
Nature Changes as We Age

Human lifetimes mirror river paths, in ways both subtle and obvious: rivers are in constant motion, always taking on new forms. Just like they bend and curve, speed up and slow down, we, too, constantly shift in relation to our environment as time goes on. We start at one point and end at another, switching course to yield to obstacles blocking our path along the way. As we go, we pick up our own debris—though it looks a little different from the silt and sediment that fresh waters carry. With rivers, as with people, the only constant is change. As the Greek philosopher Heraclitus said, "No man ever steps in the same river twice, for it's not the same river and he's not the same man." Perhaps it's no surprise that, as we'll discuss later, there is a growing movement to give rivers around the world legal personhood status as protection from threats like pollution and dams, to fully recognize these parallels and use them as forces of conservation. With their lifelike qualities, rivers ask us to consider our own journeys and reflect on our shifting relationship to nature over time, starting in childhood.

When we're kids, nature is a classroom without rules, a place we can go to build confidence, learn motor skills, tap into creativity and imagination, express ourselves, and face our fears. Nature also seems to have similar benefits on mental restoration in childhood to what it has in adulthood.[11] In his hallmark book *Last Child in the Woods*;[12] the journalist Richard Louv writes of nature-deficit disorder, a plague on children that's characterized by behavioral issues and attentional difficulties. Not a contagious virus or chronic condition, it incubates when kids spend most of their free time indoors, on screens. After analyzing the research and interviewing children across the country, Louv concluded that kids who spend more time outdoors tend to be healthier not only physically but emotionally and spiritually too. Louv agrees with Maslow's hypothesis that peak, transcendent experiences are actually the most intense in childhood—and nature is the place to have them. While research on spiritual experiences outdoors during childhood is limited ("The absence of research may suggest a certain nervousness," Louv writes in *Last Child in the Woods*; "After all, a child's spiritual experience in nature—especially in solitude—is beyond adult or institutional control"), one retrospective study on 250 adults found that most peak experiences they remembered having before age fourteen occurred in nature.[13]

Maslow theorized that these peak experiences start to soften once we hit adolescence, into what he called "plateaus." As we become more familiar with the natural world that surrounds us, it loses some (but of course not all) of its mystery. However, those teenage years are also when many of us start to become consciously aware of how nature can support us through the upheavals of life and relationships.

Anecdotally, one environmental psychologist I interviewed traced her interest in the field to the times in high school when she'd head to the woods near her house to escape problems with friends and get perspective on the stress of being a teenager. Since social interactions and relationship building are so crucial during adolescence, these seem to be areas where nature can have an outsized impact.

Most of the research on nature once we reach adulthood becomes about restoration—how nature can provide a salve for the stressors of workplace demands, family responsibilities, and so forth. The amount of time we have to spend recharging outdoors might start to decrease as we get older due to jobs, kids, and other responsibilities. We can of course still have transformative experiences outdoors, but they might be more dependent on other people's schedules.

The next significant shift in outdoor experience comes once we reach retirement age.[14] Merja Rantakokko, a principal researcher who studies older people's outdoor mobility at the JAMK University of Applied Sciences in Finland, notes that on a physical level just getting outside the home becomes more important the older we get. "That is the cornerstone for independent living, and when you're able to live an independent life, it improves your quality of life," Rantakokko tells me. And if the excursion is to safe, nearby nature, where we can comfortably observe a dynamic and restorative environment, all the better.

In many ways, our relationship with the outdoors in older adulthood most closely mimics that of childhood. At a certain point, we come full circle and see nature both as a place to fear (this time, because of potential falls or injuries and not boogey monsters) and as a portal to personal discovery. In many spiritual philosophies, with age comes the death of ego and the movement into a more collective consciousness. With years lived and wisdom gained, we can more clearly situate ourselves in relation to the wider world. We can contemplate larger questions of life, death, and legacy and in doing so invite those peak experiences of youth to find us yet again.

"Have you also learned that secret from the river; that there is no such thing as time?" reads Hermann Hesse's classic novel *Siddhartha*.[15] "That the river is everywhere at the same time, at the source and at the mouth, at the waterfall, at the ferry, at the current, in the ocean and in the mountains, everywhere and that the present only exists for it, not the shadow of the past nor the shadow of the future?" Like a river, our lives exist cyclically. At some point, endings and beginnings start to blend together, in murky waters that both obscure and reveal.

The River Delta: Measuring What's Lost as Environments Trickle Down Through Generations

Rivers are liminal spaces, always in motion, constantly teetering between old and new ways of being. Like ephemeral sunsets and passing storms, they are thresholds between before and after, past and future. As such, they symbolize not just an individual's life course but also the flow of life through generations.

In addition to depending on rivers for physical offerings, a number of Indigenous communities around the world have long extracted stories, history, and mythology from their depths. Some, like the Kukama-Kukamiria people who live in the Peruvian Amazon, consider the water a portal through which they can connect with ancestors.[16] In their community, when someone dies and their body cannot be found, it is believed that they dwell in underwater cities in the river for eternity. Others, like the Tahltan who live on Tl'abāne, the Stikine River valley in northwest Canada, consider the water home to future generations. "They believe that the people with the greatest claim to ownership of the valley are the generations as yet unborn," the anthropologist and Explorer-in-Residence at the National

Geographic Society Wade Davis writes of Tahltan elders.[17] "The Sacred Headwaters will be their nursery." When considered from these perspectives, any damage to the river is a loss that spans lifetimes.

So what do future generations lose when nature is destroyed? That question has been the subject of some speculation. A certain sect of psychologists believes it could contribute to an "extinction of experience,"[18] in which generations that have less contact with pristine nature are actually less likely to have positive experiences in it, diminishing some of its potential mental health benefits. "In this era of increased concern over climate change and global urbanization, you definitely want children to be aware of these benefits because if you're more connected to nature, generally, you're more in support of initiatives to protect or to conserve it," Ingrid Jarvis, a PhD candidate in the Department of Forest and Conservation Sciences at the University of British Columbia, explains to me.

Peter H. Kahn Jr., an environmental psychology professor and research director at the University of Washington, believes that intensely damaging "environmental generational amnesia" can occur when subsequent generations believe that the degraded world they inherit is the planet in its natural form. "A problem arises insofar as the amount of environmental degradation increases across generations, but each generation tends to take that degraded condition as the non-degraded condition: the normal experience," he and coauthor Terry Hartig write in an article in the journal *Science*.[19]

Members of future generations that do have access to pristine nature might still have to grapple with a type of embodied loss over their lifetime: solastalgia. Unlike nostalgia, which describes a desire for something that you no longer have, solastalgia is a longing for something that's right in front of you but drastically changed. Coined by the environmental philosopher and professor of sustainability at Murdoch University in Australia Glenn Albrecht in 2005, this new word describes an increasingly familiar feeling: the pain of watching a favorite natural landscape degrade in front of one's eyes. It mirrors the heartache of watching a loved one fall ill: to stand in their presence is to mourn what they used to be. Albrecht likens the distress caused by environmental change to a "homesickness you have when you are still at home."[20]

Rivers are keepers of time and memory. As portals, both spiritual and physical, they remind us to honor the past and protect the future. In their ripples lie whispers to be good ancestors: to care for this planet's resources so they can flow on to the next generation, and all those after.

The Practice

Rivers provide points of connection and pathways to discovery. These rituals can help you go with their flow, from up close and afar, and maybe enjoy a few breakthroughs along the way.

IF YOU HAVE 5–10 MINUTES:
Do a meditation on the water.

Moving waters show the beauty in impermanence. Watching them can be a reminder that to move is to be alive. They also make for good places to rest your attention and bring awareness to the fact that every thought is fleeting, and that's just the nature of life.

The next time you and the river have an uninterrupted moment, sit by its side, look to its surface waters, and let the mind go where it will, noticing as you transition from one thought to the other. This technique from Mark Coleman, a mindfulness meditation teacher and nature guide, might help: as you look at the water, label whatever sense you're thinking about from moment to moment. If you have a thought that the grass beneath you is itchy, label "touch." If your mind goes to the sound of the water, label "sound." "The idea behind this meditation is to become more mindful of how rapidly your experience changes," Coleman writes in his book *Awake in the Wild: Mindfulness in Nature as a Path of Self-Discovery*.[21] This transience applies to all aspects of life; the good and the bad are always fleeting, so the question becomes how we can more gently take the rapids in stride.

Ask what the river can teach you.

Though absent of desks, pens, and computers, rivers are realms of deep learning. Chandra Brown, the founder of the Freeflow Institute, which leads workshops for writers and creatives on rivers across the world, has seen the water breed academic discovery many times over. Brown, who also has experience teaching in a classroom setting, notes that, compared with indoor environments, rivers can strip us down to our most basic selves—who tend to be more open to novel, original thinking.

"You see that there's more receptivity; there's more reciprocity; there's more engagement," Brown tells me of leading groups outdoors. "We're forced to slow down and sort of move at the pace of the landscape, the pace of the river, and reprioritize our learning."

We can all be students of the landscape by heading out for a day on the river with the intention to learn, be it from a text you bring, a person who tags along with you, or the land you traverse.

> Just being on the river does a really nice job of offering up some perspective. And any time I'm afforded perspective, I'm grateful.
>
> —CHANDRA BROWN,
> writer, educator, and river guide

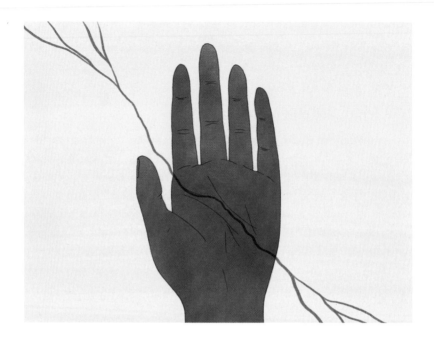

Return to a river of your past.

Spiritual moments in nature come in many forms. They can be loud and breathtaking affairs or quiet, contemplative moments. They can be spurred by views that are wildly foreign or exquisitely familiar. They can bellow their lessons right away or code them in ripple effects that reach us in time. There seem to be countless ways to experience transcendence outdoors, and rivers open the floodgates to many of them.

Whenever we revisit landscapes from our past, we invite a gentler awe, one that's bred by familiarity, to find us. Is there a river that you grew up going to, or one that, in retrospect, altered your life in some way? The next time you have an opportunity to return to that river, take it. Sit by the water, follow it downstream, and listen to its whispers of how you have changed.

CONNECTING FROM AFAR:

Don't dam your thoughts.

The constant movement of streams reveals drifts of the mind. Our thoughts flow like water, and wafting through them can feel a lot like paddling upstream, full of doubts and aches. And when we try to control them, we all know what happens: they move even faster, get even stronger.

One way to make friends with thoughts without a river by your side is by writing them down using a stream-of-consciousness (the name is fitting, no?) journaling technique. Julia Cameron, artist, author, and an authority on free-flow writing, recommends starting every morning by writing three pages by hand about whatever is on your mind that day. The end product doesn't need to be coherent: the point is to give your ideas a voice, get them out on the page, and move on with a better understanding of your true inner landscape and where you have been trying to censor it. In her book *The Artist's Way*,[22] Cameron writes that the technique allows us to "see that our moods, views, and insights are transitory. We acquire a sense of movement, a current of change in our lives. This current, or river, is a flow of grace moving us to our right livelihood, companions, destiny." By saying yes to our rivers, currents and all, Cameron says that we can flow through life with confidence and purpose, more aware of the final destination we're working toward. After doing this freewriting technique for the twelve weeks prescribed in *The Artist's Way*, I can attest to its directional value.

Remember that the only way out is through.

Tori Baird, canoeist and founder of Paddle Like a Girl, is very familiar with what she calls "type B fun"—the sort of experience that's awful at the time but awesome in retrospect. She recalls her remote whitewater rafting trips throughout Canada with a mix of nostalgia and horror: unpredictable conditions, physically demanding tasks, and the sense of accomplishment that comes when you do something you never dreamed you could do.

RIVERS & STREAMS **197**

Beyond being grounds on which to test yourself, rivers also serve as portals to more of the remote outdoors; they provide access to land that can't be reached by foot and have allowed Baird to see places that not many other humans have. The pride that comes with completing a trip makes the tough parts worth it and keeps her coming back to the boat and encouraging other women to do the same. "They give you that confidence that you can handle other challenges in everyday life," Baird tells me of river excursions. "You think: I can't believe I'm capable of doing these things—what else can I do?"

And you don't necessarily need to head to a river to access this sense of pride and accomplishment. Instead, you can use the river as a visualization tool whenever life gets choppy. Close your eyes, picture yourself flowing along the water, and remember the calm waters and the rush of relief that lies at the end of your trip.

Journal on the river's themes.

Embody the river's free-flowing nature as you answer these journaling questions, meant to help you reflect on the past, ease into the present, and dream for the future.

- What is the most transformative experience you've had outdoors? Describe how you felt in that moment, what made it so special, and any insights you walked away with.

- Rivers carry water to their rightful destination, usually a lake or ocean. Consider an end point that you're working toward. How could you embody the water and move toward this goal with more confidence and ease, trusting that you'll make your way there eventually?

- What does being a good ancestor mean to you? What kind of world do you hope to leave behind for the next generation?

- What is your favorite place in nature? (It can be a type of landscape or a particular spot that holds meaning.) Has it always been your favorite place? Draw a map tracing your favorite nature spots through your life, and consider how each one has shaped you, inspired you, or helped you come to some realization about yourself or the world around you.

The Action

Rivers nourish us not only spiritually but physically as well. They're corridors that carry fresh water for drinking and agriculture, nutrients to keep land habitable, and fish that keep us fed. Their flows keep humanity running along, but these flows are increasingly unpredictable. Rivers are becoming more prone to sudden floods and consuming droughts, less full of fish than they are of filth, largely because of the ways we are manipulating them.

More than half of the planet's freshwater river basins are now considered heavily affected by human activities.[23] Pollution, climate change, and fragmentation have caused global populations of migratory freshwater fish species to plummet by 76 percent since just 1970, an even faster clip than marine (saltwater) species.[24] As the freshwater fish researcher Guohuan Su tells *National Geographic*, "You could say we live in the arms of the rivers, and we're cutting them off."[25]

Here are a few of the most dramatic ways we are severing rivers today, and how we can begin to repair them.

Overextraction

The Colorado River is a prime example of how human thirst can disrupt a river's flows. A majesty that once steadily gushed 1,450 miles from the Rocky Mountains into the Gulf of California, the Colorado has become increasingly fragmented after years of providing drinking water to millions of people, fueling farms in surrounding drought-prone regions, powering some of the country's largest dams, and keeping tourism industries afloat. If the rate of diversion in the Colorado River Basin continues, the US Bureau of Reclamation estimates that by 2060, demand for the river's water will outpace supply by at least 3.2 million acre-feet (what it would take to cover 3.2 million acres of land in water one foot deep),[26] almost half the amount currently allocated to the states in the river's Upper Basin (parts of Colorado, New Mexico, Utah, and Wyoming) every year.[27]

Some of the river's reservoirs are already running dangerously dry, a trend compounded by unpredictable weather patterns. In normal times, snowfall in the Rockies gradually feeds the river as it melts. But in warmer winters when the Rockies get more rain than snow, that water arrives all at once and leads to flooding, then nothing. Higher temperatures also cause more evaporation. And when more water vapor is sitting in the air, less of it is available on the ground. We've essentially overdrawn the river's bank account to the point that we're living paycheck to paycheck—and climate change means that some of those checks will never come.

The status of the Colorado River is emblematic of freshwater deficits around the world—each caused by a complicated mix of human extraction and ecological pressure.

The Mindset Shift: "I recognize the rights of nature."

Environmental problems hardly ever have straightforward solutions. Ones involving rivers are particularly nebulous. Since rivers are a source of livelihood and identity, telling people that the way they're using theirs is "wrong" becomes a personal affront, an attack on existence. It's also unrealistic. Humans can't quit their river extraction habits cold turkey. We need fresh water, and the food it grows, in order to live, so the only way forward is to balance our needs with those of the river itself.

A growing international campaign seeks to give rivers a (very literal) voice in this balancing act. The Rights of Nature movement states that natural ecosystems have the same fundamental rights to life that we humans do and should have the ability to exercise them.[28] A handful of countries around the world have endorsed this idea by officially granting their rivers legal personhood status. It sounds far-fetched at first: a river dressed to impress in a courtroom, staunchly defending its right to flow freely. But when you consider that some communities' ability to live is directly dependent on the health of this natural resource, giving rivers a voice in our court of law becomes less crazy.

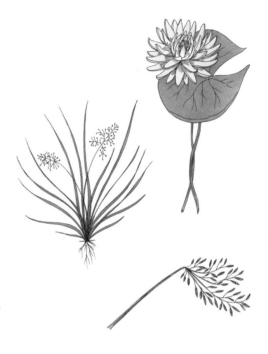

The first river to be granted personhood rights was the Whanganui River of the North Island of New Zealand, also referred to as Te Awa Tupua. A proverb among Māori tribes who live along the river is *Ko au te awa. Ko te awa ko au,* translating to "I am the river. The river is me." In 2017, after decades of battling parliament to recognize the Whanganui's cultural and spiritual value, the Māori succeeded in getting it represented in court. Any decisions directly affecting the future of the river must now be run by its two human representatives (one government-appointed, one a member of the Māori) who can "act and speak for and on behalf of Te Awa Tupua."[29] Since this landmark decision, Colombia, Bangladesh, and

India have also recognized the rights of certain rivers in their own legal systems.

There's concern that some of these rulings will prove primarily for show and sit unenforced. In the case of Colombia's framework, which recognizes that rivers have rights insofar as they can support human communities, legal scholars and environmentalists write in a 2020 review that "the Rights of Nature may be contingent on whether or not there is an immediate human cost to their exploitation."[30] But other river rights declarations have shown some real teeth. In Bangladesh, for example, where every river that flows through the country now has a legal right, over 4,000 illegal structures that encroached on riverbanks were demolished, and 231 unauthorized riverside factories were closed within a year of the new legal protections going into effect.[31] However, the free-flowing nature of rivers poses a challenge to this early progress: some of Bangladesh's larger rivers start outside the country's borders, meaning that only a percentage of them are legally "living." The fate of those rivers will depend on other countries adopting and enforcing river rights laws too.

With this in mind, the Earth Law Center is now circulating a "Universal Declaration of River Rights" far and wide to encourage governments around the world to protect all rivers in their court of law.[32] The declaration has the support of a number of environmental NGOs, legal experts, and citizens (you can add your name online at www.rightsofrivers.org). "This movement has come out of very strong social, and very, very strong cultural values," Ian Harrison, a freshwater specialist at Conservation International, tells me. "It's become one of the most interesting growing movements in the last few years around the world."

By placing rivers within a human framework, this movement acknowledges that we are not separate from them. Their life is our life. Their demise is our demise. Regardless of whether the declaration goes through, this reframing is one we could all stand to incorporate into our lives. How might you treat nature differently, if it were a person like you and me?

Pollution

In addition to extraction, pollution is also a major threat to rivers. From the Citarum River in Indonesia, completely covered by a solid layer of bottles in some areas, to the Yangtze in China, where locals can tell what the trendy colors are that fashion season by looking at the shade of waters stained with chemical dyes from garment factories, humanity's waste is dumped directly into river paths around the world. A disturbing study from eastern Britain recently found that plastic in particular is now so ingrained in local rivers that aquatic insects are settling on it at a higher rate than they are rocks and other natural features. "It shows just how poor the habitat quality of many urban rivers is, given that litter can support more diversity than other available habitats," the lead study author tells Environment and Energy Publishing.[33]

In the US, land contamination poses another threat to water safety when it's carried into rivers by rain or snowfall. Two nutrients of concern to the Environmental Protection Agency are nitrogen and phosphorus. According to the agency's latest water quality survey in 2013 to 2014,[34] 58 percent of the nation's rivers and streams contained excess phosphorus and 43 percent contained excess nitrogen—mostly originating from chemical fertilizers on farms and lawns, animal manure, or improperly treated wastewater. These nutrients, while a natural part of river ecosystems, become harmful in high numbers. That's because they create conditions for massive amounts of algae and bacteria to grow and overtake the river, blocking incoming light, messing with water flows, and starving the area of oxygen as they decompose. These "algae blooms" can lead to what's known as dead zones—patches of water void of life. In some cases, they can also make water toxic for human use, potentially deadly to swim in or consume fish from.

The largest dead zone in the US covers over five thousand square miles of the Gulf of Mexico, an area fed by the Mississippi River. The problem

> The river system is so vulnerable partly because it's a much more restricted system with a lot more species in it—so any change is going to have a much higher effect. . . . You only need to affect a small stretch of river, and you're affecting a lot of species.
>
> —IAN HARRISON,
> freshwater specialist,
> Conservation International

persists in part because it's unseen and unfelt for most people living along the Mississippi. The river starts all the way up in a glacial lake in Minnesota, accumulating nutrient runoff as it weaves through the country and carrying the runoff downstream. Those at the start of the river don't necessarily know how their activities affect the Gulf. They certainly don't see it happen. In this case, coming face-to-face with one's impact would require traveling fifteen hundred miles, dunking your head under the water, and realizing that there's not a fish in sight.

The Mindset Shift:
"I see every environmental challenge
as an opportunity."

The connectivity of rivers makes them incredibly vulnerable to contamination. Pollution in one area of a river can mean pollution downstream too. "That connectivity is a major reason why the threats are so significant. They kind of bleed on down," says Ian Harrison from Conservation International. But while this connectivity presents challenges, it can also open up opportunities. Polluting a river isn't the only thing that will have downstream effects. Cleaning it up will too.

The revitalization of rivers like the Thames and the Chicago River demonstrate that with public support, rivers can go from toxic wastelands to scenic attractions relatively quickly. "When you restore a forest, it takes a lot longer to see the primary forest come back," Natalia Piland, an urban ecologist and postdoctoral associate at the Tropical Rivers Lab at Florida International University, tells me. "But with a river, you can clean it and start having a healthy relationship with it pretty quickly. . . . I think that rivers provide a space for public participation in science in ways that many other ecosystems don't."

Citizens can become more engaged with river conservation and cleanup in their area by organizing or participating in trash pickups, researching citizen science opportunities, attending local government meetings where rivers are on the agenda, or simply walking the river more often and being vocal about any changes they see over time.

Ecosystem Fragmentation

Nothing changes the flow of a river more dramatically than a dam. Large-scale dam construction started to really boom in the twentieth century, as we scrambled to harness the power of rivers for electricity, control their floods, and redirect their waters to developing cities and farms. And the number of large dams has increased at least tenfold from 1950 to 2017.[35] There are now over eight hundred thousand dams throughout the world, manipulating two-thirds of the world's longest rivers.[36]

These dams have clear human value: they provide renewable hydropower and store water that keep cities from running dry. But any time you wedge a wall of steel and concrete in the middle of an ecosystem, it's going to affect surrounding wildlife.

By disrupting the natural flow, water level, and temperature of a river, dams lead to conditions that may no longer be suitable for native insects and fish that have adapted to a certain cadence of water to feed, breed, and stay protected from predators. Dams can also make way for nonnative, sometimes invasive species to enter waterways. And if they don't have special passageways for aquatic life, dams can block the path of migratory fish who need to swim upstream in order to reproduce. (When these fish can't get upstream to reproduce, that of course throws off the ecosystem balance even more.)

Dams can create conditions that are harmful to humans too. Free-flowing rivers carry sediments that make surrounding land more fertile, hospitable, and protected from coastal flooding. Dams can trap these sediments, leading to less livable, more vulnerable land downstream. And while dams speed up water flows in some areas, they slow it down in others, and slow water is more prone to the type of nutrient buildups that can lead to dead zones. Like all river issues, this one is a sticky battle between humanity's progress and nature's integrity.

The Mindset Shift:
"I take a downstream approach
to decision-making."

Constructing so many dams in a relatively short period of time was, in many ways, overzealous and shortsighted—and we're now dealing with the consequences. "When the Bureau of Reclamation built its dams, it didn't usually take species migration, or sedimentology, into account," Heather Hansman writes in *Downriver: Into the Future of Water in the West*,[37] her account of traveling down the Green River, a tributary of the Colorado, and learning about the threats to its flows along the way. "We need power, but we also need sustainable rivers to guarantee that we have water in the future."

Removing ill-constructed dams that have fallen into disrepair and pose an environmental threat is one way forward. While it takes planning to ensure that destroying a dam won't further harm ecosystems downstream, success stories describe fish beginning to return to the upper river shortly after dam removals.[38] Dams that need to remain intact can be retrofitted with corridors that make it possible for more fish to pass through them (in both directions, downstream and upstream) and that adjust their water release to better mimic natural cycles. Ultimately, though, the only way to maintain the intelligence of rivers is to stop obstructing them in the first place.

The interconnectedness of all things means that changes in nature reverberate, always. Saving our rivers, and in turn ourselves, will require adopting a more downstream way of thinking—one that considers the impact all our actions have beyond our immediate line of sight, beyond the river bend.

CHAPTER EIGHT

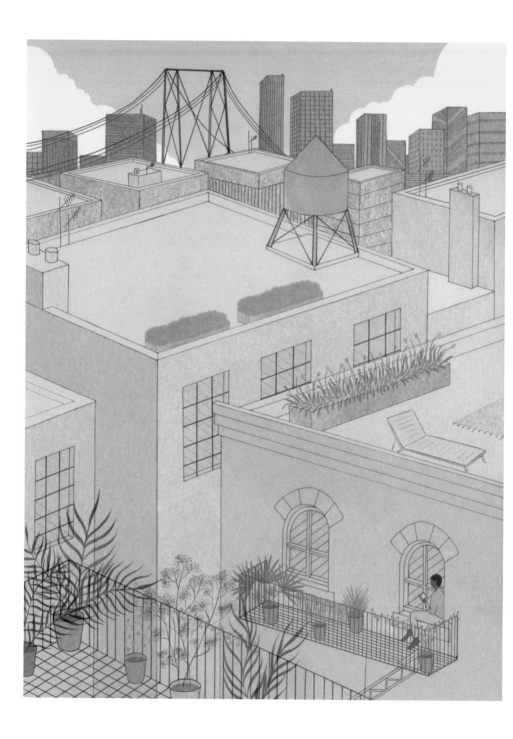

CITIES & BUILT ENVIRONMENTS

respite, reciprocity, humanity

There are plenty of reasons to love New York. The food, the culture, the shows, the first days of spring when the streets take on a new life. The grit and the twinkle; the ambition in the air during the morning commute. The freedom to laugh or cry or sing on the street without disturbing the peace (it was never there, anyway). The possibilities, the people, the endless surprise. The way the city looks during sunset, a view that could never get old.

Of course, there are trade-offs. The noise, the traffic, the rats, the smell when spring turns to summer and trash stews in the sun. The burnout and gloominess; the morning commutes when trains are delayed and you need to run to the office instead. The realization that, even surrounded by people, you can still feel totally and utterly alone. The prohibitive cost of possibilities, the crowds, the endless craving for fresh air. The way the grass and sky look when you take a weekend away from it all and ask yourself, Should I move?

These are all a part of what makes a city a city. There are reasons to love them and reasons to hate them, but, at the end of the day, they're still where we go when we want to feel alive.

The Remedy

Over half of the global population now lives in cities. By 2050, nearly 70 percent of the estimated 9.8 billion people on Earth will likely call them home.[1]

Cities are the human landscape. Of the eight landscapes we explore in this book, this is the only one that we've designed for ourselves. As such, we can shape it to display all the worst qualities the human species has to offer (greed, arrogance, delusion) or all the best (intelligence, creativity, community). How much of the natural world we let into this human environment, and how we choose to engage with it, is also up to us.

This final chapter reveals the nature that's already in our cities—and makes the case for adding more of it. It explores how we can all have expansive outdoor experiences within narrow grids of gray, the type that we used to think was reserved for remote wilderness. With a shift in perspective and a willingness to explore, we recognize that nature doesn't have to be way out there. More often than not, it's already waiting right here in front of us.

The Inherent Stressors of City Living

There are some perks to being surrounded by tons of other people: city dwellers tend to have access to higher-quality health care, better employment opportunities, and more diverse options for food, arts, culture, entertainment, and so on. But the urban existence also comes with its fair share of air pollution, noise pollution, light pollution, and hotter temperatures.

Research coming in from cities around the world shows that the cons of cities can quickly outweigh the pros when it comes to our mental health. A study in Canada found that city dwellers reported a higher prevalence of major depressive episodes than rural groups on average, even when controlling for confounding factors like income and race.[2] Another report on nearly seventy-five thousand residents of the Netherlands also associated urban living with an increased risk of depression.[3] And in the US, one pa-

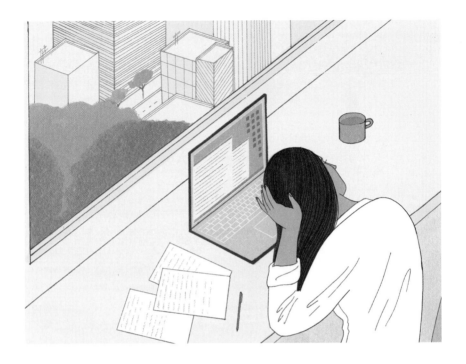

per found that suburbanites were slightly more satisfied and happy with their lives than demographically similar urbanites.[4] A scientific literature review published in 2009 supports the idea that globally, the prevalence of anxiety and depression does tend to be higher in urban environments on average.[5]

Pollution likely drives some of these outcomes. Levels of air pollutants like nitrogen dioxide and sulfur dioxide tend to be higher in cities, and they've been associated with increased rates of anxiety[6] and psychotic experiences.[7] Noise pollution is another irritant, and the cars, construction, and commotion of city streets can contribute to high blood pressure, poor sleep, and increased heart rate.[8] The bustle of city living might even somehow alter the way our brain responds to stress. When one small 2011 study put a group of thirty-two urban and rural dwellers through a stressful situation, the urban dwellers had significantly more activity in the amygdala region of the brain, which is responsible for regulating emotion and mood.[9] Since the amygdala is engaged in times of fear and anxiety, these findings suggest that city dwellers tend to feel stress more intensely than noncity dwellers.

This isn't to say that living in a city automatically guarantees poor health, but that certain stressors are built into the human landscape.

Why We Need to Close the Urban-Nature Divide

Despite the many ways that cities can harm our health, we now know a lot about how nature can help lessen the blow. Beyond providing opportunities for the fatigued brain to relax and recover, natural ecosystems can reduce air pollution, buffer noise, and provide opportunities to cool down on a hot day. For nearly every pitfall of modern urban life—social isolation and loneliness, sedentary jobs, relentless stress—getting outdoors can offer a salve.

But for so long, "getting outdoors" has been shorthand for *leaving* the city—for taking some time away from the built environment altogether. "Maybe it's rooted in the relative youth of our nation, or maybe it's manifest destiny and our relationships with the frontier and wilderness," Kathleen Wolf, a research social scientist at the University of Washington's College of the Environment, guesses as to why Americans in particular hold tight to the idea that real nature—nature with a capital N, as she puts it—needs to be beyond the city.

Wolf and many of the other researchers I've spoken with consider this view that real nature must be free of human influence to be problematic. For starters, most landscapes in nature are now influenced by humans to some degree (just consider the fact that our microplastics have been found in the deepest ocean trenches and the highest mountain peaks). Writing off the potential health benefits of all those places would be doing ourselves a disservice. The perspective harms the natural environment too. If we all keep escaping the human-made in favor of seemingly pristine, untouched landscapes, before too long, there won't be any of the latter left.

Finding respite in urban nature starts when we begin to see our cities as just another type of natural landscape. Instead of excluding humans from the nature narrative, we need to talk about nature as it includes people.

Now, it's worth noting that by setting green (nature) against gray (city) in very crude terms, a lot of the research I've presented in this book so far has been built on the very nature-urban binary I'm proposing we move away from. By asking participants to walk along a remote forest trail or a high-traffic highway, look out the window at a view of a park or a brick wall, it has stripped away all potential for an in-between experience. It's done so for a reason. To extrapolate the health benefits of the natural, researchers have needed to pit it against the unnatural—but they'll be the first to tell you that brick walls and traffic congestion are by no means all that a city can be.

In fact, the happiness, relaxation, and awe that we find in wide-open landscapes can also sit within a well-designed city block. We can start to get glimpses of these emotions by noticing the grass that pokes through our sidewalks, the lone trees that stand tall on our streets, and the blue sky that persists over our buildings. Cities are largely manufactured spaces, but that doesn't mean that the small patches of nature that do exist within them need to be any less real or any less restorative.

Taking a Walk on the Wild Side of My City

For those of us urban dwellers who always crave the feeling of oceans and forests, mountains and deserts, the solution might not be moving away from cities—but reimagining how we live in them.

Consider the city walk. It can be a time to put on headphones and tune out the world, or an opportunity to tune *in to* the relatively lush landscapes that sit within city boundaries—the open, grassy park, the patches of trees,

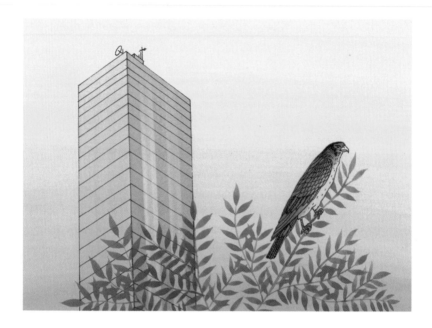

maybe even the river or salt marsh. In a well-planned city, you can find all of it within walking distance, a rarity in more spread-out rural environments. With this in mind, I set out to rediscover the nature in my own neighborhood and investigate how to engage with it in more therapeutic ways.

Tuning In to the City's Nonhuman Inhabitants: Biodiversity Still Exists in Urban Areas

I walk out of my apartment building and into one of the first warm days of the year. Though the last of winter's snow is still hanging on, spring is in the air and on my neighbors' giddy pale faces. As I make my way to the waterfront, picking up tail ends of their conversations, I notice another sound: birds chirping back and forth, as if they, too, were making plans for the new season. They all seem to be coming from a rogue bush nestled on the side of the wooden promenade. I stand next to it, watching its visitors flying in and out, singing all the while, and find it kind of amazing that such a hive of activity is always within ear's reach of this built-up throughway.

This pleasant start to my walk reminds me that some level of biodiversity—the number of species and variation within those species that exist within a given area—can still greet us in the urban environment.

While developing previously undeveloped land will always dramatically reduce biological diversity, unique native and nonnative species do exist in cities. Birds are an easier example to pick up on, but not the only one. Cities can actually have a higher species richness of vascular plants[10] and insects like bees[11] in some cases too, thanks in part to their diverse smattering of natural and seminatural spaces. In his "Four Natures" framework,[12] the ecologist and professor of ecosystem science and plant ecology at the Technical University of Berlin Ingo Kowarik emphasizes the different kinds of nature possible in a city, each one with its own potential for biological richness: patches of protected remnants of old-growth nature like forests or wetlands; rural landscapes like fields and grasslands; constructed green spaces like gardens and parks; and vacant industrial sites that have been left to develop their own urban wilderness.

Compared with low-density residential neighborhoods where the majority of the green space is privately owned, cities also tend to have a higher proportion of public spaces where you can see biodiversity up close. Another plus: these public places can be managed in ways that are appealing and approachable to lots of different people. There are plenty of urban dwellers who are unable or uninterested in heading to the untamed wilderness but would be happy to spend the day in a well-kept city park with comfortable seating and plenty of shade, and get their biodiversity fix that way.

You'll remember from the mountain chapter that biodiversity adds to the complexity of an environment and might therefore promote mental restoration according to attention restoration theory. On a more personal level, Richard Louv theorizes that we feel pulled to urban biodiversity because, as he said on his book tour for *Our Wild Calling: How Connecting with*

Animals Can Transform Our Lives—and Save Theirs, "we are desperate not to feel alone in the universe."[13]

A handful of researchers have headed to cities to test biodiversity's restorative capacity in the urban context. And sure enough, results from Georgetown, the capital city of Guyana,[14] to Bari, Florence, Rome, and Padua in Italy[15] have found that the more species richness people perceive, the more restorative they judge a place to be. Even when situated next to a built environment, then, biodiversity seems to help promote well-being.

Seeking Shade:
The Many Benefits of a Lone Street Tree

After paying the birds a visit, I make my way over to the neighborhood park. To get there, I need to pass through a busy street lined with restaurants and bars. About ten blocks later, the happy hour signs and folding tables are replaced by a row of street trees, and I know I'm getting close. There can't be more than five of them in front of me, but their thick trunks and effusive branches span the entire city block. Their fallen leaves, now dull and decaying, crinkle underfoot and smell like wet earth. Walking underneath them always feels like passing through a regal corridor; my shoulders relax, my pace slows, and my gaze opens up to take it all in.

We now know how a walk through damp, fragrant woodlands soothes the mind by engaging all five senses. And while these old-growth street trees don't have quite the same force, they do carry their own quiet calm.

For people who don't have access to a full-on forest, city trees can be the next best thing, as evidenced by one study on 77 residents of Helsinki, Finland,[16] who had reduced cortisol levels after a stroll through urban woodlands—which they considered even more restorative than a walk through an urban park. Over in Iceland, another study presented 188 adults with digitally manipulated images of a city street and asked them to rate the likelihood that they'd feel restored walking home from work along each one.[17] The more street trees that were present in the image, the more restorative it appeared to participants, suggesting that street trees give people the feeling of being away from the cognitive demands of the urban environment (work, to-do lists, etc.).

These small studies suggest that city trees can make us feel at ease. Larger, city-scale analyses show they can also set a shaded path for population-wide health benefits. In one study from Leipzig, Germany, the environmental psychology lecturer Melissa Marselle, now at the University of Surrey, and her team studied two data points from nearly ten thousand people: antidepressant use and proximity to street trees.[18] They found that those city dwellers who lived within one hundred meters (about one football field length) of trees had a lower likelihood of being prescribed antidepressants than those who lived farther away from canopy, suggesting that close-to-home trees can support mental well-being. This association was especially strong for socially deprived groups.

A model of 276 metropolitan areas in the US found something similar: those who lived in areas with more green land cover, specifically edge environments where trees stood next to built spaces, were less likely to report frequent mental distress.[19] Another survey of green space and mental health outcomes in Wisconsin goes so far as to say that "results indicate that the difference in depressive symptoms between an individual living in an environment with no tree canopy and an environment with 100% tree canopy is larger than the difference in symptoms associated with an individual who is uninsured compared to an individual with private insurance."[20]

Researchers can't fully explain the mood-boosting powers of street trees just yet. They probably have at least something to do with greenery's ability to help people restore from mental fatigue more generally. But trees also come with unique ecosystem services—like casting shade on hot days and removing carbon dioxide and volatile organic compounds from polluted city air—which can only help. Clusters of trees can also dampen surrounding commotion, reducing the health threats of noise pollution.

Beyond reducing our mental strain, these qualities might improve our overall health. A 2016 study in California associated neighborhood tree cover with lower rates of obesity, type 2 diabetes, high blood pressure, and asthma.[21] These sorts of studies have led some to consider trees increasingly life-saving infrastructure in the age of climate change.

Here Today, Gone Tomorrow: How We Can Get Lost in Ephemeral Urban Environments

I walk into the park as the late afternoon sun starts to climb to its luminous, golden peak. A place that I've walked through countless times takes on a new quality at this time of day; the spacious light reveals nooks and crannies I hadn't noticed before. Every minute somehow becomes more saturated until the grass, dirt, and sky all shimmer gold.

You never know exactly when these fleeting moments of beauty will arrive. Nature doesn't follow an agenda; it shows off on a whim, and its displays always have a way of making me question why I stick so tightly to my own schedule. Clearly, they tell me, the best things in life are unplanned.

The ephemerality of nature is part of its charm. Even the most mundane parts of it have an endless capacity to change in ways that capture our attention. This means that when you love a certain tree, for example, you don't just love the tree itself. You love the way its leaves take on color throughout the year, the shadows it casts in morning light, the sound it makes when the wind passes through its canopy.

In qualitative research, when participants are asked to describe why they feel connected to certain environments, these fleeting moments almost always come up. Alex Smalley, the researcher we met in the ocean chapter who studies people's reactions to digital re-creations of the natural world, thinks that this ephemerality, beyond being memorable, is also innately restorative.

"If I spend time in a landscape that I know well, I become attuned to its cycles," he tells me. "If I get caught out in a sudden rainbow or sunset or snowfall, that's something I will connect with very differently that I will remember and possibly try to relive. I will find it restorative because of its scarcity and ephemerality."

Nature's ability to surprise, delight, and restore is very welcome in the rigid city environment. The bud of a flower, the color of a sunset, the arc of a rainbow look somehow even more fascinating against an otherwise concrete canvas.

Katherine Irvine, from the James Hutton Institute, explains that when people look out for all these different attributes in their city's nature, they might find that they no longer feel the need to escape it for something more grand. "When you start thinking about nature that way, you don't have to go to the wilderness. You realize there's a wilderness right there in the urban environment," she tells me over video chat from her home in Scotland.

As we're talking, Irvine's eyes veer outside her window, to where a raptor has decided to perch. She smiles at the serendipity. A rare bird has found its way to her yard in the middle of the city: what better sign that moments of awe and elation can find us in the urban environment? Maybe our job is just to catch them before they fly away.

Meet Me in the Park: Why City Nature Is Better When We're Together

As I walk the perimeter of the park, I pass groups of friends, rec sport teams, families, and couples inhabiting the space in their own ways. The grassy lawn is a gathering spot for the community, and folks head there to celebrate, play, and just be together.

So far, most nature-health research has looked at individual experiences of the outdoors. By and large, it's found that heading out into nature (urban nature very much included) solo can help us relax, reflect, and recover from some of life's demands. But what about when we're not alone? Can we still reap the benefits of outdoor time when we spend it with other people? Can getting outside with others strengthen our relationships in turn?

The relational restoration theory[22] suggests the answer is yes. Humans are, after all, social creatures, so it would make sense that something that's good for us is also good for our relationships. Have you ever taken a walk outside with a romantic partner and found that it's suddenly easier to verbalize what you need to work on as a couple? Or met with a coworker outside and come up with a creative idea faster than you ever have in a conference room?

According to this relational theory, this might happen because nature lightens our individual mental loads and, in turn, increases our capacity to put energy into strengthening our connections with other people. Beyond restoring us on an individual level, it can restore some element of our relationships too—especially the ones that we've neglected. "We have these adaptive resources that do not dwell only within us, but dwell within our relationships. Like our individual cognitive and physiological resources, our relational resources are limited," Terry Hartig, a professor of environmental psychology at Uppsala University and thought leader on restorative environments, tells me. "A relationship can eventually deteriorate as relational resources like trust, respect, and liking get depleted."

This potential of nature to support relationship building is underexamined. It's difficult to measure quantitatively, in part because every relationship is different. But it's clear that there is at least some benefit to getting outside with other people, if only in the sense that it's enjoyable—especially in the urban context. While quiet woods and rivers lend themselves to solo contemplation, a city park is a place to gather with friends. "Generally, spending time in urban green space is not a solitary endeavor," Melissa Marselle at the University of Surrey tells me. "It's a social endeavor, and so we need to do more research on the social context of being in green space." In one study, Marselle did find that those who took part in nature-based group walks tended to have fewer symptoms of depression, stress, and negative emotions than those who didn't take part in nature-based group walks, a promising start to a relatively untapped area of research.[23]

If researchers can prove that getting outside with others restores the mind and somehow helps facilitate and strengthen social bonds, it would be an influential discovery—especially in the context of the increasing loneliness epidemic in cities and the world at large.

Human Nature:
The Beauty That Lives Where
Humans and Nature Meet

I take the long way home from the park to go down to the water, underneath the Brooklyn side of the Williamsburg Bridge, where people love to go to take photos around sunset.

I follow where their cameras around me are pointing: up, up, up at the looming steel towers of the bridge, imposing themselves against the open sky and Manhattan beyond. It's the ultimate contrast: the burly bridge has been around for over a century. The soft clouds and sun behind it will be there for only a moment before disappearing for the night. Headlights and honking and bikers keep the bridge alive; the sky is subdued by comparison. The bridge's clean and meticulous lines cut the wispy shapes of the clouds. Yet, for all their differences, the bridge and sky meeting is always the shot that people are after. And for good reason.

Humans have evolved to find certain aspects of nature innately inviting: certain views to register as safe, familiar, and nourishing. But we've also evolved to find some of those same qualities in each other. The laughter of our friends, the loving touch of our family; I'd argue that these things offer a similar sense of comfort and escape. Just as we find awe and wonder in sweeping natural vistas, we can be awestruck by tremendous architecture, music, and art. Long forest paths provide the opportunity for restoration, but so do long dinners that we never want to end.

"I define a restorative environment as one that *promotes* and not only permits restoration," Hartig tells me. "Those of us who study restorative environments recognize it's not just a matter of taking away what people find stressful and demanding in an environment. It's also a matter of the environment offering some possibility for positive engagement that keeps people there, psychologically as well as physically."

In other words, a cornerstone aspect of a restorative place is that it doesn't just capture our attention but holds it. Cities are literally built to grab, and hold, our attention. And when they're infused with restorative bits of nature, they can create a landscape that appeals to both our innate longings and current curiosities.

For its ephemerality and capacity for diverse experiences, its ability to provide solo refuge and support social bonds, we now know that urban nature is healing in its own right. It has the calming qualities of wilderness we seek, made all the more therapeutic by the human touch.

So just as nature can bring beautiful things to humans, I like to think that humans can bring beauty into nature too. Maybe that's why people are always photographing where the bridge meets the sky. Or why my eye gets lost in the wake the ferry leaves on the river as I make my way back home. These areas where humans and nature meet remind us that we are inherently part of nature, always existing in relation to it. I hold on to this thought as I walk back inside the lobby of my apartment building, press the up button, and stand in the small, dark elevator, and am reminded of a moment listening to the environmentalist Paul Hawken reflect on an idea by Ralph Waldo Emerson. "What would we do if the stars only came out once every thousand years?" Hawken wondered, thinking we would probably stay up all night, celebrate, be joyous, dance like kids. "Instead," he said, "the stars come out every night, and we watch television."[24]

I travel up, getting farther from the park and the river and the trees with each floor that ticks by. From my new-construction apartment's picture window, I can't see the stars. Tonight, like every night, they're masked by the city lights. And yet, maybe it's because I live in conditions that leave me inherently separate from nature that the time I do get in it does feel so special, so celebratory.

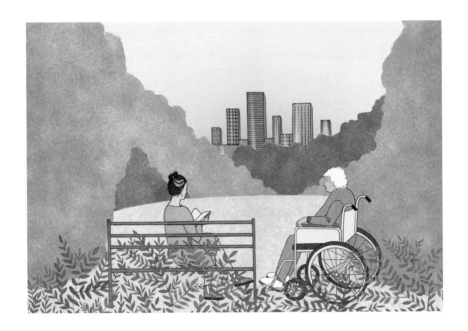

The last of the day's light streaming through my window; the shade of the street trees; the birds by the water: this is my nature. It may not be grand, but that's what makes it great. It's a retreat from inner life, and coming back to it every day, even if just for a moment, feels like a reunion a thousand years in the making.

The Practice

Finding the nature in cities often requires a little extra effort, but it's well worth it. Here are some ways to uncover new sides of your city, or any human-made community, through urban hikes, naturalist errands, and time-expanding strolls.

Look for moments of micro-restoration.

Getting your nature fix in a city often means filling up on smaller moments of restoration. The peaceful sit on a park bench, the gaze up at the sky, the glance into a canal or fountain . . . when done regularly, these activities can add up to nourishment that, as Kathleen Wolf puts it, can hold you over until your next, more decadent nature outing.

Enclosed, private spaces like under the shade of a tree are great for facilitating these moments, since this greenery can also help buffer some surrounding noise and further separate you from the action. But in a pinch, you can also make your surroundings feel more intimate by narrowing your frame of view. Homing in on a small patch of waves in the East River, for example, always puts my mind at ease. If I keep my gaze on the surface of the water immediately in front of me, and not the concrete jungle that sits beyond it, it's easier to get lost in the gentle, contained, yet expansive rhythm of the waves.

In my everyday life, I seek quality food for nutrients, energy, sustenance—but I enjoy a Thanksgiving feast with my family or a nice dinner out with a group of friends too. Nature is like that: we need that everyday sustenance with nearby nature, then, the bold, dramatic, national park experiences and time away. All of it serves a purpose.

—KATHLEEN WOLF,
research social scientist, University of
Washington's College of the Environment

Take pictures you have no intention of sharing.

I'm guilty of spending time outdoors glued to my phone's camera, especially when I'm visiting a new place. I've long wondered if taking so many pictures also takes me out of the moment itself, if it keeps me from fully engaging with that space. But funnily enough, this concern disappears when I set out with my DSLR camera instead of my iPhone. There's just something about the camera that changes the intentionality. It makes taking pictures more about noticing a place and less about proving that I was in it. I've also realized that I tend to remember experiences better when I've brought my camera into them, which might be a function of the increased mindfulness.

This realization has nudged me to approach my everyday walks from a more observant photographer's perspective, even if I don't have a fancy camera on me. And before I stop to whip out my phone, I ask myself whether this is something I'm capturing for my own memory or out of the urge to share. This more selective approach helps me feel more tuned in to the city, and myself.

Slow down time.

City life can be all about the grind: its pace fast, hard, and unforgiving. Escaping the demands of the clock is one reason that people head out into nature, where time seems to move slower somehow.

In one study in which thirty-three residents of southwest England were interviewed about therapeutic landscapes, many referenced the more expansive sense of time that the outdoors provided. Nature's unpredictable rhythms seemed to help people become less tethered to the minutiae of their own schedules and take a wider view on life. According to the study, "through allowing the mind and body to temporarily escape from pressured time in this way, study participants were able to perform important emotion work, proactively regulating and trying to dissipate negative emotions before they escalate or spill over into other spheres of their everyday lives."[25]

When I spoke with Sarah Bell, a lecturer in health geography at the University of Exeter and author on the study, she told me that the ancient Greeks actually have a name for this deeper sense of time: *kairos*. Compared with our clock time, *chronos*, *kairos* reveals itself slowly and cyclically.

For your next walk through a city environment, see if you can leave your watch at home and let yourself embrace *kairos* instead. As you go, take note of all the other elements around you that don't follow the same cadence as our human clocks.

IF YOU HAVE AN HOUR:

Find a patch of green and go.

Of the 8.4 million people who reside in New York City, Susan Hewitt has logged the most nature observations in iNaturalist, a popular phone app that lets users identify and share the nonhuman species around them.[26]

With over sixty thousand observations of 2,169 species within city limits under her belt, she tells me about impressive marine mollusks on Randall's Island and wild plants in Tompkins Square Park, but also the more commonplace stuff that usually gets overlooked. "I'm not a snob about how wild my wildlife is," Hewitt says. "I don't turn my nose up at weeds." Over her nearly forty years in New York, this laissez-faire approach has worked out well for her. It's shown her that nature always persists, even in the built environment, to remind her of her place in the wider world. "There's no question that it draws you out of yourself. Whenever you're thinking about other organisms, you're not thinking about yourself—and generally, that's a good thing."

Hewitt's advice for anyone interested in discovering the wild side of their city? Keep your definition of nature broad and stay curious about new places. Take a page from her book, and every time you need to run an errand in another part of town, consult the map first. Look for any little squares or triangles of green nearby, and go check them out to see what wild things you can uncover.

I always say that I find it very touching that nature is absolutely everywhere if you keep your eyes open and you're
interested. . . . The city gives me what I need to feel happy
in terms of nature.

—SUSAN HEWITT,
urban naturalist and citizen scientist
based in Manhattan

Seek out the oldest and tallest trees in your neighborhood.

The next time you're up for a longer city adventure, look up the oldest tree
in your area and pay it a visit. (The 133-foot-tall poplar in Queens, with
350 to 400 years under its roots, is calling my name.) Doing so will connect
you with times long gone, and research has found that old-growth trees
also tend to be considered more restorative to be around due in part to
their size and complexity.

Once you've hit up the oldest, move on to the tallest. According to
some fascinating research by the landscape architect Rob Kuper, taller
trees, in conjunction with taller groundcover plants, may also have greater
restorative potential than shorter plants, possibly due to their more obvious presence in the landscape and greater potential to attract people's attention in a variety of ways.[27]

Take an "I Spy" walk with someone.

Apply the nascent research on how sharing nature experiences can help
bring people closer together by taking a walk through some green with a

friend, partner, or family member. (Terry Hartig notes this can be a great thing parents can do with young kids too.) Notice how you feel going into it, and ask your walking buddy how they're doing too. Then, along the way, share what in your city's nature is sticking out to you that day—the tree's shade, the birds, the plant-covered balconies—almost like a game of I Spy that trains you to look out for the more natural spaces in your area. Compare notes when you get back on how you both feel after the walk. If you like the way you feel, why not make it a tradition?

IF YOU HAVE LONGER:
Go on an urban hike.

Liz Thomas, a professional hiker and adventure conservationist who holds a speed record on the Appalachian Trail, has also "hiked" over a dozen cities in her day, from New York to Chicago to Grand Rapids, Michigan.

Thomas tells me about her urban treks slightly breathlessly (she is, of course, on a walk during our call): in Los Angeles, she followed the Inman 300, a challenging city course that took her over hundreds of public stairways scattered across thirty-six zip codes—and made her question her choice of footwear with each step. Her Denver route was more relaxed: one hundred miles over eight days, with stops strategically placed at sixty-five local breweries. Her New York map passed through one hundred "playground-parks," previously asphalt schoolyards that had been greened by the Trust for Public Land and stayed open to the public when classes weren't in session.

Urban hiking started as a way for thru-hikers like Thomas to train and find a sense of adventure after returning home from trail life, but it's a concept anyone can try. Thomas says the main difference between urban hiking and just taking a walk in your neighborhood is the intention to visit places you don't usually go.

"Instead of walking the one street that you always walk, walk one street over," she tells me. "Be really deliberate about your choice to make it so you're experiencing places that are a little bit different than where you normally go."

After deciding how many miles you want to hit in a day (or over multiple days) and what landmarks you want to hit along the way (bookstores? parks? coffee shops?), you can map your trail ahead of time (Thomas likes using Google My Maps to make hers) so that all you need to do once you get started is have fun and pay attention. Bring a backup battery for your phone if you're heading out for a longer day, just in case, along with some water, sun protection, and good walking shoes.

Exploring your city on foot is a great way to notice more of its features, both natural and human-made, and learn new things about the culture and history of your place. Thomas tells me these hikes have given her a new outlook on the throughlines that unite various neighborhoods. They've shown her that the "other side of town" is never that far away after all; it's all within walking distance.

Conserve the nature of your city.

In an urban environment that can feel isolated from people and nature, community conservation projects take on a whole new appeal.

Kathleen Wolf refers to city stewardship as an expression of gratitude: a way to acknowledge the natural elements that are around us—even in an environment that often divorces us from them. It's also a way to practice a more reciprocal human-nature relationship and remember the positive influence that people can have on place. And as it brings you closer to the natural areas in your neighborhood, volunteering can also bring you closer to its people. Based on what we suspect of social cohesion, outdoor conservation work can be an easy entry for forming connections with others.

So the next weekend you're hoping to spend outdoors, instead of visiting a new place, consider seeing your own neighborhood in a new way by volunteering for a local cleanup, restoration project, or community gardening initiative.

Bring the outside in.

Interestingly enough, many of the nature health researchers I've talked to live in relatively urban environments. Studying the health benefits of nature for a living keeps them busy, and they often lament feeling somewhat removed from their subject in their everyday lives. Their science-backed solution? When you can't get outside, bring the outside in.

Buying houseplants is far from the only way to do so. Sarah Bell shared one creative idea for how to invite more nature into the built environment, inspired by her work researching how people living with sight impairment perceive and engage with the natural world: hold a multisensory nature visualization by popping on a nature soundtrack, lighting a candle, or diffusing some landscape-inspired oils, closing your eyes, and imagining being in a favorite outdoor place in order to, as Bell describes, cocoon yourself in an "overcoat of nature" for a while.

Or, take a cue from Katherine Irvine and orient your home toward nature for those busy days when longer trips outside aren't in the cards. "Doing this kind of research has really made me think about how I can bring nature into my world when I live in an urban environment," she tells me. "I've tried to integrate regular and ongoing microdoses rather than a single macrodose on a periodic basis."

For Irvine, this looks like planting spring-blooming bulbs outside so they're visible from her window, and positioning her desk so she can watch their big reveal as she works. For you, it might look like buying lace curtains with details that remind you to take a mindful moment when the sunlight streams into them and paints patterns on your walls. Or it can mean getting a small indoor fountain and setting it to start running at night to help you relax if you're an ocean lover, or hanging a photograph of a bare horizon above your workspace to help you daydream of the desert. Model your built environment after a favorite landscape, and see if it can deliver any similar effects.

Designate a "break window."

According to the original formulators of attention restoration theory, the Kaplans, it is possible to recover from mental fatigue by simply looking at nature through a window.[28] This can hold true even if your view is of the cityscape—as long as it has some element of green.

For example, a study from China pitted two urban high-rises against each other—one that looked out onto built space and one that overlooked a part of the city that had a park—and measured people's physiological responses to gazing out of each.[29] Sure enough, the city view that included a bit of green led to a significant increase in parasympathetic activity, signaling relaxation. In a separate study from Iran, city views that included more sky were rated as more restorative.[30]

City dwellers can apply this intel by picking a window at home that has a view of the most green, sky blue, or both to designate as a "relax" zone—a place to go to let your mind recover with the view of the city, without actually needing to step out into it. If all your windows look out onto other buildings (been there), a window box, situated inside or outside, can do the trick.

Journal on the city's themes.

These questions can help you get into a city state of mind by considering how you and the outdoors meet, what nature brings to you, and what you bring to it.

- Consider your relationship with time. What are you doing when you feel like time moves the slowest? What are you doing when you feel time moves the fastest? How can you find more of a balance between the two?

- What's one part of your neighborhood or immediate surroundings that you have yet to explore, and what's keeping you from it?

- What does nature give to you? What do you give to it in return?

- What are your skills and passions? What would it look like to apply them to the environmental movement?

Action

Home to most of the world's people, urban areas are also ground zero for the majority of the world's carbon emissions.[31] As human populations continue to expand, cities will need to thoughtfully grow in ways that protect the health of their people and the planet. While not a panacea, *greening* (a term I'm using loosely in this section to describe investing in any type of nature: trees, grass, flowers, coastal pathways, etc.) certainly helps achieve both goals.

Research has consistently shown that people who live in urban areas with more green space tend to report fewer days of mental health complaints[32] and higher overall well-being[33] than those who live in less green areas—and this holds true across socioeconomic groups.[34] From a sustainability perspective, urban greenery provides important ecosystem services such as air pollution removal, heat reduction, stormwater protection, and carbon storage. Building opportunities for nature contact into cities might also encourage more residents to become invested in conservation.

So for this section, instead of describing the threats to our cities, we're ending on a high note and exploring the opportunities to improve them using greenery. The best way to distribute nature will vary by city, but these four principles of successful green design are universal.

Design for decentralized experiences.

Massive parks are often the gold standard in green city design, but smaller slices of nature are important too. After all, unless you live right next door,

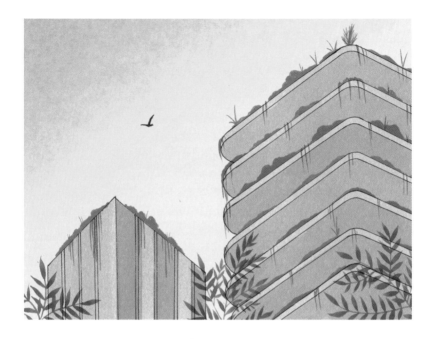

visiting a large urban park requires some level of effort on your end. You need to set aside the time during your day, figure out how to get there, and muster up the energy to actually go. For some people, taking these steps is no big deal and a small price to pay for a day outdoors. But for others—say, older people, people who are sick, people who don't have access to consistent transportation, people with limited mobility, and so on—the logistics can prove prohibitory, so it's essential that some level of greenery exists to meet them where they are.

"If you have nature where people are living, then you get over that motivational bit. You're already bringing it to their doorsteps," Melissa Marselle tells me. In the study from Germany where she found that people who lived near tree-lined streets were less likely to be prescribed antidepressants, Marselle also looked into where those street trees were planted: How close did they need to be to someone's home to provide this potential mental health boost? In the end, it was the nature that was right near where people lived, that they unintentionally passed by every day, that had the most significant effect.

This suggests that unconnected patches of green aren't the best use of city space from a human health perspective. Instead, most of the researchers I spoke with agree that linked networks of greenery offered more opportunities for meaningful nature contact. Think larger parks connected by tree-lined streets, green traffic medians, and small pocket parks in abandoned lots or railways. "If you have a network of spaces of different kinds, then you can satisfy a whole variety of demands," Rich Mitchell, the epidemiologist from Glasgow we met in the ice and snow chapter, tells me. In this sense, the city becomes a landscape in itself—rather than home to a few insulated parks. Green passageways are also safer for city wildlife, and the Nature Conservancy estimates that less than 2 percent of natural lands in the eastern US are currently connected in a way that lets animals move freely through them.[35]

Kathleen Wolf envisions a world in which there is some level of consistency in how these spaces are rolled out in different cities. If we were all literate in a universal language of urban greening, getting outdoors in cities could become more second nature.

Design for biodiversity.

The conservation biologist Richard Fuller is quick to say that urbanization of any type is intensely damaging to nature. Any time you build on a piece of land, you're stripping that place of some level of natural variation. But, at the same time, he says that urbanization has also *saved* the world's biodiversity. "Urbanization concentrates people into small areas. It deletes biodiversity from those areas, but it minimizes the spatial footprint of human occupation of the Earth," Fuller tells me from Australia. In other words, concentrated human settlements are bad for all the other life on our planet—but human sprawl is even worse.

This, Fuller says, is the central dilemma of designing the human habitat. When you stack a lot of people on top of each other in boxes of concrete, the compact living damages our health but protects the natural environment we've spared from development in the process. But when you give everyone the green that is so good for them, expanding their footprint to include a backyard and garden, you might make people healthier, but you make nature miserable. "If we all lived on our own five-acre block," he says, "the world's biodiversity would already be gone."

From a biodiversity perspective, the best thing we can do is stop developing new human habitats and instead maximize the cities we already have to be as compact and rich in therapeutic landscapes as possible.

These human landscapes need to be conducive to human whims. That is, urban green space should be designed to facilitate different experiences, depending on what visitors are in the mood for. I'll admit that a part of me started this project wanting to find that unicorn landscape: that universally pleasing combination of trees and water and field that could be deployed in cities with abandon. But maybe it's better that it doesn't exist. Imagine how boring it would be to travel to a new park already knowing what you'll find there—the same type of trees, arranged in the same pattern, surrounding the same birdbath. There is, after all, no one way to be outside, and it's unlikely that one place can ever be perfect for everyone, every day.

Design for lasting equity.

In addition to making way for diverse wildlife and experiences, urban greenery needs to be designed for a diversity of people. As it stands now, urban green space is clustered in wealthier, predominantly white areas. Yet all signs point to the fact that, when rolled out more equally, it can reduce health disparities between disadvantaged populations and privileged groups.[36]

When deciding where to place new multiuse green networks, less affluent areas should take priority. But simply adding new green space to underserved areas of cities is not enough. Policies also need to be put in place to ensure that it doesn't uproot the residents of that area in the long run.

"Green gentrification" (also known as ecological or environmental gentrification) describes how greening projects can contribute to physical and/or cultural displacement. Alessandro Rigolon, an assistant professor in the Department of City and Metropolitan Planning at the University of Utah whose research focuses on the equitable distribution of urban greenery, gives the Chicago 606 and the Atlanta BeltLine as examples: these green walkways, which span miles of their respective cities, have both spurred an increase in development and a surge in housing prices in surrounding low-income communities. You can't peg gentrification to one park alone. But since greening projects tend to make an area more desirable to live in, if protections aren't put in place for the community's current residents, such projects can be used as another way to drive people out. "Many cities have chosen to move forward with urban sustainability initiatives under the assumption that they benefit all residents equally, when in reality the greatest gains tend to accrue for the most well-off," Rigolon and coauthor Jeremy Németh wrote in a 2019 study.[37]

This raises the question of how cities can bring green spaces to the people who could most benefit from them without driving those same people away. Rigolon has a few ideas: "What is increasingly clear is that low-income communities of color don't need to have one of their needs met at a time. Projects that are just addressing one need can backfire," he tells me. "There needs to be a more deliberate and holistic approach wherein we try to address multiple needs at the same time—for example, housing, jobs, and good transportation, in addition to green space." His research has found that when green space is included in a wider community revitalization plan, alongside the creation of affordable housing, property tax freezes for existing homeowners, better-paying jobs, small business support, and so on, it seems to be less likely to contribute to gentrification over time.[38] These larger plans also do more to support community health than even the most restorative park ever could. "For most people, at the end of the day, it's probably more important that they've got a roof over their head and some money in the bank than contact with nature," Mitchell tells me. "But of course, these things are connected."

These parks-related antidisplacement strategies should be implemented early in a project, as should the process of consulting community members about any proposed changes. "It's not that people of color don't care about their parks. Sometimes, it's that no one has ever asked them what they think," Carolyn Finney, a cultural geographer and the author of *Black Faces, White Spaces: Reimagining the Relationship of African Americans to the Great Outdoors*, told the Trust for Public Land for a report on the inequities of urban green space.[39] "Cities need to make space for their voices."

People of different ages and physical abilities should also be invited to the planning process. Sarah Bell, who has worked with individuals who have various degrees of sight impairment, gives sensory gardens as a prime example of why. "Often that sensory garden is in a tiny little corner of an otherwise expansive sensory-rich parkland, which, if it just had the right adjustments (e.g., accessible path networks, inclusive interpretation, etc.), could be a place for people with varied sensory priorities and interests to experience the pleasures of movement and exploration," she tells me.

Collaboration with community members from different backgrounds and needs is essential for ensuring that green space is a useful and usable amenity for all.

Design for a changing climate.

Greening can help make cities more resilient and livable in the age of climate change—though we can't just plant some trees and call it a day. Greening needs to be combined with solutions like carbon reductions, energy reform, and cleaner transportation options. And from a sustainability perspective, preserving existing nature is just as important, if not more so, as bringing new nature into cities.

To understand why, we can look to the work of GreenEquityHEALTH, an ongoing five-year interdisciplinary project exploring how urban green space provides ecosystem services with a particular focus on health and environmental justice.[40] One of its projects in Leipzig, Germany, measured the potential health benefits of an old-growth urban park and a newer park over the course of a particularly hot, dry summer in the city. They found that the older park provided more ecosystem services compared with the new park and was considered a more comfortable destination overall.[41] Its denser canopy provided more cooling shade and its covered grasses and soil held up better in the hot sun. Presumably, its more established network of trees also provided more carbon capture than the new park and allowed for more biodiversity. This finding is a reminder that rich ecosystems take decades to grow, and the ones that have withstood the test of time should be protected, especially as our cities get hotter.

It's impossible to know what's in store for our cities—but it's hard to imagine a future in which nature doesn't make them a more pleasant place to be. Of course, the nature in cities doesn't render more remote wilderness expendable. All nature, both nearby and far away, is essential and must be protected with all of our might.

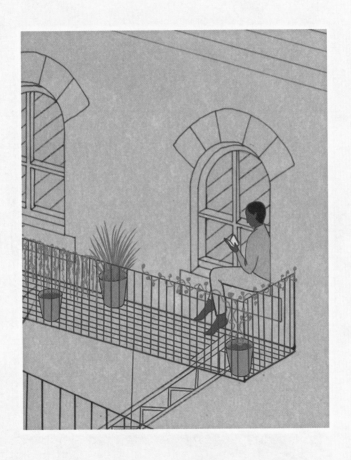

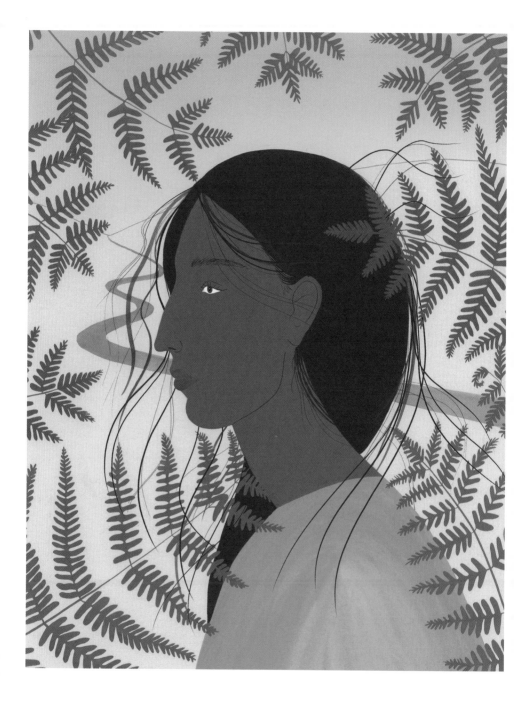

EPILOGUE

I had big plans to write this book from the road. I imagined weeks spent sweating in the desert, long stints in wood cabins, maybe a trip to icy climes if I was really feeling daring. I wanted to immerse myself in every landscape, settle into their grasp, and write about what I found there. COVID-19 had other plans for me, as it did for all of us.

I wrote the majority of *Return to Nature* from April 2020 to April 2021. When I first got the news that this book was going to come to life, the world was just settling into the loss of the pandemic. That bleak early spring, when days were spent wondering aloud what the future would bring, is a time of vivid, if fragmented, memory for me. One moment that I distinctly recall is listening to a podcast hosted by Cheryl Strayed, her voice holding the uncertainty we all felt as she worked through things in real time.[1] She said: "We have to take a step back from each other, but maybe there are other things we can step closer to." Looking back, she was right. And for many people, those things were found outdoors.

I can only imagine how many authors will go on to write books about this past year, attempting to make sense and meaning of what sits in the rearview. I'm not going to try to parse out the lessons of a time that has been so painful and continues to be as I write these words. What I will say is that, since that dreary April in 2020, I've seen friends gabbing on park benches, makeshift picnics of sparkling water and cheese wedged as a barrier between them. I've seen grassy fields turn into workout studios, yoga mats placed in sprawling rows six feet apart. I've seen people laugh, cry, shout, eat, share, love, and do all the other things that make us human, on the sidewalk. I've seen more dogs being walked than I ever thought possible. I've seen people play out their lives outside. And I've seen us better for it.

Forced to stand still for all these months, we've learned to simply watch the world move around us. And move it has: the cycling of leaves through all four seasons, the daily dance of clouds, the minute-by-minute shifts in sun and shadow . . . these are the modest dramas we've taken in from our windows, seen on our walks. When we've had to lean on our nearby nature to stand in for the faraway, we found it to be up to the challenge every time.

Even when we are able to immerse ourselves in foreign and wild and wonderful wilderness yet again, I hope we remember these window journeys, these armchair travels. I hope we all continue to seek smaller moments of wonder and surprise in the outdoors, the kinds that make those larger ones feel all the more grand. I hope we remember what a world cut off from nature could look like. I hope we do everything in our power to keep it from becoming reality. I hope this book can help.

As I write this, spring is in bloom and the human world is also starting to open up with the flowers. Vaccination rollouts and easing travel restrictions have me wondering how to put all that I've learned in the past year into practice in the real albeit reconstructed world.

Where do we go from here? Outside, sure. While the experts I spoke with for this book acknowledged that there are still particulars we don't know about how nature influences our health, they shouldn't keep us indoors. I used to naively hope that through writing this book I would find some ideal landscape, the perfect mix of relaxing and awe-inspiring that makes everyone walk away with a restored body and renewed mind. The bad news is that such a place does not exist. But isn't that great news too? It means we can create it for ourselves. Our relationship with nature is, after all, deeply personal. Ultimately, it's our inner landscape that will go on to shape our outer discovery.

The guest that Strayed was talking to all those months ago was the pro-lific writer and thinker Pico Iyer. He, too, shared words that I have held with me through this time: "Life is about a joyful participation in a world of sorrows," he said, and "every life ends in death, every meeting ends in a separation, but that's not a reason to grieve. It's actually a reason to find our beauty and joy right now."

Our world is, as it has ever been, fraught with sorrows. We're standing at the precipice of daunting social and environmental crises, ones that we can't solve just by forest bathing. But if there's anything I've learned while writing this, it's that getting outside can support us as we search within ourselves for the solutions we so need.

Nature, like us, is full of joy and pain. In it we see ourselves clearly. We recognize our capacity to be as forceful and domineering as the snow, as unpredictable as waves, as resolute as rivers. We are reminded of our own nuance, our own human nature. I started this project looking for a way to return to a childhood in the trees despite being an adult living in concrete. Along the way, I have found that there are more shades between green and gray than I could have possibly imagined, and they all sit outside my front door, as they do within me. I look out on the city and see vibrant blues and purples, deep reds and yellows, burnt oranges. I open my window and breathe them all in, drinking the fresh air as if for the first time.

Acknowledgments

When I work on a big project like this, I tend to put the rest of my life on hold. Thank you to Phil, June, Emily, John, and the rest of the quarantine pod for being patient with me as I did. You're my favorites. I'm forever grateful to my mom for offering up her house, fridge, and coffeemaker in the mountains for writing weekends and Pops for all the calls to tell me I could do it. I love you both endlessly. Lindsay, I'm so lucky to call you my forever coauthor and friend. Thank you for your mentorship and encouragement. Many thanks to team mbg for allowing me the time and space to do this book right.

Return to Nature would not have been possible without my wonderful editor Anna Paustenbach, who kept me on a clear path through a project that could have veered down a million side trails; my supportive agent Amy Hughes, who got this idea into the right hands; and my talented illustrator, Harriet Lee-Merrion, who brought these words to life so beautifully. Special thanks to Chelsea Szmania for her rigorous fact-checking. Lisa Zuniga, Janet Evans-Scanlon, Paula Dragosh, Makenna Holfold, Yvonne Chan, Katie Shepherd, Daniel Rovzar, and Judith Curr at HarperCollins, thank you for taking this book from idea to reality.

I'd pictured my interviews for this book taking place on a boat or on a hike (or at least in a lab with a nice view). Instead, they all happened over Zoom. I'm grateful for the technology that's allowed me to "travel" tens of thousands of miles over this past year, connecting me to the mountains of Bhutan and the coast of England, to people as far away as Melbourne and

Nairobi and as close as across the East River. A heartfelt thank-you to all the researchers, adventurers, and nature lovers who were generous enough to speak to me for this project:

Keenan Adams, Tori Baird, Jo Barton, Sarah Bell, Easkey Britton, Cassandra Brooks, Chandra Brown, Robin Chazdon, Susan Chomba, Douglas E. Christie, Jeannette (Nette) Compton, Tashi Dorji, Jason Duvall, Mollie Engelhart, Chris Fagan, Lora Fleming, Rich Fuller, Timothy Gallati, Caroline Hägerhäll, Nicole A. Hall, Ian Harrison, Terry Hartig, Reginaldo Haslett-Marroquín, Jill Heinerth, Gordon Hempton, Susan Hewitt, Katherine Irvine, M Jackson, Sonya Jakubec, Ingrid Jarvis, Nadja Kabisch, Emi Koch, Kalevi Korpela, Laura Kottlowski, Rob Kuper, Susannah Lerman, Julia Lucas (and Irine Polyzogopoulos), Freddie Lymeus, George MacKerron, Melissa Marselle, Rich Mitchell, Denise Mitten, Yoshifumi Miyazaki, James W. Navalta, Sumant Nigam, Emily Penn, Natalia Piland, Julia Plevin, Gavin Pretor-Pinney, Merja Rantakokko, Eleanor Ratcliffe, Dani Reyes-Acosta, Alessandro Rigolon, Jennifer D. Roberts, Melanie Rudd, Connor Ryan, David Sabgir, Judith Sadora, Carola Salvi, Roz Savage, Tashi Sherpa (and his son for translating!), Manuela Siegfried, Natalie Small, Alex Smalley, William Sullivan, Liz Thomas, Catharine Ward Thompson, Elsye "Chardonnay" Walker, Dan Wenk, Matthew Wichrowski, Kathryn Williams, Kathleen Wolf, and Youmin Yap. Your minds make this book what it is. I've never enjoyed interviews more, and I hope I did you proud.

I wrote most of this book on unceded Native territory and would like to acknowledge the first stewards of this land, the Canarsee tribe.

Writing is about finding, accepting, and working within your own limitations. Thank you to Florence Williams, Robert Macfarlane, Richard Louv, and all the other writers before me who have given voice to nature. Your words inspire me to push my own limits a bit farther.

Finally, thank you to the Manhattan skyline, the Green Mountains of Vermont, the Massachusetts horizon, the coast of Maine, and the other views that kept me going during long book days. You made the work so worth it.

Notes

Any quote that doesn't have an endnote was told to me directly over a phone or video interview.

INTRODUCTION

1. N. Klepeis, W. Nelson, W. Ott, J. Robinson, A. Tsang, P. Switzer, J. Behar, et al., *The National Human Activity Pattern Survey (NHAPS)*, 2001, https://indoor.lbl.gov/sites/all/files/lbnl-47713.pdf.
2. S. Kellert, D. Case, D. Escher, D. Witter, J. Mikels-Carrasco, and P. Seng, *The Nature of Americans: Disconnection and Recommendations for Reconnection*, 2017, https://natureofamericans.org/sites/default/files/reports/Nature-of-Americans_National_Report_1.3_4-26-17.pdf.
3. Nielsen, "Time Flies: U.S. Adults Now Spend Nearly Half a Day Interacting with Media," July 31, 2018, https://www.nielsen.com/us/en/insights/article/2018/time-flies-us-adults-now-spend-nearly-half-a-day-interacting-with-media/.
4. World Health Organization, "Depression," January 30, 2020, https://www.who.int/news-room/fact-sheets/detail/depression.
5. National Institute of Mental Health, "Mental Illness," January 2021, https://www.nimh.nih.gov/health/statistics/mental-illness.shtml; Anxiety and Depression Association of America, "Facts and Statistics," n.d., https://adaa.org/understanding-anxiety/facts-statistics.
6. Oliver Milman, "Heating Arctic May Be to Blame for Snowstorms in Texas, Scientists Argue," *Guardian*, February 17, 2021, https://www.theguardian.com/science/2021/feb/17/arctic-heating-winter-storms-climate-change.
7. A. Tyson and B. Kennedy, "Two-Thirds of Americans Think Government Should Do More on Climate," Pew Research Center Science & Society, June 23, 2020, https://

www.pewresearch.org/science/2020/06/23/two-thirds-of-americans-think-govern ment-should-do-more-on-climate/.

8. C. Knecht, "Urban Nature and Well-Being: Some Empirical Support and Design Implications," *Berkeley Planning Journal* 17, no. 1 (2004): 1, https://doi.org/10.5070 /bp317111508.

9. R. W. Kimmerer, *Braiding Sweetgrass: Indigenous Wisdom, Scientific Knowledge, and the Teachings of Plants* (Minneapolis, Minnesota: Milkweed Editions, 2013).

10. Wilderness Act of 1964, Public Law 88-577 (16 U.S.C. 1131-1136), Wilderness Connect, https://wilderness.net/learn-about-wilderness/key-laws/wilderness-act/default.php.

11. L. M. Fredrickson and D. H. Anderson, "A Qualitative Exploration of the Wilderness Experience as a Source of Spiritual Inspiration," *Journal of Environmental Psychology* 19, no. 1 (1999): 21–39, https://doi.org/10.1006/jevp.1998.0110.

12. E. Ratcliffe, B. Gatersleben, and P. T. Sowden, "Bird Sounds and Their Contributions to Perceived Attention Restoration and Stress Recovery," *Journal of Environmental Psychology* 36 (2013): 226, https://doi.org/10.1016/j.jenvp.2013.08.004.

13. Paul Griffin, *The Carbon Majors Database: CDP Carbon Majors Report 2017*, July 2017, https://b8f65cb373b1b7b15feb-c70d8ead6ced550b4d987d7c03fcdd1d.ssl.cf3 .rackcdn.com/cms/reports/documents/000/002/327/original/Carbon-Majors- Report-2017.pdf?1499691240.

14. J. Whitburn, W. Linklater, and W. Abrahamse, "Meta-analysis of Human Connection to Nature and Proenvironmental Behavior," *Conservation Biology* 34, no. 1 (2019): 180–93, https://doi.org/10.1111/cobi.13381.

15. I. Alcock, M. P. White, S. Pahl, R. Duarte-Davidson, and L. E. Fleming, "Associations Between Pro-environmental Behaviour and Neighbourhood Nature, Nature Visit Frequency, and Nature Appreciation: Evidence from a Nationally Representative Survey in England," *Environment International* 136 (2020), https://doi.org/10.1016 /j.envint.2019.105441.

CHAPTER ONE: PARKS & GARDENS

1. J. Marinelli, "Forgotten Landscapes: Bringing Back the Rich Grasslands of the Southeast," Yale Environment 360, June 20, 2019, https://e360.yale.edu/features /forgotten-landscapes-bringing-back-the-rich-grasslands-of-the-southeast.

2. D. Rojas-Rueda, M. J. Nieuwenhuijsen, M. Gascon, D. Perez-Leon, and P. Mudu, "Green Spaces and Mortality: A Systematic Review and Meta-analysis of Cohort Studies," *Lancet Planetary Health* 3, no. 11 (2019): e469–e477, https://doi.org/10 .1016/s2542-5196(19)30215-3.

3. E. A. Richardson, N. K. Shortt, R. Mitchell, and J. Pearce, "A Sibling Study of Whether

Maternal Exposure to Different Types of Natural Space Is Related to Birthweight," *International Journal of Epidemiology* 47, no. 1 (2017c: 146–55, https://doi.org/10 .1093/ije/dyx258.

4. J. Casey, P. James, K. Rudolph, C. D. Wu, B. Schwartz, "Greenness and Birth Outcomes in a Range of Pennsylvania Communities," *International Journal of Environmental Research and Public Health* 13, no. 3 (2016): 311, https://doi.org/10.3390/ijerph13030311.

5. American Heart Association, "More Green Spaces Can Help Boost Air Quality, Reduce Heart Disease Deaths," ScienceDaily, 2020, https://www.sciencedaily.com /releases/2020/11/201109074111.htm.

6. C. Ward Thompson, J. Roe, P. Aspinall, R. Mitchell, A. Clow, and D. Miller, "More Green Space Is Linked to Less Stress in Deprived Communities: Evidence from Salivary Cortisol Patterns," *Landscape and Urban Planning* 105, no. 3 (2012): 221– 29, https://doi.org/10.1016/j.landurbplan.2011.12.015.

7. J. Maas, R. A. Verheij, S. de Vries, P. Spreeuwenberg, F. G. Schellevis, and P. P. Groenewegen, "Morbidity Is Related to a Green Living Environment," *Journal of Epidemiology and Community Health* 63, no. 12 (2009): 967–73, https://doi.org /10.1136/jech.2008.079038.

8. H. Frumkin, "Building the Science Base: Ecopsychology Meets Epidemiology," in P. H. Kahn Jr. and P. H. Hasbach, eds., *Ecopsychology: Science, Totems, and the Technological Species* (Cambridge, MA: MIT Press, 2012).

9. C. M. Hägerhäll, Å. Ode Sang, J.-E. Englund, F. Ahlner, K. Rybka, J. Huber, and N. Burenhult, "Do Humans Really Prefer Semi-open Natural Landscapes? A Cross-Cultural Reappraisal," *Frontiers in Psychology* 9, no. 1 (2018), https://doi.org/10 .3389/fpsyg.2018.00822.

10. R. L. Coley, W. C. Sullivan, and F. E. Kuo, "Where Does Community Grow?: The Social Context Created by Nature in Urban Public Housing," *Environment and Behavior* 29, no. 4 (1997): 468–94, https://doi.org/10.1177/001391659702900402.

11. F. E. Kuo, W. C. Sullivan, R. L. Coley, and L. Brunson, "Fertile Ground for Community: Inner-City Neighborhood Common Spaces," *American Journal of Community Psychology* 26, no. 6 (1998): 823–51, https://doi.org/10.1023/a:10222 94028903.

12. L. Brunson, F. E. Kuo, W. C. Sullivan, "Resident Appropriation of Defensible Space in Public Housing: Implications for Safety and Community," *Environment and Behavior* 33, no. 5 (2001): 626–52, https://doi.org/10.1177/00139160121973160.

13. F. E. Kuo, "The Role of Arboriculture in a Healthy Social Ecology," *Journal of Arboriculture* 29, no. 3 (2003): 148–55, http://www.globalbioenergy.org/uploads /media/The_role_of_arboriculture_in_a_healthy_social_ecology.pdf.

14. G.-W. Kim, G.-W. Jeong, T.-H. Kim, H.-S. Baek, S.-K. Oh, H.-K. Kang, S.-G. Lee, et al., "Functional Neuroanatomy Associated with Natural and Urban Scenic Views in the Human Brain: 3.0T Functional MR Imaging," *Korean Journal of Radiology* 11, no. 5 (2010): 507–13, https://doi.org/10.3348/kjr.2010.11.5.507.

15. D. Umberson and J. Karas Montez, "Social Relationships and Health: A Flashpoint for Health Policy," supplement, *Journal of Health and Social Behavior* 51, no. 1 (2010): S54–S66, https://doi.org/10.1177/0022146510383501.

16. C. P. Fagundes, J. M. Bennett, H. M. Derry, and J. K. Kiecolt-Glaser, "Relationships and Inflammation Across the Lifespan: Social Developmental Pathways to Disease," *Social and Personality Psychology Compass* 5, no. 11 (2011): 891–903, https://doi.org/10.1111/j.1751-9004.2011.00392.x.

17. T. Miyazaki, T. Ishikawa, H. Iimori, A. Miki, M. Wenner, I. Fukunishi, and N. Kawamura, "Relationship Between Perceived Social Support and Immune Function," *Stress and Health* 19, no. 1 (2003): 3–7, https://doi.org/10.1002/smi.950.

18. G. Hempton, *On Being* (podcast), August 29, 2019, https://onbeing.org/programs/gordon-hempton-silence-and-the-presence-of-everything/.

19. Ratcliffe, Gatersleben, and Sowden, "Bird Sounds and Their Contributions."

20. J. Lubbock, *The Pleasures of Life* (Kent, England: Dorley House Books, Inc., 1887).

21. Kate Marvel, "Can Clouds Buy Us More Time to Solve Climate Change?," TED, July 17, 2017, https://www.ted.com/talks/kate_marvel_can_clouds_buy_us_more_time_to_solve_climate_change#t-317845.

22. G. Pretor-Pinney, *The Cloudspotter's Guide: The Science, History, and Culture of Clouds* (New York: TarcherPerigee, 2007).

23. T. Sugiyama, E. Leslie, B. Giles-Corti, and N. Owen, "Associations of Neighbourhood Greenness with Physical and Mental Health: Do Walking, Social Coherence, and Local Social Interaction Explain the Relationships?," *Journal of Epidemiology and Community Health* 62, no. 5 (2008): e9, https://doi.org/10.1136/jech.2007.064287.

24. C. Song, H. Ikei, M. Igarashi, M. Takagaki, and Y. Miyazaki, "Physiological and Psychological Effects of a Walk in Urban Parks in Fall," *International Journal of Environmental Research and Public Health* 12, no. 11 (2015): 14216–28, https://doi.org/10.3390/ijerph121114216.

25. K. Horton and J. Loyo, *Walk with a Doc 2017 Evaluability Assessment*, Limetree Research, 2017, https://walkwithadoc.org/wp-content/uploads/Evaluability-Report-2018.pdf.

26. Institute at the Golden Gate, *Healthy Parks Healthy People: Bay Area, A Roadmap and Case Study for Regional Collaboration*, 2017, https://instituteatgoldengate.org/resources/hphp-bay-area-roadmap-case-studies.

27. F. Lymeus, P. Lindberg, and T. Hartig, "Building Mindfulness Bottom-Up: Medita-tion in Natural Settings Supports Open Monitoring and Attention Restoration," *Consciousness and Cognition* 59 (2018): 40–56, https://doi.org/10.1016/j.concog.2018.01.008.

28. F. Lymeus, P. Lindberg, and T. Hartig, "A Natural Meditation Setting Improves Compliance with Mindfulness Training," *Journal of Environmental Psychology* 64 (2019): 98–106, https://doi.org/10.1016/j.jenvp.2019.05.008.

29. F. Lymeus, M. Ahrling, J. Apelman, C. de Mander Florin, C. Nilsson, J. Vincenti, A. Zetterberg, et al., "Mindfulness-Based Restoration Skills Training (ReST) in a Natural Setting Compared to Conventional Mindfulness Training: Psychological Functioning After a Five-Week Course," *Frontiers in Psychology* 11, no. 1 (2020), https://doi.org/10.3389/fpsyg.2020.01560.

30. S. Kaplan, "Meditation, Restoration, and the Management of Mental Fatigue," *Environment and Behavior* 33, no. 4 (2001): 480–506, https://doi.org/10.1177/00139160121973106.

31. K. E. Lee, K. J. H. Williams, L. D. Sargent, N. S. G. Williams, and K. A. Johnson, "Forty-Second Green Roof Views Sustain Attention: The Role of Micro-breaks in Attention Restoration," *Journal of Environmental Psychology* 42 (2015): 182–89, https://doi.org/10.1016/j.jenvp.2015.04.003.

32. S. W. Kress and J. D. Dawson, *Bird Life* (New York: St. Martin's, 2001).

33. D. A. Luther and E. P. Derryberry, "Birdsongs Keep Pace with City Life: Changes in Song over Time in an Urban Songbird Affects Communication," *Animal Behaviour* 83, no. 4 (2012): 1059–66, https://doi.org/10.1016/j.anbehav.2012.01.034.

34. B. Kempenaers, P. Borgström, P. Loës, E. Schlicht, and M. Valcu, "Artificial Night Lighting Affects Dawn Song, Extra-Pair Siring Success, and Lay Date in Songbirds," *Current Biology* 20, no. 19 (2010): 1735–39, https://doi.org/10.1016/j.cub.2010.08.028.

35. J. Duvall, "Using Engagement-Based Strategies to Alter Perceptions of the Walking Environment," *Environment and Behavior* 45, no. 3 (2011): 303–22, https://doi.org/10.1177/0013916511423808.

36. S.-A. Park, A.-Y. Lee, H.-G. Park, and W.-L. Lee, "Benefits of Gardening Activities for Cognitive Function According to Measurement of Brain Nerve Growth Factor Levels," *International Journal of Environmental Research and Public Health* 16, no. 5 (2019): 760, https://doi.org/10.3390/ijerph16050760.

37. A. E. Van Den Berg and M. H. G. Custers, "Gardening Promotes Neuroendocrine and Affective Restoration from Stress," *Journal of Health Psychology* 16, no. 1 (2010): 3–11, https://doi.org/10.1177/1359105310365577.

38. L. A. Simons, J. Simons, J. McCallum, and Y. Friedlander, "Lifestyle Factors and Risk of Dementia: Dubbo Study of the Elderly," *Medical Journal of Australia* 184, no. 2 (2006): 68–70, https://doi.org/10.5694/j.1326-5377.2006.tb00120.x.

39. M. Wichrowski, J. Whiteson, F. Haas, A. Mola, and M. J. Rey, "Effects of Horticultural Therapy on Mood and Heart Rate in Patients Participating in an Inpatient Cardiopulmonary Rehabilitation Program," *Journal of Cardiopulmonary Rehabilitation* 25, no. 5 (2005): 270–74, https://doi.org/10.1097/00008483-200509000-00008.

40. D. A. Cohen, B. Han, K. P. Derose, S. Williamson, T. Marsh, L. Raaen, and T. L. McKenzie, "The Paradox of Parks in Low-Income Areas : Park Use and Perceived Threats," *Environment and Behavior and Prevention* 48, no. 1 (2016): 230–45, https://doi.org/10.1177/0013916515614366.

41. National Wildlife Federation, *Reversing America's Wildlife Crisis*, 2018, https://wildlife.org/wp-content/uploads/2018/03/Reversing-Americas-Wildlife-Crisis-032918.pdf.

42. United Nations, *"UN Report: Nature's Dangerous Decline 'Unprecedented'; Species Extinction Rates 'Accelerating,'"* May 2019, https://www.un.org/sustainabledevelopment/blog/2019/05/nature-decline-unprecedented-report/.

43. A. J. Eichenwald, M. J. Evans, and J. W. Malcom, "US Imperiled Species Are Most Vulnerable to Habitat Loss on Private Lands," *Frontiers in Ecology and the Environment* 18, no. 8 (2020): 439–46, https://doi.org/10.1002/fee.2177.

44. US Department of Agriculture Forest Service, "Bee Abundance and Diversity in Suburban Yards," June 23, 2020, https://www.nrs.fs.fed.us/urban/landscape_change/bee-habitat/.

45. E. Marris, "Nature Is Everywhere—We Just Need to Learn to See It," TED, June 2016 https://www.ted.com/talks/emma_marris_nature_is_everywhere_we_just_need_to_learn_to_see_it?language=en#t-752970.

46. Erica Cirino, "More Plastic in the World Means More Plastic in Osprey Nests," Audubon, September 6, 2017, https://www.audubon.org/news/more-plastic-world-means-more-plastic-osprey-nests.

47. L. V. Moore, A. V. Diez Roux, K. R. Evenson, A. P. McGinn, and S. J. Brines, "Availability of Recreational Resources in Minority and Low Socioeconomic Status Areas," *American Journal of Preventive Medicine* 34, no. 1 (2008): 16–22, https://doi.org/10.1016/j.amepre.2007.09.021.

48. Trust for Public Land, "The Heat Is On," 2020, https://www.tpl.org/the-heat-is-on.

49. I. Mikati, A. F. Benson, T. J. Luben, J. D. Sacks, and J. Richmond-Bryant, "Disparities in Distribution of Particulate Matter Emission Sources by Race and Poverty Status," *American Journal of Public Health* 108, no. 4 (2018): 480–85, https://doi.org/10.2105/ajph.2017.304297.

50. Mapping Inequality, "Redlining in New Deal America," n.d.,. https://dsl.richmond
.edu/panorama/redlining/#loc=5/39.1/-94.58.

51. K. M. Shaw, K. A. Theis, S. Self-Brown, D. W. Roblin, and L. Barker, "Chronic Disease
Disparities by County Economic Status and Metropolitan Classification, Behavioral
Risk Factor Surveillance System, 2013," *Preventing Chronic Disease* 13, no. 1 (2016),
https://doi.org/10.5888/pcd13.160088.

52. B. Plumer, N. Popovich, and B. Palmer, "How Decades of Racist Housing Policy Left
Neighborhoods Sweltering," *New York Times*, November 16, 2020, https://www
.nytimes.com/interactive/2020/08/24/climate/racism-redlining-cities-global
-warming.html.

53. R. J. Mitchell, E. A. Richardson, N. K. Shortt, and J. R. Pearce, "Neighborhood
Environments and Socioeconomic Inequalities in Mental Well-Being," *American
Journal of Preventive Medicine* 49, no. 1 (2015): 80–84, https://doi.org/10.1016/j
.amepre.2015.01.017.

54. Trust for Public Land, "Parks and the Pandemic," 2020, https://www.tpl.org/parks-
and-the-pandemic.

55. Trust for Public Land, "The ParkScore Index: Methodology and FAQ," 2020, https://
www.tpl.org/parkscore/about.

CHAPTER TWO: OCEANS & COASTS

1. United Nations, "Percentage of Total Population Living in Coastal Areas," June 2007,
https://www.un.org/esa/sustdev/natlinfo/indicators/methodology_sheets/oceans
_seas_coasts/pop_coastal_areas.pdf.

2. B. W. Wheeler, M. White, W. Stahl-Timmins, and M. H. Depledge, "Does Living by
the Coast Improve Health and Wellbeing?," *Health & Place* 18, no. 5 (2012): 1198–
201, https://doi.org/10.1016/j.healthplace.2012.06.015.

3. J. K. Garrett, T. J. Clitherow, M. P. White, B. W. Wheeler, and L. E. Fleming, "Coastal
Proximity and Mental Health Among Urban Adults in England: The Moderating
Effect of Household Income," *Health & Place* 59 (September 2019), https://doi.org
/10.1016/j.healthplace.2019.102200.

4. G. MacKerron and S. Mourato, "Happiness Is Greater in Natural Environments,"
Global Environmental Change 23, no. 5 (2013): 992–1000, https://doi.org/10.1016/j
.gloenvcha.2013.03.010.

5. M. P. White, S. Pahl, K. Ashbullby, S. Herbert, and M. H. Depledge, "Feelings of
Restoration from Recent Nature Visits," *Journal of Environmental Psychology* 35
(2013): 40–51, https://doi.org/10.1016/j.jenvp.2013.04.002.

6. S. Dempsey, M. T. Devine, T. Gillespie, S. Lyons, and A. Nolan, "Coastal Blue Space

and Depression in Older Adults," *Health & Place* 54 (2018): 110–17, https://doi
.org/10.1016/j.healthplace.2018.09.002.

7. C. Peng, K. Yamashita, and E. Kobayashi, "Effects of the Coastal Environment on
Well-Being," *Journal of Coastal Zone Management* 19, no. 2 (2016): 1, https://www
.longdom.org/open-access/effects-of-the-coastal-environment-on-wellbeing-jczm
-1000421.pdf.

8. I.-C. Tang, Y.-P. Tsai, Y.-J. Lin, J.-H. Chen, C.-H. Hsieh, S.-H. Hung, W. C. Sullivan, et
al., "Using Functional Magnetic Resonance Imaging (fMRI) to Analyze Brain Region
Activity When Viewing Landscapes," *Landscape and Urban Planning* 162 (2017):
137–44, https://doi.org/10.1016/j.landurbplan.2017.02.007.

9. L. Mandolesi, A. Polverino, S. Montuori, F. Foti, G. Ferraioli, P. Sorrentino, and G.
Sorrentino, "Effects of Physical Exercise on Cognitive Functioning and Wellbeing:
Biological and Psychological Benefits," *Frontiers in Psychology* 9, no. 1 (2018), https:
//doi.org/10.3389/fpsyg.2018.00509.

10. T. P. Pasanen, M. P. White, B. W. Wheeler, J. K. Garrett, and L. R. Elliott, "Neighbourhood Blue Space, Health, and Wellbeing: The Mediating Role of Different Types of
Physical Activity," *Environment International* 131 (2019), https://doi.org/10.1016
/j.envint.2019.105016.

11. M. Marselle, K. Irvine, A. Lorenzo-Arribas, and S. L. Warber, "Moving Beyond Green:
Exploring the Relationship of Environment Type and Indicators of Perceived Environmental Quality on Emotional Well-Being Following Group Walks," *International
Journal of Environmental Research and Public Health* 12, no. 1 (2014): 106–30,
https://doi.org/10.3390/ijerph120100106.

12. S.-Y. Jiang, A. Ma, and S. Ramachandran, "Negative Air Ions and Their Effects on
Human Health and Air Quality Improvement," *International Journal of Molecular
Sciences* 19, no. 10 (2018), https://doi.org/10.3390/ijms19102966.

13. B. Bowers, R. Flory, J. Ametepe, L. Staley, A. Patrick, and H. Carrington, "Controlled
Trial Evaluation of Exposure Duration to Negative Air Ions for the Treatment of
Seasonal Affective Disorder," *Psychiatry Research* 259 (2018): 7–14, https://doi
.org/10.1016/j.psychres.2017.08.040.

14. R. Yamada, S. Yanoma, M. Akaike, A. Tsuburaya, Y. Sugimasa, S. Takemiya, H.
Motohashi, et al., "Water-Generated Negative Air Ions Activate NK Cell and Inhibit
Carcinogenesis in Mice," *Cancer Letters* 239, no. 2 (2006): 190–97, https://doi
.org/10.1016/j.canlet.2005.08.002.

15. A. Braun, "The Historic Healing Power of the Beach," *The Atlantic*, August 29, 2013,
https://www.theatlantic.com/health/archive/2013/08/the-historic-healing-power
-of-the-beach/279175/.

16. D. Cracknell, *By the Sea: The Therapeutic Benefits of Being in, on, and by the Water* (London, England: Aster, 2019).

17. E. Hunt, "Blue Spaces: Why Time Spent near Water Is the Secret of Happiness," *Guardian*, November 3, 2019, https://www.theguardian.com/lifeandstyle/2019/nov/03/blue-space-living-near-water-good-secret-of-happiness.

18. T. Xia, L. Song, T. T. Wang, L. Tan, and L. Mo, "Exploring the Effect of Red and Blue on Cognitive Task Performances," *Frontiers in Psychology* 7, no. 1 (2016), https://doi.org/10.3389/fpsyg.2016.00784.

19. W. J. Nichols and C. Cousteau, *Blue Mind: The Surprising Science That Shows How Being Near, In, On, or Under Water Can Make You Happier, Healthier, More Connected, and Better at What You Do* (New York: Back Bay Books, 2015).

20. K. H. Walter, N. P. Otis, T. N. Ray, L. H. Glassman, B. Michalewicz-Kragh, A. L. Powell, and C. J. Thomsen, "Breaking the Surface: Psychological Outcomes Among U.S. Active Duty Service Members Following a Surf Therapy Program," *Psychology of Sport and Exercise* 45 (2019), https://doi.org/10.1016/j.psychsport.2019.101551.

21. Waves for Change, *Waves for Change: 2019/20 Reflections*, 2020, https://www.waves-for-change.org/wp-content/uploads/2020/09/Waves-for-Change_2019-Annual-Report.pdf.

22. E. Britton, G. Kindermann, and C. Carlin, "Surfing and the Senses: Using Body Mapping to Understand the Embodied and Therapeutic Experiences of Young Surfers with Autism," *Global Journal of Community Psychology Practice* 11, no. 2 (2020): 1, https://www.researchgate.net/publication/341214795_Surfing_and_the_Senses_Using_Body_Mapping_to_Understand_the_Embodied_and_Therapeutic_Experiences_of_Young_Surfers_with_Autism.

23. National Trust, "A Coastal Walk Helps You Sleep Longer," April 4, 2019, https://nt.global.ssl.fastly.net/documents/sleep-mood-and-coastal-walking---a-report-by-eleanor-ratcliffe.pdf.

24. J. S. Feinstein, S. S. Khalsa, H. Yeh, C. Wohlrab, W. K. Simmons, M. B. Stein, and M. P. Paulus, "Examining the Short-Term Anxiolytic and Antidepressant Effect of Floatation-REST," *PLOS ONE* 13, no. 2 (2018), https://doi.org/10.1371/journal.pone.0190292.

25. W. Browning, C. Ryan, and J. Clancy, *Fourteen Patterns of Biophilic Design: Improving Health and Well-Being in the Built Environment* (New York: Terrapin Bright Green LLC, 2014), http://www.terrapinbrightgreen.com/wp-content/uploads/2014/04/14-Patterns-of-Biophilic-Design-Terrapin-2014p.pdf.

26. C. D. Gould van Praag, S. N. Garfinkel, O. Sparasci, A. Mees, A. O. Philippides, M. Ware, C. Ottaviani, and H. D. Critchley, "Mind-Wandering and Alterations to Default

Mode Network Connectivity When Listening to Naturalistic Versus Artificial Sounds," *Scientific Reports* 7, no. 1 (2017): 1, https://doi.org/10.1038/srep45273.

27. P. H. Kahn, R. L. Severson, and J. H. Ruckert, "The Human Relation with Nature and Technological Nature," *Current Directions in Psychological Science* 18, no. 1 (2009): 37–42, https://doi.org/10.1111/j.1467–8721.2009.01602.x.

28. M. Kuo, "Our Better Nature: How the Great Outdoors Can Improve Your Life," *Hidden Brain* (podcast), NPR, September 10, 2018, https://www.npr.org/2018/09/10/6464 13667/our-better-nature-how-the-great-outdoors-can-improve-your-life.

29. K. J. Wyles, S. Pahl, K. Thomas, and R. C. Thompson, "Factors That Can Undermine the Psychological Benefits of Coastal Environments, Exploring the Effect of Tidal State, Presence, and Type of Litter," *Environment and Behavior* 48, no. 9 (2016): 1095–126, https://doi.org/10.1177/0013916515592177.

30. D. Cracknell, M. P. White, S. Pahl, W. J. Nichols, and M. H. Depledge, "Marine Biota and Psychological Well-Being : A Preliminary Examination of Dose-Response Effects in an Aquarium Setting," *Environment and Behavior* 48, no. 10 (2016): 1242–69, https://doi.org/10.1177/0013916515597512.

31. J. R. Jambeck, R. Geyer, C. Wilcox, T. R. Siegler, M. Perryman, A. Andrady, R. Narayan, and K. L. Law, "Plastic Waste Inputs from Land into the Ocean," *Science* 347, no. 6223 (2015): 768–71, https://doi.org/10.1126/science.1260352.

32. J. Cohen, "An Ocean of Plastic," *Current*, University of California, Santa Barbara, February 12, 2015, https://www.news.ucsb.edu/2015/014985/ocean-plastic.

33. E. Loewe, "An Expert Debunks the Most Common Myths About Microplastics," mindbodygreen, August 31, 2019, https://www.mindbodygreen.com/articles/microplastics-101-how-they-impact-our-health-and-the-environment.

34. Food and Agriculture Organization of the United Nations, *The State of World Fisheries and Aquaculture*, 2018, http://www.fao.org/3/i9540en/i9540en.pdf.

35. B. Worm, "Averting a Global Fisheries Disaster," *Proceedings of the National Academy of Sciences* 113, no. 18 (2016): 4895–97, https://doi.org/10.1073/pnas.1604008113.

36. N. Gruber, D. Clement, B. R. Carter, R. A. Feely, S. van Heuven, M. Hoppema, M. Ishii, et al., "The Oceanic Sink for Anthropogenic CO_2 from 1994 to 2007," *Science* 363, no. 6432 (2019): 1193–99, https://doi.org/10.1126/science.aau5153.

37. C. Gutsch, "The Diver: Sylvia Earle," *Atmos*, May 21, 2020, https://atmos.earth/sylvia-earle-cyrill-gutsch-ocean-interview/.

CHAPTER THREE: MOUNTAINS & HIGHLANDS

1. Food and Agriculture Organization of the United Nations, *Mapping the Vulnerability of Mountain Peoples to Food Insecurity*, 2015, http://www.fao.org/3/i5175e/i5175e.pdf.

2. V. F. Gladwell, D. K. Brown, C. Wood, G. R. Sandercock, and J. L. Barton, "The Great Outdoors: How a Green Exercise Environment Can Benefit All," *Extreme Physiology and Medicine* 2, no. 1 (2013): 1, https://doi.org/10.1186/2046-7648-2-3.

3. J. J. Wooller, M. Rogerson, J. Barton, D. Micklewright, and V. Gladwell, "Can Simulated Green Exercise Improve Recovery from Acute Mental Stress?," *Frontiers in Psychology* 9, no. 1 (2018), https://doi.org/10.3389/fpsyg.2018.02167.

4. M. Rogerson, V. Gladwell, D. Gallagher, and J. Barton, "Influences of Green Outdoors Versus Indoors Environmental Settings on Psychological and Social Outcomes of Controlled Exercise," *International Journal of Environmental Research and Public Health* 13, no. 4 (2016): 363, https://doi.org/10.3390/ijerph13040363.

5. J. Pretty, J. Peacock, M. Sellens, and M. Griffin, "The Mental and Physical Health Outcomes of Green Exercise," *International Journal of Environmental Health Research* 15, no. 5 (2005): 319–37, https://doi.org/10.1080/09603120500155963.

6. D. Mitten, J. R. Overholt, F. I. Haynes, C. C. D'Amore, and J. C. Ady, "Hiking: A Low-Cost, Accessible Intervention to Promote Health Benefits," *American Journal of Lifestyle Medicine* 12, no. 4 (2016): 302–10, https://doi.org/10.1177/1559827 616658229.

7. G. N. Bratman, J. P. Hamilton, K. S. Hahn, G. C. Daily, and J. J. Gross, "Nature Experience Reduces Rumination and Subgenual Prefrontal Cortex Activation," *Proceedings of the National Academy of Sciences* 112, no. 28 (2015): 8567–72, https://doi.org/10.1073/pnas.1510459112.

8. S. Kaplan, "The Restorative Benefits of Nature: Toward an Integrative Framework," *Journal of Environmental Psychology* 15, no. 3 (1995): 169–82, https://doi.org/10 .1016/0272-4944(95)90001-2.

9. University of Copenhagen, "Why Is Earth So Biologically Diverse? Mountains Hold the Answer," ScienceDaily, September 12, 2019, 1, https://www.sciencedaily.com /releases/2019/09/190912140454.htm.

10. P. Wester, A. Mishra, A. Mukherji, and A. B. Shrestha, eds., *The Hindu Kush Himalaya Assessment: Mountains, Climate Change, Sustainability, and People,* (Cham, Switzerland: Springer, 2019), 1, https://doi.org/10.1007/978-3-319-92288-1.

11. E. Bertuzzo, F. Carrara, L. Mari, F. Altermatt, I. Rodriguez-Iturbe, and A. Rinaldo, "Geomorphic Controls on Elevational Gradients of Species Richness," *Proceedings of the National Academy of Sciences* 113, no. 7 (2016): 1737–42, https://doi.org/10 .1073/pnas.1518922113.

12. R. A. Fuller, K. N. Irvine, P. Devine-Wright, P. H. Warren, and K. J. Gaston, "Psychological Benefits of Greenspace Increase with Biodiversity," *Biology Letters* 3, no. 4 (2007): 390–94, https://doi.org/10.1098/rsbl.2007.0149.

13. M. N. Shiota, D. Keltner, and A. Mossman, "The Nature of Awe: Elicitors, Appraisals, and Effects on Self-Concept," *Cognition and Emotion* 21, no. 5 (2007): 944–63, https://doi.org/10.1080/02699930600923668.

14. J.-J. Li, K. Dou, Y.-J. Wang, and Y.-G. Nie, "Why Awe Promotes Prosocial Behaviors? The Mediating Effects of Future Time Perspective and Self-Transcendence Meaning of Life," *Frontiers in Psychology* 10 (2019), https://doi.org/10.3389/fpsyg.2019.01140.

15. A. B. Cohen, J. Gruber, and D. Keltner, "Comparing Spiritual Transformations and Experiences of Profound Beauty," *Psychology of Religion and Spirituality* 2, no. 3 (2010): 127–35, https://doi.org/10.1037/a0019126.

16. L. C. Bethelmy and J. A. Corraliza, "Transcendence and Sublime Experience in Nature: Awe and Inspiring Energy," *Frontiers in Psychology* 10 (2019): 1, https://doi.org/10.3389/fpsyg.2019.00509.

17. N. Morgan, "Do Mountains Inspire Creativity?," *Psychology Today*, September 14, 2019, https://www.psychologytoday.com/us/blog/in-the-mountains/201909/do-mountains-inspire-creativity.

18. M. Rudd, K. D. Vohs, and J. Aaker, "Awe Expands People's Perception of Time, Alters Decision Making, and Enhances Well-Being," *Psychological Science* 23, no. 10 (2012): 1130–36, https://doi.org/10.1177/0956797612438731.

19. M Shiota, "Let's Talk About 'Awe,'" YouTube, October 4, 2018, https://www.youtube.com/watch?v=1o2XkcftsMQ.

20. C. L. Anderson, M. Monroy, and D. Keltner, "Awe in Nature Heals: Evidence from Military Veterans, At-Risk Youth, and College Students," *Emotion* 18, no. 8 (2018): 1195–202, https://doi.org/10.1037/emo0000442.

21. "What Awe in Nature Does for Us," *Outside Podcast*, July 23, 2019, https://www.outsideonline.com/2400026/science-of-awe-nature-mental-health.

22. F. Williams, *The Nature Fix: Why Nature Makes Us Happier, Healthier, and More Creative* (New York: W. W. Norton, 2018).

23. Chief J. Snow, *These Mountains Are Our Sacred Places: The Story of the Stoney People* (Allston, Massachusetts: Fifth House, 2005).

24. C. G. Jung and R. Hull, *The Archetypes and the Collective Unconscious*, vol. 9, pt. 1 of *Collected Works of C. G. Jung*, 2nd ed. (Princeton, NJ: Princeton Univ. Press, 1981).

25. N. Morgan, *In the Mountains: The Health and Wellbeing Benefits of Spending Time at Altitude* (London, England: Octopus Publishing Group, 2019).

26. Williams, *The Nature Fix*.

27. R. Moor, *On Trails: An Exploration* (New York: Simon & Schuster, 2017).

28. M. Rudd, "Expand Your Breath, Expand Your Time: Slow Controlled Breathing

Boosts Time Affluence," *NA–Advances in Consumer Research* 42 (2014): 163–67, https://www.acrwebsite.org/volumes/1017176/volumes/v42/NA-42.

29. E. Loewe, "How to Make Your Midday Walk a More Mindful Experience, from a 'Walking Professor,'" mindbodygreen, May 22, 2019, https://www.mindbodygreen.com/articles/how-to-make-your-midday-walk-a-more-mindful-experience-from-a-walking-professor.

30. Y. A. W. de Kort, A. L. Meijnders, A. A. G. Sponselee, and W. A. IJsselsteijn, "What's Wrong with Virtual Trees? Restoring from Stress in a Mediated Environment," *Journal of Environmental Psychology* 26, no. 4 (2006): 309–20, https://doi.org/10.1016/j.jenvp.2006.09.001.

31. B. Gurubacharya, "Nepal Everest Cleanup Drive Yields Garbage, Bodies," AP News, June 5, 2019, https://apnews.com/article/f8dc96c20a304590838c47c599f82585.

32. P. R. Elsen, W. B. Monahan, and A. M. Merenlender, "Topography and Human Pressure in Mountain Ranges Alter Expected Species Responses to Climate Change," *Nature Communications* 11, no. 1 (2020): 1, https://doi.org/10.1038/s41467-020-15881-x.

33. Congressional Research Service, *Federal Land Ownership: Overview and Data*, February 2020, https://fas.org/sgp/crs/misc/R42346.pdf.

34. B. G. Freeman, M. N. Scholer, V. Ruiz-Gutierrez, and J. W. Fitzpatrick, "Climate Change Causes Upslope Shifts and Mountaintop Extirpations in a Tropical Bird Community," *Proceedings of the National Academy of Sciences* 115, no. 47 (2018): 11982–87, https://doi.org/10.1073/pnas.1804224115.

CHAPTER FOUR: FORESTS & TREES

1. Food and Agriculture Organization of the United Nations, *FRA 2000: On Definitions of Forest and Forest Change*, 2000, http://www.fao.org/3/ad665e/ad665e03.htm.

2. World Bank, "Forest Area (% of Land Area): Data," 2016, https://data.worldbank.org/indicator/AG.LND.FRST.ZS.

3. United Nations Sustainable Development Goals, "Goal 15: Biodiversity, Forests, Desertification," 2020, https://www.un.org/sustainabledevelopment/biodiversity/.

4. Q. Li, *Forest Bathing: How Trees Can Help You Find Health and Happiness* (New York: Viking, 2018).

5. Li, *Forest Bathing*.

6. A. Furuyashiki, K. Tabuchi, K. Norikoshi, T. Kobayashi, and S. Oriyama, "A Comparative Study of the Physiological and Psychological Effects of Forest Bathing (Shinrin-yoku) on Working Age People with and without Depressive Tendencies," *Environmental Health and Preventive Medicine* 24, no. 1 (2019): 1, https://doi.org/10.1186/s12199-019-0800-1.

7. E. Morita, M. Imai, M. Okawa, T. Miyaura, and S. Miyazaki, "A Before and After Comparison of the Effects of Forest Walking on the Sleep of a Community-Based Sample of People with Sleep Complaints," *BioPsychoSocial Medicine* 5, no. 1 (2011): 13, https://doi.org/10.1186/1751-0759-5-13.

8. S. W. Simard, D. A. Perry, M. D. Jones, D. D. Myrold, D. M. Durall, and R. Molina, "Net Transfer of Carbon Between Ectomycorrhizal Tree Species in the Field," *Nature* 388, no. 6642 (1997): 579–82, https://doi.org/10.1038/41557.

9. J. Lee, K. S. Cho, Y. Jeon, J. B. Kim, Y. Lim, K. Lee, and I.-S. Lee, "Characteristics and Distribution of Terpenes in South Korean Forests," *Journal of Ecology and Environment* 41, no. 1 (2017): 1, https://doi.org/10.1186/s41610-017-0038-z.

10. D. Joung, C. Song, H. Ikei, T. Okuda, M. Igarashi, H. Koizumi, B. J. Park, et al., "Physiological and Psychological Effects of Olfactory Stimulation with D-limonene," *Advances in Horticultural Science* 28, no. 2 (2014): 1, https://doi.org/10.13128ahs-22808.

11. H. Ikei, C. Song, and Y. Miyazaki, "Effects of Olfactory Stimulation by α-pinene on Autonomic Nervous Activity," *Journal of Wood Science* 62, no. 6 (2016): 568–72, https://doi.org/10.1007/s10086-016-1576-1.

12. S. Dayawansa, K. Umeno, H. Takakura, E. Hori, E. Tabuchi, Y. Nagashima, H. Oosu, et al., "Autonomic Responses During Inhalation of Natural Fragrance of 'Cedrol' in Humans," *Autonomic Neuroscience* 108, nos. 1–2 (2003): 79–86, https://doi.org/10.1016/j.autneu.2003.08.002.

13. Li, *Forest Bathing*.

14. T.-M. Tsao, M.-J. Tsai, J.-S. Hwang, W.-F. Cheng, C.-F. Wu, C.-C. K. Chou, and T.-C. Su, "Health Effects of a Forest Environment on Natural Killer Cells in Humans: An Observational Pilot Study," *Oncotarget* 9, no. 23 (2018): 16501–11, https://doi.org/10.18632/oncotarget.24741.

15. C. Song, H. Ikei, T. Kagawa, and Y. Miyazaki, "Effect of Viewing Real Forest Landscapes on Brain Activity," *Sustainability* 12, no. 16 (2020): 6601, https://doi.org/10.3390/su12166601.

16. R. Ulrich, "View Through a Window May Influence Recovery from Surgery," *Science* 224, no. 4647 (1984): 420–21, https://doi.org/10.1126/science.6143402.

17. C. M. Hägerhäll, T. Laike, R. P. Taylor, M. Küller, R. Küller, and T. P. Martin, "Investigations of Human EEG Response to Viewing Fractal Patterns," *Perception* 37, no. 10 (2008): 1488–94, https://doi.org/10.1068/p5918.

18. Y. Joye, L. Steg, A. B. Ünal, and R. Pals, "When Complex Is Easy on the Mind: Internal Repetition of Visual Information in Complex Objects Is a Source of Perceptual Fluency," *Journal of Experimental Psychology: Human Perception and Performance* 42, no. 1 (2016): 103–14, https://doi.org/10.1037/xhp0000105.

19. H. Namazi, V. V. Kulish, and A. Akrami, "The Analysis of the Influence of Fractal Structure of Stimuli on Fractal Dynamics in Fixational Eye Movements and EEG Signal," *Scientific Reports* 6, no. 1 (2016): 1, https://doi.org/10.1038/srep26639.

20. R. P. Taylor and B. Spehar, "Fractal Fluency: An Intimate Relationship Between the Brain and Processing of Fractal Stimuli," in *The Fractal Geometry of the Brain*, edited by A. Di Ieva (New York: Springer, 2016), 485–96, https://link.springer.com/chap ter/10.1007%2F978-1-4939-3995-4_30.

21. P. Wohlleben, T. Flannery, J. Billinghurst, and S. Simard, *The Hidden Life of Trees* (Vancouver, British Columbia: Greystone Books, 2016).

22. D. J. Nowak, S. Hirabayashi, A. Bodine, and E. Greenfield, "Tree and Forest Effects on Air Quality and Human Health in the United States," *Environmental Pollution* 193 (2014): 119–29, https://doi.org/10.1016/j.envpol.2014.05.028.

23. Nowak, Hirabayashi, Bodine, and Greenfield, "Tree and Forest Effects on Air Quality and Human Health in the United States."

24. J. Shin, J. Y. Park, and J. Choi, "Long-Term Exposure to Ambient Air Pollutants and Mental Health Status: A Nationwide Population-Based Cross-Sectional Study," *PLOS ONE* 13, no. 4 (2018): e0195607, https://doi.org/10.1371/journal.pone .0195607.

25. M. Lõhmus, "Possible Biological Mechanisms Linking Mental Health and Heat—a Contemplative Review," *International Journal of Environmental Research and Public Health* 15, no. 7 (2018): 1515, https://doi.org/10.3390/ijerph15071515.

26. H. Jo, C. Song, H. Ikei, S. Enomoto, H. Kobayashi, and Y. Miyazaki, "Physiological and Psychological Effects of Forest and Urban Sounds Using High-Resolution Sound Sources," *International Journal of Environmental Research and Public Health* 16, no. 15 (2019): 2649, https://doi.org/10.3390/ijerph16152649.

27. H. Ochiai, C. Song, H. Jo, M. Oishi, M. Imai, and Y. Miyazaki, "Relaxing Effect Induced by Forest Sound in Patients with Gambling Disorder," *Sustainability* 12, no. 15 (2020): 5969, https://doi.org/10.3390/su12155969.

28. M. Annerstedt, P. Jönsson, M., Wallergård, G. Johansson, B. Karlson, P. Grahn, Å. M. Hansen, and P. Währborg, "Inducing Physiological Stress Recovery with Sounds of Nature in a Virtual Reality Forest—Results from a Pilot Study," *Physiology & Behavior* 118 (2013): 240–50, https://doi.org/10.1016/j.physbeh.2013.05.023.

29. H. Ikei, C. Song, and Y. Miyazaki, "Physiological Effects of Touching Wood," *International Journal of Environmental Research and Public Health* 14, no. 7 (2017): 801, https://doi.org/10.3390/ijerph14070801.

30. D. R. Montgomery and A. Biklé, *The Hidden Half of Nature: The Microbial Roots of Life and Health* (New York: W. W. Norton, 2016).

31. R. E. Creamer, S. E. Hannula, J. P. Van Leeuwen, D. Stone, M. Rutgers, R. M. Schmelz, P. C. de Ruiter, et al., "Ecological Network Analysis Reveals the Inter-connection Between Soil Biodiversity and Ecosystem Function as Affected by Land Use Across Europe," *Applied Soil Ecology* 97 (2016): 112–24, https://doi.org/10.1016/j.apsoil.2015.08.006.

32. D. G. Smith, R. Martinelli, G. S. Besra, P. A. Illarionov, I. Szatmari, P. Brazda, M. A. Allen, et al., "Identification and Characterization of a Novel Anti-inflammatory Lipid Isolated from *Mycobacterium vaccae*, a Soil-Derived Bacterium with Immunoregulatory and Stress Resilience Properties," *Psychopharmacology* 236, no. 5 (2019): 1653–70, https://doi.org/10.1007/s00213-019-05253-9.

33. M. G. Frank, L. K. Fonken, S. D. Dolzani, J. L. Annis, P. H. Siebler, D. Schmidt, L. R. Watkins, et al., "Immunization with *Mycobacterium vaccae* Induces an Anti-Inflammatory Milieu in the CNS: Attenuation of Stress-Induced Microglial Priming, Alarmins and Anxiety-Like Behavior," *Brain, Behavior, and Immunity* 73 (2018): 352–63, https://doi.org/10.1016/j.bbi.2018.05.020.

34. J. Plevin, *The Healing Magic of Forest Bathing: Finding Calm, Creativity, and Connection in the Natural World* (Berkeley, California: Ten Speed Press, 2019).

35. D. Martens, H. Gutscher, and N. Bauer, "Walking in 'Wild' and 'Tended' Urban Forests: The Impact on Psychological Well-Being," *Journal of Environmental Psychology* 31, no. 1 (2011): 36–44, https://doi.org/10.1016/j.jenvp.2010.11.001.

36. D. Joung, G. Kim, Y. Choi, H. J. Lim, S. Park, J.-M. Woo, and B.-J. Park, "The Prefrontal Cortex Activity and Psychological Effects of Viewing Forest Landscapes in Autumn Season," *International Journal of Environmental Research and Public Health* 12, no. 7 (2015): 7235–43, https://doi.org/10.3390/ijerph120707235.

37. C. Song, H. Ikei, T. Kagawa, and Y. Miyazaki, "Effect of Viewing Real Forest Landscapes on Brain Activity," *Sustainability* 12, no. 16 (2020): 6601, https://doi.org/10.3390/su12166601.

38. E. Loewe, "Jane Goodall Talks COVID, Conservation, and Her Hope for the Future," mindbodygreen, October 30, 2020, https://www.mindbodygreen.com/articles/jane-goodall-covid-q-and-a.

39. G. Popkin, "Cure Yourself of Tree Blindness," *New York Times*, August 26, 2017, https://www.nytimes.com/2017/08/26/opinion/sunday/cure-yourself-of-tree-blindness.html.

40. R. Powers, *The Overstory* (New York: W. W. Norton, 2018).

41. E. John, "Richard Powers: 'We're Completely Alienated from Everything Else Alive,'" *Guardian*, June 16, 2018, https://www.theguardian.com/books/2018/jun/16/richard-powers-interview-overstory.

42. Li, *Forest Bathing.*
43. Q. Li, M. Kobayashi, Y. Wakayama, H. Inagaki, M. Katsumata, Y. Hirata, K. Hirata, et al., "Effect of Phytoncide from Trees on Human Natural Killer Cell Function," *International Journal of Immunopathology and Pharmacology* 22, no. 4 (2009): 951–59, https://doi.org/10.1177/039463200902200410.
44. Project Drawdown, "Forest Protection," August 7, 2020, https://drawdown.org/solutions/forest-protection.
45. T. W. Crowther, H. B. Glick, K. R. Covey, C. Bettigole, D. S. Maynard, S. M. Thomas, J. R. Smith, et al., "Mapping Tree Density at a Global Scale," *Nature* 525, no. 7568 (2015): 201–5, https://doi.org/10.1038/nature14967.
46. R. L. Chazdon, "Protecting Intact Forests Requires Holistic Approaches," *Nature Ecology & Evolution* 2, no. 6 (2018): 915, https://doi.org/10.1038/s41559-018-0546-y.
47. Regreening Africa home page, n.d., https://regreeningafrica.org/.
48. K. A. Duffy, C. R. Schwalm, V. L. Arcus, G. W. Koch, L. L. Liang, and L. A. Schipper, "How Close Are We to the Temperature Tipping Point of the Terrestrial Biosphere?," *Science Advances* 7, no. 3 (2021), https://doi.org/10.1126/sciadv.aay1052.

CHAPTER FIVE: ICE & SNOW

1. A. L. Wagner, F. Keusch, T. Yan, and P. J. Clarke, "The Impact of Weather on Summer and Winter Exercise Behaviors," *Journal of Sport and Health Science* 8, no. 1 (2019): 39–45, https://doi.org/10.1016/j.jshs.2016.07.007.
2. Vice President for Communications, "Going Outside—Even in the Cold—Improves Memory, Attention," University of Michigan News, December 16, 2008, https://news.umich.edu/going-outsideeven-in-the-coldimproves-memory-attention/.
3. Wim Hof Method, "Who Is 'The Iceman' Wim Hof," n.d., https://www.wimhofmethod.com/iceman-wim-hof.
4. Wim Hof, TEDxAmsterdam, December 1, 2010, TED Talks, https://www.youtube.com/watch?v=L9Cgaa8U4eY.
5. Harvard Health Publishing, "The Wonders of Winter Workouts," Harvard Medical School, December 1, 2018, https://www.health.harvard.edu/staying-healthy/the-wonders-of-winter-workouts.
6. N. A. Shevchuk, "Adapted Cold Shower as a Potential Treatment for Depression," *Medical Hypotheses* 70, no. 5 (2008): 995–1001, https://doi.org/10.1016/j.mehy.2007.04.052.
7. One Square Inch of Silence home page, n.d., https://onesquareinch.org/.
8. L. M. Kuehne and J. D. Olden, "Military Flights Threaten the Wilderness Soundscapes of the Olympic Peninsula, Washington," *Northwest Science* 94, no. 2 (2020): 1, https://doi.org/10.3955/046.094.0208.

9. World Health Organization, Regional Office for Europe, *Burden of Disease from Environmental Noise: Quantification of Healthy Life Years Lost in Europe*, 2011, https://apps.who.int/iris/bitstream/handle/10665/326424/9789289002295-eng.pdf.

10. Order of Cistercians of the Strict Observance, *Constitutions of the Monks*, 2016, https://ocso.org/wp-content/uploads/2016/05/1-Const-Monks-Oct-2016-EN.pdf.

11. Bureau of Labor Statistics, US Department of Labor, "American Time Use Survey—2012 Results," June 20, 2013, 20–24, https://www.bls.gov/news.release/archives/atus_06202013.pdf.

12. T. D. Wilson, D. A. Reinhard, E. C. Westgate, D. T. Gilbert, N. Ellerbeck, C. Hahn, C. L. Brown, and A. Shaked, "Just Think: The Challenges of the Disengaged Mind," *Science* 345, no. 6192 (2014): 75–77, https://doi.org/10.1126/science.1250830.

13. L. Bernardi, C. Porta, and P. Sleight, "Cardiovascular, Cerebrovascular, and Respiratory Changes Induced by Different Types of Music in Musicians and Non-musicians: The Importance of Silence," *Heart* 92, no. 4 (2005): 445–52, https://doi.org/10.1136/hrt.2005.064600.

14. B. Lopez, *Arctic Dreams* (New York: Vintage, 2001).

15. J. McPhee, *Basin and Range* (New York: Farrar, Straus and Giroux, 1982), http://web.mit.edu/allanmc/www/mcphee.pdf.

16. NASA, "Global Temperature," Global Climate Change: Vital Signs of the Planet, n.d., https://climate.nasa.gov/vital-signs/global-temperature/; Z. Hausfather, "State of the Climate: 2020 on Course to Be Warmest Year on Record," Carbon Brief, October 23, 2020, https://www.carbonbrief.org/state-of-the-climate-2020-on-course-to-be-warmest-year-on-record.

17. National Oceanic and Atmospheric Administration, US Department of Commerce, "The Changing Arctic: A Greener, Warmer, and Increasingly Accessible Region," December 15, 2017, https://www.noaa.gov/explainers/changing-arctic-greener-warmer-and-increasingly-accessible-region#.

18. D. Dunne, "Interactive: When Will the Arctic See Its First Ice-Free Summer?," Carbon Brief, 2020, https://interactive.carbonbrief.org/when-will-the-arctic-see-its-first-ice-free-summer/.

19. D. Jamail, *The End of Ice: Bearing Witness and Finding Meaning in the Path of Climate Disruption* (New York: New Press, 2019).

20. T. Schuur, "Permafrost and the Global Carbon Cycle," NOAA Arctic Program, 2019, https://arctic.noaa.gov/Report-Card/Report-Card-2019/ArtMID/7916/ArticleID/844/Permafrost-and-the-Global-Carbon-Cycle.

21. K. Hansen, "Okjökull Remembered," NASA Earth Observatory, 2019, https://earthobservatory.nasa.gov/images/145439/okjokull-remembered.

22. P. Hawken, ed., *Drawdown* (New York: Penguin Books, 2017).

23. F. Jabr, "How the Antarctic Icefish Lost Its Red Blood Cells but Survived Anyway," Scientific American Blog Network, August 3, 2012, https://blogs.scientificamerican .com/brainwaves/how-the-antarctic-icefish-lost-its-red-blood-cells-but-survived -anyway/.

CHAPTER SIX: DESERTS & DRYLANDS

1. V. Menon, S. K. Kar, N. Suthar, and N. Nebhinani, "Vitamin D and Depression: A Critical Appraisal of the Evidence and Future Directions," *Indian Journal of Psychological Medicine* 42, no. 1 (2020): 11–21, https://doi.org/10.4103/ijpsym.ijpsym_160_19.

2. J. W. Navalta, N. G. Bodell, E. A. Tanner, C. D. Aguilar, and K. N. Radzak, "Effect of Exercise in a Desert Environment on Physiological and Subjective Measures," *International Journal of Environmental Health Research* 31, no. 2 (2019): 121–31, https://doi.org/10.1080/09603123.2019.1631961.

3. T. Laukkanen, S. Kunutsor, J. Kauhanen, and J. A. Laukkanen, "Sauna Bathing Is Inversely Associated with Dementia and Alzheimer's Disease in Middle-Aged Finnish Men," *Age and Ageing* 46, no. 2 (2016): 245–49, https://doi.org/10.1093/ageing/afw212.

4. S. Hayasaka, Y. Nakamura, E. Kajii, M. Ide, Y. Shibata, T. Noda, C. Murata, et al., "Effects of Charcoal Kiln Saunas (Jjimjilbang) on Psychological States," *Complementary Therapies in Clinical Practice* 14, no. 2 (2008): 143–48, https://doi.org/10.1016/j .ctcp.2007.12.004.

5. J. Sarris, M. de Manincor, F. Hargraves, and J. Tsonis, "Harnessing the Four Elements for Mental Health," *Frontiers in Psychiatry* 10, no. 1 (2019), https://doi.org/10.3389/ fpsyt.2019.00256.

6. V. J. Robertson, A. R. Ward, and P. Jung, "The Effect of Heat on Tissue Extensibility: A Comparison of Deep and Superficial Heating," *Archives of Physical Medicine and Rehabilitation* 86, no. 4 (2005): 819–25, https://doi.org/10.1016/j.apmr.2004.07.353.

7. C. Salvi and E. M. Bowden, "Looking for Creativity: Where Do We Look When We Look for New Ideas?," *Frontiers in Psychology* 7, no. 1 (2016), https://doi.org/10.3389 /fpsyg.2016.00161.

8. J. Drori and L. Clerc, *Around the World in Eighty Plants* (London, England: Laurence King, 2021).

9. G. P. Nabhan, *The Nature of Desert Nature* (Tucson: Univ. of Arizona Press, 2020).

10. E. Abbey, *Desert Solitaire* (New York: Touchstone, 1990).

11. United Nations, "Why Now?," United Nations Decade for Deserts and the Fight Against Desertification, 2020, https://www.un.org/en/events/desertification_decade /whynow.shtml.

12. Sow a Heart Farm home page, n.d., https://www.sowaheart.com/.

13. Environmental Working Group, "USDA Subsidies in the United States Totaled $424.4 Billion from 1995–2020," EWG's Farm Subsidy Database, 2020, https://farm.ewg.org/progdetail.php?fips=00000&progcode=totalfarm°ionname=theUnitedStateS.

14. Environmental Working Group, "Commodity Subsidies in the United States Totaled $240.5 Billion from 1995–2020," EWG's Farm Subsidy Database, 2020, https://farm.ewg.org/progdetail.php?fips=00000&progcode=totalfarm&page=conc°ionname=theUnitedStates.

15. USDA, *Farm Producers: Revised Census Questions Provide Expanded Demographic Information*, 2017, https://www.nass.usda.gov/Publications/Highlights/2019/2017 Census_Farm_Producers.pdf.

16. Regenerative Agriculture Alliance home page, n.d., https://www.regenagalliance.org/.

17. United Nations University, "World Losing 2,000 Hectares of Farm Soil Daily to Salt-Induced Degradation," October 28, 2014, https://unu.edu/media-relations/releases/world-losing-2000-hectares-of-farm-soil-daily-to-salt-induced-degradation.html.

18. World Bank, "Curbing Desertification in China," July 4, 2019, https://www.worldbank.org/en/news/feature/2019/07/04/china-fighting-desertification-and-boosting-incomes-in-ningxia.

19. N. Thomas and S. Nigam, "Twentieth-Century Climate Change over Africa: Seasonal Hydroclimate Trends and Sahara Desert Expansion," *Journal of Climate* 31, no. 9 (2018): 3349–70, https://doi.org/10.1175/jcli-d-17–0187.1.

20. J. Haner, E. Wong, D. Watkins and J. White, "Living in China's Expanding Deserts," *New York Times*, October 24, 2016, https://www.nytimes.com/interactive/2016/10/24/world/asia/living-in-chinas-expanding-deserts.html.

21. S. Mallone, M. Stafoggia, A. Faustini, S. Gobbi, F. Forastiere, and C. A. Perucci, "Effect of Saharan Dust on the Association Between Particulate Matter and Daily Mortality in Rome, Italy," *Epidemiology* 20 (2009): S66–S67, https://doi.org/10.1097/01.ede.0000362907.77717.07.

22. T. Yunkaporta, *Sand Talk: How Indigenous Thinking Can Save the World* (New York: HarperOne, 2020).

23. S. Wunder and R. Bodle, "Achieving Land Degradation Neutrality in Germany: Implementation Process and Design of a Land Use Change Based Indicator," *Environmental Science & Policy* 92 (2019): 46–55, https://doi.org/10.1016/j.envsci.2018.09.022.

CHAPTER SEVEN: RIVERS & STREAMS

1. A. E. Stamps, "Mystery, Complexity, Legibility, and Coherence: A Meta-analysis,"

Journal of Environmental Psychology 24, no. 1 (2004): 1–16, https://doi.org/10.1016/s0272-4944(03)00023-9.

2. R. Kaplan and S. Kaplan, *The Experience of Nature: A Psychological Perspective* (Cambridge, England: Cambridge Univ. Press, 1989).

3. O. Laing, *To the River: A Journey Beneath the Surface* (Edinburgh: Canongate Books, 2017).

4. L. Miller, I. M. Balodis, C. H. McClintock, J. Xu, C. M. Lacadie, R. Sinha, and M. N. Potenza, "Neural Correlates of Personalized Spiritual Experiences," *Cerebral Cortex* 29, no. 6 (2019): 2331–38, https://doi.org/10.1093/cercor/bhy102.

5. K. Williams and D. Harvey, "Transcendent Experience in Forest Environments," *Journal of Environmental Psychology* 21, no. 3 (2001): 249–60, https://doi.org/10.1006/jevp.2001.0204.

6. A. H. Maslow, *Religions, Values, and Peak-Experiences* (New York: Penguin Books, 1994).

7. Edmund Burke, *A Philosophical Enquiry into the Origin of Our Ideas of the Sublime and Beautiful*, 1759, University of Pennsylvania, https://web.english.upenn.edu/%7Emgamer/Etexts/burkesublime.html.

8. L. M. Fredrickson and D. H. Anderson, "A Qualitative Exploration of the Wilderness Experience as a Source of Spiritual Inspiration," *Journal of Environmental Psychology* 19, no. 1 (1999): 21–39, https://doi.org/10.1006/jevp.1998.0110.

9. K. N. Irvine, D. Hoesly, R. Bell-Williams, and S. L. Warber, "Biodiversity and Spiritual Well-Being," in *Biodiversity and Health in the Face of Climate Change*, edited by M. R. Marselle, J. Stadler, H. Korn, K. N. Irvine, and A. Bonn (Cham, Switzerland: Springer, 2019), 213–47, https://doi.org/10.1007/978-3-030-02318-8_10.

10. M. P. White, I. Alcock, J. Grellier, B. W. Wheeler, T. Hartig, S. L. Warber, A. Bone, et al., "Spending at Least 120 Minutes a Week in Nature Is Associated with Good Health and Wellbeing," *Scientific Reports* 9, no. 1 (2019): 1, https://doi.org/10.1038/s41598-019-44097-3.

11. S. Collado and H. Staats, "Contact with Nature and Children's Restorative Experiences: An Eye to the Future," *Frontiers in Psychology* 7, no. 1 (2016), https://doi.org/10.3389/fpsyg.2016.01885.

12. R. Louv, *Last Child in the Woods: Saving Our Children from Nature-Deficit Disorder* (New York: Algonquin Books, 2008).

13. E. Hoffman, "Peak Experiences in Childhood: An Exploratory Study," *Journal of Humanistic Psychology* 38, no. 1 (1998): 109–20, https://doi.org/10.1177/00221678980381011.

14. K. Colley, M. J. B. Currie, and K. N. Irvine, "Then and Now: Examining Older People's Engagement in Outdoor Recreation Across the Life Course," *Leisure Sciences* 41, no. 3 (2017): 186–202, https://doi.org/10.1080/01490400.2017.1349696.

15. H. Hesse, *Siddhartha: A Novel*, translated by H. Rosner (New York: Bantam, 1982).

16. R. Vallejos, "The Kukama-Kukamiria Documentation Project," Department of Linguistics, University of New Mexico, 2017, http://www.unm.edu/%7Ervallejos/kukamaproject.html.

17. W. Davis and D. Suzuki, *The Sacred Headwaters: The Fight to Save the Stikine, Skeena, and Nass* (Vancouver, Canada: Greystone Books, 2015).

18. M. Soga and K. J. Gaston, "Extinction of Experience: The Loss of Human-Nature Interactions," *Frontiers in Ecology and the Environment* 14, no. 2 (2016): 94–101, https://doi.org/10.1002/fee.1225.

19. T. Hartig and P. H. Kahn, "Living in Cities, Naturally," *Science* 352, no. 6288 (2016): 938–40, https://doi.org/10.1126/science.aaf3759.

20. G. Albrecht, G. M. Sartore, L. Connor, N. Higginbotham, S. Freeman, B. Kelly, H. Stain, et al., "Solastalgia: The Distress Caused by Environmental Change," supplement, *Australasian Psychiatry* 15, no. 1 (2007): S95–S98, https://doi.org/10.1080/10398560701701288.

21. M. Coleman and J. Kornfield, *Awake in the Wild: Mindfulness in Nature as a Path of Self-Discovery* (Novato, California: New World Library, 2006).

22. J. Cameron, *The Artist's Way: A Spiritual Path to Higher Creativity* (New York: TarcherPerigee, 2016).

23. G. Su, M. Logez, J. Xu, S. Tao, S. Villéger, and S. Brosse, "Human Impacts on Global Freshwater Fish Biodiversity," *Science* 371, no. 6531 (2021): 835–38, https://doi.org/10.1126/science.abd3369.

24. S. Deinet, K. Scott-Gatty, H. Rotton, W. M. Twardek, V. Marconi, L. McRae, L. J. Baumgartner, et al., *Living Planet Index: Technical Report*, IUCN, WWF, World Fish Migration Foundation, Nature Conservancy, and ZSL, 2020, https://worldfishmigrationfoundation.com/wp-content/uploads/2020/07/LPI_report_2020.pdf.

25. S. Lovgren, "Rivers and Lakes Are the Most Degraded Ecosystems in the World," *National Geographic*, March 1, 2021, https://www.nationalgeographic.com/environment/article/rivers-and-lakes-are-most-degraded-ecosystems-in-world-can-we-save-them.

26. American Rivers and Western Resource Advocates, *The Hardest Working River in the West: Common-Sense Solutions for a Reliable Water Future for the Colorado River Basin*, July 2014, https://westernresourceadvocates.org/wp-content/uploads/dlm_uploads/2015/07/CO_River_Solutions_Whitepaper.pdf.

27. H. Hansman, *Downriver: Into the Future of Water in the West* (Chicago: Univ. of Chicago Press, 2019).

28. Global Alliance for the Rights of Nature, "What Is Rights of Nature?," n.d., https://www.therightsofnature.org/what-is-rights-of-nature/.
29. Te Awa Tupua (Whanganui River Claims Settlement) Act 2017, No 7 (as at 30 January 2021), New Zealand Legislation, https://www.legislation.govt.nz/act/public/2017/0007/latest/whole.html.
30. Cyrus R. Vance Center for International Justice, Earth Law Center, and International Rivers, *Rights of Rivers: A Global Survey of the Rapidly Developing Rights of Nature Jurisprudence Pertaining to Rivers*, 2020, https://static1.squarespace.com/static/559 14fd1e4b01fb0b851a814/t/5f760119bde1f0691fc7c7e0/1601569082236/Rights +of+Rivers+Report_Final.pdf.
31. Agence France-Presse, "Bangladesh High Court Declares Country's Rivers 'Legal Persons,'" NDTV, July 2, 2019, https://www.ndtv.com/world-news/bangladesh -high-court-declares-countrys-rivers-legal-persons-2063061.
32. Earth Law Center, "Universal Declaration of the Rights of Rivers," 2020, https://static1.squarespace.com/static/55914fd1e4b01fb0b851a814/t/5c93e932ec212 d197abf81bd/1553197367064/Universal+Declaration+of+the+Rights+of+Rivers _Final.pdf.
33. V. Yurk, "Water Pollution: River Bugs Find New Homes on Trash—Study," *Greenwire*, E&E News, January 27, 2021, https://www.eenews.net/greenwire/stories/1063723673/.
34. United States Environmental Protection Agency, "National Rivers and Streams Assessment 2013–14 Key Findings," 2014, https://www.epa.gov/national-aquatic -resource-surveys/national-rivers-and-streams-assessment-2013-14-key-findings.
35. C. Zarfl, A. Lumsdon, J. Berlekamp, L. Tydecks, and K. Tockner, "A Global Boom in Hydropower Dam Construction," *Aquatic Sciences* 77, no. 1 (2015), https://doi.org /10.1007/s00027–014–0377–0.
36. G. Grill, B. Lehner, M. Thieme, B. Geenen, D. Tickner, F. Antonelli, S. Babu, et al., "Mapping the World's Free-Flowing Rivers," *Nature* 569, no. 7755 (2019): 215–21, https://doi.org/10.1038/s41586-019-1111-9.
37. Hansman, *Downriver*.
38. NOAA, "Barriers to Fish Migration," 2020, https://www.fisheries.noaa.gov/insight /barriers-fish-migration.

CHAPTER EIGHT: CITIES & BUILT ENVIRONMENTS

1. "Sixty-Eight Percent of the World Population Projected to Live in Urban Areas by 2050, Says UN," United Nations Department of Economic and Social Affairs, May 16, 2018, https://www.un.org/development/desa/en/news/population/2018-revision -of-world-urbanization-prospects.html.

2. J. L. Wang, "Rural-Urban Differences in the Prevalence of Major Depression and Associated Impairment," *Social Psychiatry and Psychiatric Epidemiology* 39, no. 1 (2004): 19–25, https://doi.org/10.1007/s00127–004–0698–8.

3. W. L. Zijlema, B. Klijs, R. P. Stolk, and J. G. M. Rosmalen, "(Un)Healthy in the City: Respiratory, Cardiometabolic, and Mental Health Associated with Urbanity," *PLOS ONE* 10, no. 12, https://doi.org/10.1371/journal.pone.0143910.

4. E. A. Morris, "Do Cities or Suburbs Offer Higher Quality of Life? Intrametropolitan Location, Activity Patterns, Access, and Subjective Well-Being," *Cities* 89 (2019): 228–42, https://doi.org/10.1016/j.cities.2019.02.012.

5. J. Peen, R. A. Schoevers, A. T. Beekman, and J. Dekker, "The Current Status of Urban-Rural Differences in Psychiatric Disorders," *Acta Psychiatrica Scandinavica* 121, no. 2 (2010): 84–93, https://doi.org/10.1111/j.1600–0447.2009.01438.x.

6. M. C. Power, M.-A. Kioumourtzoglou, J. E. Hart, O. I. Okereke, F. Laden, and M. G. Weisskopf, "The Relation Between Past Exposure to Fine Particulate Air Pollution and Prevalent Anxiety: Observational Cohort Study," *BMJ* 350 (2015), https://doi.org/10.1136/bmj.h1111.

7. J. B. Newbury, L. Arseneault, S. Beevers, N. Kitwiroon, S. Roberts, C. M. Pariante, F. J. Kelly, and H. L. Fisher, "Association of Air Pollution Exposure with Psychotic Experiences During Adolescence," *JAMA Psychiatry* 76, no. 6 (2019): 614, https://doi.org/10.1001/jamapsychiatry.2019.0056.

8. R. Chepesiuk, "Decibel Hell: The Effects of Living in a Noisy World," *Environmental Health Perspectives* 113, no. 1 (2005): 1, https://doi.org/10.1289/ehp.113-a34.

9. Douglas Mental Health University Institute, "Stress in the City: Brain Activity and Biology Behind Mood Disorders of Urbanites," ScienceDaily, June 23, 2011, https://www.sciencedaily.com/releases/2011/06/110622135216.htm.

10. N. Müller, M. Ignatieva, C. H. Nilon, P. Werner, and W. C. Zipperer, "Patterns and Trends in Urban Biodiversity and Landscape Design," in *Urbanization, Biodiversity, and Ecosystem Services: Challenges and Opportunities*, edited by T. Elmqvist, M. Fragkias, J. Goodness, B. Güneralp, P. J. Marcotullio, R. I. McDonald, S. Parnell, et al. (Dordrecht, Netherlands: Springer, 2013), 123–74, https://doi.org/10.1007/978–94–007–7088–1_10.

11. P. Theodorou, R. Radzevičiūtė, G. Lentendu, B. Kahnt, M. Husemann, C. Bleidorn, J. Settele, et al., "Urban Areas as Hotspots for Bees and Pollination but Not a Panacea for All Insects," *Nature Communications* 11, no. 1 (2020): 1, https://doi.org/10.1038/s41467-020-14496-6.

12. I. Kowarik, "Cities and Wilderness: A New Perspective," *International Journal of Wilderness* 19 (2013): 32–36, https://www.researchgate.net/publication/259389620_Cities_and_wilderness_A_new_perspective.

13. "Richard Louv Wants You to Bond with Wild Animals," *Outside Podcast*, November 13, 2019, https://www.outsideonline.com/2405410/our-wild-calling-richard-louv -book-podcast.

14. J. C. Fisher, K. N. Irvine, J. E. Bicknell, W. M. Hayes, D. Fernandes, J. Mistry, and Z. G. Davies, "Perceived Biodiversity, Sound, Naturalness, and Safety Enhance the Restorative Quality and Wellbeing Benefits of Green and Blue Space in a Neotropical City," *Science of the Total Environment* 755 (2021), https://doi.org/10.1016/j.scit otenv.2020.143095.

15. G. Carrus, M. Scopelliti, R. Lafortezza, G. Colangelo, F. Ferrini, F. Salbitano, M. Agrimi, et al., "Go Greener, Feel Better? The Positive Effects of Biodiversity on the Well-Being of Individuals Visiting Urban and Peri-urban Green Areas," *Landscape and Urban Planning* 134 (2015): 221–28, https://doi.org/10.1016/j.landurbplan .2014.10.022.

16. L. Tyrväinen, A. Ojala, K. Korpela, T. Lanki, Y. Tsunetsugu, and T. Kagawa, "The Influence of Urban Green Environments on Stress Relief Measures: A Field Experiment," *Journal of Environmental Psychology* 38 (2014): 1–9, https://doi.org/10.1016/j.jenvp .2013.12.005.

17. P. J. Lindal and T. Hartig, "Effects of Urban Street Vegetation on Judgments of Restoration Likelihood," *Urban Forestry & Urban Greening* 14, no. 2 (2015): 200– 209, https://doi.org/10.1016/j.ufug.2015.02.001.

18. M. R. Marselle, D. E. Bowler, J. Watzema, D. Eichenberg, T. Kirsten, and A. Bonn, "Urban Street Tree Biodiversity and Antidepressant Prescriptions," *Scientific Reports* 10, no. 1 (2020): 1, https://doi.org/10.1038/s41598-020-79924-5.

19. W.-L. Tsai, M. R. McHale, V. Jennings, O. Marquet, J. A. Hipp, Y.-F. Leung, and M. F. Floyd, "Relationships Between Characteristics of Urban Green Land Cover and Mental Health in U.S. Metropolitan Areas," *International Journal of Environmental Research and Public Health* 15, no. 2 (2018): 340, https://doi.org/10.3390/ijerph15020340.

20. K. M. M. Beyer, A. Kaltenbach, A. Szabo, S. Bogar, F. J. Nieto, and K. M. Malecki, "Exposure to Neighborhood Green Space and Mental Health: Evidence from the Survey of the Health of Wisconsin," *International Journal of Environmental Research and Public Health* 11, no. 3 (2014): 3453–72, https://doi.org/10.3390/ijerph110303453.

21. J. M. Ulmer, K. L. Wolf, D. R. Backman, R. L. Tretheway, C. J. A. Blain, J. P. M. O'Neil-Dunne, and L. D. Frank, "Multiple Health Benefits of Urban Tree Canopy: The Mounting Evidence for a Green Prescription," *Health & Place* 42 (2016): 54–62, https://doi.org/10.1016/j.healthplace.2016.08.011.

22. T. Hartig, "Restoration in Nature: Beyond the Conventional Narrative," in *Nature and Psychology: Biological, Cognitive, Developmental, and Social Pathways to Well-Being,*

edited by A. R. Schutte, J. Torquati, and J. R. Stevens (Proceedings of the Sixty-Seventh Annual Nebraska Symposium on Motivation) (Cham, Switzerland: Springer Nature, in press).

23. M. Marselle, K. Irvine, and S. Warber, "Examining Group Walks in Nature and Multiple Aspects of Well-Being: A Large-Scale Study," *Ecopsychology* 6, no. 3 (2014): 1, https://www.liebertpub.com/doi/abs/10.1089/eco.2014.0027.

24. The *mindbodygreen Podcast* (podcast), "Acclaimed Environmentalist Paul Hawken on Trump, Greenwashing & the Future of Our Planet," January 22, 2018, https://podcasts.apple.com/us/podcast/the-mindbodygreen-podcast.

25. S. L. Bell, B. W. Wheeler, and C. Phoenix, "Using Geonarratives to Explore the Diverse Temporalities of Therapeutic Landscapes: Perspectives from 'Green' and 'Blue' Settings," *Annals of the American Association of Geographers* 107, no. 1 (2016): 93–108, https://doi.org/10.1080/24694452.2016.1218269.

26. Susan J. Hewitt's profile, iNaturalist, n.d., https://www.inaturalist.org/users/50920.

27. R. Kuper, "Restorative Potential, Fascination, and Extent for Designed Digital Landscape Models," *Urban Forestry & Urban Greening* 28 (2017): 118–30, https://doi.org/10.1016/j.ufug.2017.10.002.

28. R. Kaplan, "The Nature of the View from Home: Psychological Benefits," *Environment and Behavior* 33, no. 4 (2001): 507–42, https://doi.org/10.1177/00139160121972 3115.

29. M. Elsadek, B. Liu, and J. Xie, "Window View and Relaxation: Viewing Green Space from a High-Rise Estate Improves Urban Dwellers' Wellbeing," *Urban Forestry & Urban Greening* 55 (2020), https://doi.org/10.1016/j.ufug.2020.126846.

30. S. Masoudinejad and T. Hartig, "Window View to the Sky as a Restorative Resource for Residents in Densely Populated Cities," *Environment and Behavior* 52, no. 4 (2018): 401–36, https://doi.org/10.1177/0013916518807274.

31. United Nations, "Cities and Pollution," 2018, https://www.un.org/en/climatechange /climate-solutions/cities-pollution.

32. A. Akpinar, C. Barbosa-Leiker, and K. R. Brooks, "Does Green Space Matter? Exploring Relationships Between Green Space Type and Health Indicators," *Urban Forestry & Urban Greening* 20 (2016): 407–18, https://doi.org/10.1016/j.ufug.2016.10.013.

33. M. P. White, I. Alcock, B. W. Wheeler, and M. H. Depledge, "Would You Be Happier Living in a Greener Urban Area? A Fixed-Effects Analysis of Panel Data," *Psychological Science* 24, no. 6 (2013): 920–28, https://doi.org/10.1177/0956797612464659.

34. J. R. Olsen, N. Nicholls, and R. Mitchell, "Are Urban Landscapes Associated with Reported Life Satisfaction and Inequalities in Life Satisfaction at the City Level? A

Cross-Sectional Study of Sixty-Six European Cities," *Social Science & Medicine* 226 (2019): 263–74, https://doi.org/10.1016/j.socscimed.2019.03.009.

35. J. L. McGuire, J. J. Lawler, B. H. McRae, T. A. Nuñez, and D. M. Theobald, "Achieving Climate Connectivity in a Fragmented Landscape," *Proceedings of the National Academy of Sciences* 113, no. 26 (2016): 7195–200, https://doi.org/10.1073/pnas.1602817113.

36. A. Rigolon, M. H. E. M. Browning, O. McAnirlin, and H. V. Yoon, "Green Space and Health Equity: A Systematic Review on the Potential of Green Space to Reduce Health Disparities," *International Journal of Environmental Research and Public Health* 18, no. 5 (2021): 2563, https://doi.org/10.3390/ijerph18052563.

37. A. Rigolon and J. Németh, "Green Gentrification or 'Just Green Enough': Do Park Location, Size, and Function Affect Whether a Place Gentrifies or Not?," *Urban Studies* 57, no. 2 (2019): 402–20, https://doi.org/10.1177/0042098019849380.

38. A. Rigolon and J. Christensen, *Greening Without Gentrification: Learning from Parks-Related Anti-Displacement Strategies Nationwide*, August 2019, https://www.ioes.ucla.edu/wp-content/uploads/Greening-without-Gentrification-report-2019.pdf.

39. Trust for Public Land, *The Heat Is On*, 2020, https://www.tpl.org/sites/default/files/The-Heat-is-on_A-Trust-for-Public-Land_special-report_r10.pdf.

40. Humboldt-Universität Zu Berlin, "GreenEquityHEALTH," n.d., https://www.geographie.hu-berlin.de/en/Members-en/1684583/Greenequityhealth.

41. N. Kabisch, R. Krämer, J. Hemmerling, O. Masztalerz, M. Adam, M. Brenck, et al., *GreenEquityHEALTH Factsheet II: The Value of Urban Parks for Health and Wellbeing*, June 30, 2020, https://www.researchgate.net/publication/343473722_GreenEquity Health_Factsheet_II_-_The_Value_of_Urban_Parks_for_Health_and_Well being.

EPILOGUE

1. "Joyful Participation in a World of Sorrows," *Sugar Calling* (podcast), April 29, 2020, https://www.nytimes.com/2020/04/15/podcasts/sugar-calling-pico-iyer-corona virus.html.

Further Reading by Landscape

PARKS & GARDENS

The Cloudspotter's Guide: The Science, History, and Culture of Clouds, by Gavin Pretor-Pinney

The Hidden Half of Nature: The Microbial Roots of Life and Health, by David R. Montgomery and Anne Biklé

OCEANS & COASTS

Blue Mind: The Surprising Science That Shows How Being Near, In, On, or Under Water Can Make You Happier, Healthier, More Connected, and Better at What You Do, by Wallace J. Nichols

By the Sea: The Therapeutic Benefits of Being in, on, and by the Water, by Dr. Deborah Cracknell

Deep: Freediving, Renegade Science, and What the Ocean Tells Us About Ourselves, by James Nestor

Why We Swim, by Bonnie Tsui

The Beach: The History of Paradise on Earth, by Lena Lenček and Gideon Bosker

MOUNTAINS & HIGHLANDS

In the Mountains: The Health and Wellbeing Benefits of Spending Time at Altitude, by Ned Morgan

On Trails: An Exploration, by Robert Moor

Mountains of the Mind, by Robert Macfarlane

These Mountains Are Our Sacred Places: The Story of the Stoney People, by Chief John Snow

FORESTS & TREES

Forest Bathing: How Trees Can Help You Find Health and Happiness, by Dr. Qing Li

Gathering Moss: A Natural and Cultural History of Mosses, by Robin Wall Kimmerer

The Healing Magic of Forest Bathing: Finding Calm, Creativity, and Connection in the Natural World, by Julia Plevin

The Hidden Life of Trees: What They Feel, How They Communicate— Discoveries from a Secret World, by Peter Wohlleben

ICE & SNOW

Arctic Dreams, by Barry Lopez

One Square Inch of Silence: One Man's Quest to Preserve Quiet, by Gordon Hempton and John Grossmann

Silence: In the Age of Noise, by Erling Kagge

The Secret Lives of Glaciers, by M Jackson

Underland: A Deep Time Journey, by Robert Macfarlane

DESERTS & DRYLANDS

Desert Solitaire: A Season in the Wilderness, by Edward Abbey

Erosion: Essays of Undoing, by Terry Tempest Williams

The Nature of Desert Nature, by Gary Paul Nabhan

RIVERS & STREAMS

Downriver: Into the Future of Water in the West, by Heather Hansman

To the River: A Journey Beneath the Surface, by Olivia Laing

CITIES & BUILT ENVIRONMENTS

Lo—TEK: Design by Radical Indigenism, by Julia Watson

The Ideal City: Exploring Urban Futures, by gestalten and Space10

The Sustainable City, Steven Cohen

LANDSCAPE-AGNOSTIC

The Nature Fix: Why Nature Makes Us Happier, Healthier, and More Creative, by Florence Williams

Braiding Sweetgrass: Indigenous Wisdom, Scientific Knowledge, and the Teachings of Plants, by Robin Wall Kimmerer

Last Child in the Woods: Saving Our Children from Nature-Deficit Disorder, by Richard Louv

All We Can Save: Truth, Courage, and Solutions for the Climate Crisis, edited by Ayana Elizabeth Johnson and Katharine K. Wilkinson

Drawdown: The Most Comprehensive Plan Ever Proposed to Reverse Global Warming, edited by Paul Hawken

Spiritual Ecology: The Cry of the Earth, edited by Llewellyn Vaughan-Lee

Ecopsychology: Science, Totems, and the Technological Species, edited by Peter H. Kahn Jr. and Patricia H. Hasbach

Black Faces, White Spaces: Reimagining the Relationship of African Americans to the Great Outdoors, by Carolyn Finney

Tales of Two Planets: Stories of Climate Change and Inequality in a Divided World, edited by John Freeman

The Rise of the American Conservation Movement: Power, Privilege, and Environmental Protection, by Dorceta E. Taylor

War and Trade in Northern Seas

Anglo-Scandinavian economic relations in the mid-eighteenth century

H. S. K. KENT
University of Adelaide

CAMBRIDGE
AT THE UNIVERSITY PRESS 1973

Published by the Syndics of the Cambridge University Press
Bentley House, 200 Euston Road, London NW1 2DB
American Branch: 32 East 57th Street, New York, N.Y. 10022

© Cambridge University Press 1973

Library of Congress Catalogue Card Number: 72-75304

ISBN: 0 521 08579 9

Printed in Great Britain
at the University Printing House, Cambridge
(Brooke Crutchley, University Printer)

Contents

List of Appendixes   *page* vii

Preface   ix

Notes   xiii

Abbreviations   xv

1 MERCANTILIST POLICIES AND ANGLO-
   SCANDINAVIAN TRADE   1

2 THE ORGANISATION OF TRADE   14

3 THE TIMBER-TRADE   39

4 THE IRON-TRADE   59

5 MISCELLANEOUS IMPORTS FROM SCANDINAVIA   80

6 THE EXPORT TRADE   89

7 TEA-SMUGGLING AND THE BALANCE OF TRADE   112

8 THE FIRST ARMED NEUTRALITY: ANGLO-
   SCANDINAVIAN DISPUTES OVER NEUTRAL RIGHTS   130

9 TRADE AND DIPLOMACY   162

   APPENDIXES   178

   Bibliography   206

   Index of Statutes   230

   General Index   231

Appendixes

1 *The Timber-Trade*

Fig. 1 Imports of ordinary deals into England from all sources, 1750–1770   *page* 178

Fig. 2 The distribution of shipping in the timber-trade: deal imports into London from Norway, 1750–1770   179

Fig. 3 The distribution of shipping in the timber-trade: deal imports into the English out-ports from Norway, 1750–1770   179

Fig. 4 The distribution of shipping in the timber-trade: imports of 'fir timber' into England from Norway, 1750–1770   180

Table 1 Imports of masts into England from all sources, 1750–1770   181

Table 2 Timber prices at London, 1757–1770   182

Table 3 Cost of importing deals from Christiania to London, 1764   183

2 *The Iron-Trade*

Fig. 5 Imports of bar-iron into England from all sources, 1750–1770   184

Fig. 6 The distribution of shipping in the iron-trade: imports of bar-iron into London from Sweden, 1750–1770   185

Fig. 7 The distribution of shipping in the iron-trade: imports of bar-iron into the English out-ports from Sweden, 1750–1770   185

Table 4 Imports of bar-iron into England showing the percentage imported from Sweden, 1750–1770   186

3 *The Pitch- and Tar-Trade*

Fig. 8 Imports of pitch and tar into England from Sweden and the American colonies, 1750–1770   187

Appendixes

4 *Report on the Norwegian Timber-Trade and the
   Swedish and Norwegian Iron-Trade to England, 1759*   page 188

Introduction   188

On the Timber-Trade   188

On the Iron-Trade   198

5 *The emigration of British workers to Scandinavia*   202

viii

Preface

British trade with Scandinavia was constantly under attack by pamphleteers and in Parliament as a 'losing trade'. The balance of trade, so the argument ran, was heavily weighted against Britain who imported timber from Norway and iron from Sweden in large quantities, while the Scandinavian kingdoms admitted few British goods. Moreover, industry, the merchant fleet, and above all the Royal Navy depended on Norwegian timber and Swedish iron, and had early in the century depended as well on Swedish pitch and tar. For reasons both of economic well-being and national security Britain would be well advised to cut her Scandinavian trade links and obtain vital iron and timber supplies from her North American colonies. Cabinet agreed with all these arguments and Parliament passed a number of Acts to encourage the growth of colonial iron, timber, and pitch and tar exports to the mother-country. The bounties given to pitch and tar imports from North America worked well enough: the Swedish near-monopoly of supplies to Britain was broken. The encouragement given to North American timber and iron exports to Britain produced no significant result, and Britain remained dependent on Scandinavia for supplies.

This was galling and, in time of war, dangerous. To make matters worse, England as a tea-drinking country was dependent for her tea supplies on two sources: legally imported tea from the East India Company which was expensive and fell short of requirements, and smuggled tea imports which were cheap, abundant, and, it was suspected quite rightly at the time, supplied largely by the Scandinavian East India Companies. These illicit imports affected still further the balance of trade. Reasons of national security and of mercantilist policy, a potent argument when taken together, counselled therefore political action to minimise dependence on Scandinavia. Yet when England entered on a world-wide war with France in 1755, a war that was to become the Seven

Years War when it spilled over into Europe the following year, she was still as dependent as ever on Scandinavian timber and iron and, moreover, on shipping services, let alone tea to keep the home-front content.

In this study I have examined the organisation of this trade in peace and in war, starting with an analysis of commercial treaties and legislation which provided a framework within which Anglo-Scandinavian economic relations were meant to move. The various treaties came to be of particular importance during the Seven Years War when Sweden and the double kingdom of Denmark–Norway formed an Armed Neutrality League to defend ostensible treaty-rights against alleged British infringements. Treaties or no treaties, Britain was determined to ruin French trade even if that meant risking war with the Scandinavian kingdoms, which were of some consequence as naval powers. In the end, Denmark remained neutral, Sweden entered the war on the side of France against Prussia but remained non-belligerent *vis-à-vis* Britain, and the Neutrality League soon collapsed. Trade was only marginally affected, and iron, timber and tea from Scandinavia continued to reach Britain in required quantities.

The extent of this trade was in fact far larger and more vital than contemporary observers and statisticians believed it to be. Statistics of the time are largely misleading, and of course neglect the smuggling trade. Comparisons of statistics and observations in British and Scandinavian archives, and deductions from trade practices allowed me to reach conclusions on the legitimate trade in timber and iron, as well as on the range and extent of the smuggling trade.

Considering the importance and volume of Anglo-Scandinavian trade, it was remarkable that government in England had so little influence on it. On the surface, England appeared to regulate trade by legislation and treaties. In fact, it was the merchants themselves in their lawful or illicit enterprises who directed trade in blissful disregard of government whenever and wherever regulations bore too heavily on them. How this was done I have shown.

This study is based on a doctoral dissertation presented to the University of Cambridge in 1955. I am most grateful to Sir Herbert

Butterfield and to Professor Charles Wilson for their supervision at the time, and to Professor M. M. Postan for many fruitful discussions. Parts of the chapter on the timber trade appeared in an article in the *Economic History Review*, and some sections on the First Armed Neutrality in the *American Journal of International Law*. I acknowledge gratefully the assistance I received from the Scandinavian Studies Fund and the Tennant Fund of the University of Cambridge, and my thanks are due to Professor B. W. Downs, then Master of Christ's College, for his encouragement of my studies. I have since received assistance from the Scandinavian Cultural Fund, Canberra, for which I am grateful. The University of Cambridge awarded this work the Ellen McArthur Prize in 1969. I want to thank the Managers of the Ellen McArthur Fund for recommending the award and for generously assisting in the publication of the present book.

My indebtedness to many archivists and librarians in England and Scandinavia has been great. Their unfailing kindness and helpfulness in making material available to me is amply demonstrated in the bibliography. Special thanks are due to the late Lensgreve Christian Moltke of Bregentved and to Count Moltke's family who allowed me the use of the archives at Bregentved Castle.

I wish to record my gratitude to the late Professor David Joslin whose encouragement and friendship I valued.

H.S.K.K.

Notes

1. *The Calendar in the Eighteenth Century*

Denmark–Norway adopted the New Style in 1700, Great Britain in 1752, and Sweden in 1753. The New Year began in Denmark–Norway and Sweden under the Old Style on 1 January, and in Great Britain on Lady Day, 25 March. Envoys generally dated their letters in the Style of the country to which they were accredited, while receiving instructions dated in the Style of the country of despatch. I have given an indication of the Style used in correspondence prior to 1753 to avoid confusion. No particular reference to the two calendars appeared necessary in the case of treaties, Acts, regulations and the like, for which the appropriate calendar of the country of signature or origin is used, except that Gregorian calendar years are shown where required by British dates, thus: 6/2/1749–50.

2. *The dating of Diplomatic and other Official Correspondence*

Unless otherwise indicated, despatches, reports etc. from envoys and diplomatic and consular officers were dated as from the capital or provincial city in which they were stationed; instructions, memoranda etc. from cabinet ministers and government departments were dated from their respective capitals. It should be noted that Goodricke, while envoy-designate to Sweden, was stationed at Copenhagen.

3. *Spelling and place-names*

Just as English, so Swedish, Danish and Norwegian spelling was not standardized in the eighteenth century. It could and did happen that the same word was spelt in different ways within the space of a single sentence. The titles or headings of contemporary documents and publications and all quotations from them are given as they actually appeared. Place-names are also in their contemporary form.

Abbreviations

Ad.	Admiralty Papers
B.M.	British Museum, London
Bergen Arch.	Bergen City Archives
C.O.	Colonial Office Records
Cust.	Custom and Excise Records
D.N.B.	*Dictionary of National Biography*
Dan. S. Arch.	Danish State Archives, Copenhagen
E.	Exchequer Papers
F.O.	Foreign Office Records
H.C.A.	High Court of Admiralty Records
J.H.C.	*Journals, House of Commons*
Moltke Arch.	Archives of the Counts Moltke, Bregentved Castle, Denmark
Nor. S. Arch.	Norwegian State Archives, Oslo
P.R.O.	Public Record Office, London
R.H.C.	*Reports, House of Commons*
Sjaelland Arch.	Sjaelland Provincial Archives, Copenhagen
S.P.	State Papers
Swed. S. Arch.	Swedish State Archives, Stockholm
T.	Treasury Papers
T.K.U.A.	Tyske Kancellis Udenlandske Afdeling
U.L.	University Library

1 *Mercantilist Policies and Anglo-Scandinavian trade*

The large forests and productive mines of the Scandinavian peninsula had early attracted the attention of British merchants seeking timber and wood products, iron and copper, to supplement native resources of these essential materials for domestic building, naval construction, and manufacture. Both the Scandinavian powers, Sweden and the double kingdom of Denmark–Norway, had a surplus of forest and mine produce for export to England and Scotland, while themselves requiring manufactured and colonial goods that Britain could supply. On this basis of complementary needs was built an extensive trade which, from the mid-seventeenth[1] to the late eighteenth century, was meant to be protected by the Anglo-Swedish treaty of 1661 and the Anglo-Danish treaty of 1670.

The Treaty of Peace and Commerce between Great Britain and Sweden signed at Whitehall on 11 April 1661, was a short document of only seventeen articles.[2] The first two stipulated that the treaty should be binding in perpetuity, and that neither of the contracting parties would assist rebels or traitors of the other. The final article dealt with ratification of the treaty which had already come into

---

[1] Cursory information on seventeenth-century Anglo-Scandinavian trade is given by E. F. Heckscher, *Sveriges ekonomiska historia från Gustav Vasa*, pt 1, *Före Frihetstiden* (Stockholm, 1935), 2, *passim*; and A. Bugge, *Den norske Traelasthandels Historie* (Skien, 1925) vol. 2, *passim*.

[2] The ratified treaty is preserved in P.R.O., S.P. 108/518. A complete translation from the original Latin into English is printed in N. Magens, *Essay on Insurances* (London, 1755), vol. 2, pp. 599ff., and an abridged translation in *British and Foreign State Papers* (London, 1841), vol. 1, pt 1, pp. 701ff. This perpetual treaty was supplemented for short periods, but never superseded, by several treaties and conventions of limited duration which had all expired by the time of the Seven Years War, leaving the treaty of 1661 as the only agreement in force between Sweden and Great Britain.

force on signature. The remaining fourteen articles were solely concerned with the conditions under which commerce and navigation were to be carried on. Their entire liberty was assured by the third article, and respect for ancient privileges was promised in the fourth which also stated that merchants might trade in what goods and merchandises they please, and may freely import and export the same, paying the customs which are due.[1] Ships and their crews were to be safe from molestation, and to receive help when in distress; the transit of men and of goods was not to be impeded; justice should be impartial and swift; and the breaking of the law by the subjects of the one signatory in the domains of the other was not to be a pretext for the abrogation of the treaty.[2] A further and final series of articles dealt with commerce in time of war. Trade with the enemy of one or the other contracting power was allowed in all merchandise except contraband, which was specified in the eleventh article as money, arms and munitions, horses and their accoutrements, and warships. The freedom to carry goods of the enemy was implicitly excepted, however, in article twelve which sought to prevent that 'goods of Enemies should pass concealed under the name of Friends' by the institution of a passport system embodying a sworn declaration of ownership of merchandise carried. Presentation of the passport protected the ship and her crew from search which was only permissible if no passport was produced, and there was cause to suspect the carrying of enemy or contraband goods. Crews and passengers of ships which were taken prize and brought by an enemy into the harbours of either power remaining neutral were to be set free and the prize was not allowed to remain in the territorial waters of either country.[3]

The Anglo-Danish Treaty of Alliance and Trade, signed at Copenhagen on 12 July 1670, was a lengthier document of forty-two articles[4] in which the negotiators had attempted to allow for any

[1] *British and Foreign State Papers*, vol. 1, pt 1, p. 702.
[2] *Ibid.*, articles 5–10, and article 14.
[3] *Ibid.*, articles 11–13, 15 and 16.
[4] The treaty is preserved in P.R.O., S.P. 108/35, and its complete text in the original Latin is printed in L. Laursen (ed.), *Danmark–Norges Traktater, 1523–1750, med dertil hørende Aktstykker* (Copenhagen, 1923), vol. 6, pp. 317ff. An abridged text

contingency in the section dealing with commerce in peace or war. Freedom of trade, residence and transit was assured to the subjects of either signatory in the domains of the other, except in colonial territories and in certain areas of the Danish–Norwegian kingdom.[1] Merchants were to ship to the other country only produce or manufactures of their own, merchants from Denmark having the privilege, though, of sending to Britain commodities also from the Elbe region.[2] British ships had a privilege in the Norway trade in that they were exempt from search for such timber – in fact, oak – the export of which was prohibited.[3] Several articles dealt with the passage of the Sound and with the customs at the mouth of the Elbe. No duties were to be levied on British ships at Glückstadt, while at the Sound quick despatch of shipping was promised and goods landed at Elsinore for transhipment were charged only the same duties as were paid by the Dutch. Payment of the Sound Tolls could be deferred by eastward-bound ships till their return from the Baltic or for three months, whichever was the shorter period.[4] British merchants resident in Denmark – no mention was made of Norway or the royal possessions in Germany – were not allowed to engage in retail-trade, whereas no such restriction was laid on Danish merchants in Britain. Should a merchant die intestate while not in his homeland, his possessions were safeguarded and his business papers could not be examined.[5]

Articles dealing with commerce in war-time were numerous. Trade with the enemy of the other was permitted except in merchandise regarded as contraband[6] which, however, was not specified

in translation, lacking several articles, is printed in *British and Foreign State Papers*, vol. 1, pt 1, pp. 381ff.

[1] *Danmark–Norges Traktater*, Laursen (ed.), vol. 6, pp. 320, 322, 329–30, articles 5, 6, 9 and 30.

[2] *Ibid.*, pp. 320f., article 7: 'merces ex universo fluvio Albi provenientes'. Danish possessions near the mouth of the river, and her special position thereby in the Elbe trade, explain this provision.

[3] *Ibid.*, p. 322, article 9: 'domini regis Magnae Britanniae etc. naves...nulli amplius visitatione subjecta erunt'.

[4] *Ibid.*, pp. 323 and 327, articles 12–14 and 21.

[5] *Ibid.*, pp. 324f., article 17 and p. 324, article 15: 'quod nullae cartae aut rationum libri...inspectioni exponentur'.

[6] *Ibid.*, p. 324, article 16: 'prohibitis solummodo quas contrabandas vocant exceptis'.

directly and could only be inferred from the provision that neither would furnish the enemy of the other, if that enemy was the aggressor, with provisions of war such as soldiers, arms, implements, guns, ships, or other necessaries of war.[1] Passports were required to prevent enemy goods passing as those of friends, visit of a vessel being permitted if the passport was not presented or if there was just cause of suspicion.[2] Ships or goods of either power could not be adjudged good prize except by a prize court which was to give speedy justice; merchantmen of the one were permitted to take advantage of the protection of convoys of the other; letters of marque were not allowed to be taken from a third power at war with Great Britain or Denmark–Norway; territorial waters should be safeguarded to commerce; crews of ships which had been taken prize and brought into harbour were to be released, and only the cargo detained.[3] In general most-favoured-nation treatment was promised except that Sweden alone was permitted to retain established privileges.[4]

Two assumptions underlay the articles on commerce in peace and war in both these perpetual treaties. The one, that the commercial policies of the powers engaged would remain constant and the free exchange of goods stay permitted; the other, that warfare would not change and with it the rules on contraband of war, and trade with an enemy. Both assumptions proved to be incorrect. Sweden and Denmark, mainly primary producers when the treaties were signed, and lacking the means to obtain colonial

[1] Laursen (ed.), *Danmark–Norges Traktater*, vol. 6, p. 319, article 3: 'Praedicti iidem reges…se alterutrius hostibus, qui aggressores fuerint, nihil subsidii bellici, veluti milites, arma, machinas, bombardas, naves aut alia bello gerendo apta et necessaria subministraturos, aut a suis subditis subministari passuros.'

[2] *Ibid.*, pp. 325–7, article 20: 'Quod si vero solemnis haec et stata salvi conductus et certificationis formula non exhibeatur, aut alia aliqua justa atque urgens suspitionis causa sit, tum navis visitari debet.'
   It will be noted that this treaty gives wider rights to the belligerent in the matter of visit at sea than the Anglo-Swedish treaty by which visit could only be made when no passport was presented.

[3] *Ibid.*, pp. 328–31, articles 23, 24, 28 and 31–4.

[4] *Ibid.*, pp. 320–2, and 332f., articles 7, 8 and 40. The Swedish privileges related to the Sound Toll. They fell into desuetude in 1710 during the Great Northern War, and were abolished at the peace of Frederiksborg in 1720 – see E. F. Heckscher, *Sveriges ekonomiska historia från Gustav Vasa*, pt II, *Det moderna Sveriges grundläggning* (Stockholm, 1949), 2, p. 645.

goods directly, came to embark on policies designed to foster manufacture and to protect it by high duties and prohibitions against foreign competition. Denmark gained tropical colonies in the West Indies and established settlements in Africa and India from which she imported produce that had, in part, been furnished by British merchants. In Sweden, a company to trade with India and China was formed and given privileges that precluded other nations from supplying merchandise imported directly by Swedish merchants in Swedish ships. The necessity of denying an enemy supplies in war came to be more widely acted upon and led to an extension of the range of articles regarded as contraband, while the competition for trade and empire in the Anglo-French wars of the mid-century altered British views on what was lawful trade with her adversary. The rights, enumerated in the two treaties as belonging to merchant and state, could not escape from being called in question when policies of trade and warfare changed, and the undertakings given in the treaties were progressively disregarded.

Sweden began to discriminate sharply against British trade in favour of her nascent textile manufacture, within a few years of the treaty being signed, by laying a heavy duty on British woollens which were the main article of export to Sweden.[1] Limitations on trade were followed by restrictions on shipping with an edict of 1724[2] which, modelled on the British Navigation Acts, was to prevent foreign ships from carrying to Sweden any produce or articles but that of their own country and its colonies.[3] Further duties on a wider range of imports were imposed when the Swedish Diet of 1726–7 decided on a policy to foster home manufacture and protect it by heavy imposts on competing foreign goods.[4] These mercantilist devices of customs and navigation acts were continued in decrees of 1734 and 1735, by which the import of many British

---

[1] J. F. Chance, 'England and Sweden in the time of William III and Queen Anne', *Engl. Hist. Review*, 16, 679, quoting a report of the Commissioners of Trade, 1697, that the duties were imposed about the year 1680.

[2] Swed. S. Arch., Kungl. Mai:ts Förordningar, 1724, Produkt placatet.

[3] The implications of this edict on the activities of British merchants and shippers are discussed in E. F. Heckscher, *Ekonomi och historia* (Stockholm, 1922), pp. 218ff.

[4] Heckscher, *Sveriges ekonomiska historia*, II, 2, p. 588.

War and Trade in Northern Seas

goods, including practically all textiles, was either prohibited outright or made virtually impossible through prohibitive duties.[1] The coming into power of the Hat Party in 1739 led to an intensification of protectionist policies until by the middle of the century most British goods were excluded from the Swedish market.[2] The exclusion of British colonial produce had been made possible by the formation of a Swedish East India Company in 1731 which, after serving at first as a cloak for British interlopers in the English Company's preserves, came under Swedish control and supplied the home-market with merchandise formerly obtained through British merchant-houses.[3] A slight relaxation in import-regulations on a small list of goods came about only in 1761[4] by which time the Swedish company had struck some financial difficulties.[5]

Denmark–Norway took a similar course to that of Sweden in protecting her growing industries and thus also infringed incidentally the provisions of her commercial treaty with England. Textile manufacture was the first to be fostered by regulations in 1705 affecting adversely the import of British cloth.[6] A series of edicts further restricted the market for British goods,[7] but Danish protectionist policy was for a short while halted by the Customs Roll of 1732 which contained no further import-restrictions, attempting,

---

[1] Swed. S. Arch., Kungl. Mai:ts Förordningar, 1734: Kungl. Maj:ts nådiga förordning hvarmedelst wisse utrikes waror förbiudas at i Riket införas, 11 Dec 1734 [O.S.] and *ibid.*, 1735, Taxa hvarefter Landthielpen...at erläggas af de inkommande wahror, som uti följande förteckning äro upförde, 1 January 1735 [O.S.].

[2] L. Stavenow, *Sveriges historia till våra dagar*, vol. 9, *Frihetstiden, 1718–1772* (Stockholm, 1922), pp. 281–5 and Heckscher, *Sveriges ekonomiska historia*, II, 2, pp. 592f. and 654f.; and see also R. V. Eagly, 'Monetary policy and politics in Mid-Eighteenth Century Sweden', *Journal of Economic History*, 29, no 4 (1969).

[3] N. H. Quiding, *Svenskt allmänt författningsregister för tiden från år 1522 till och med år 1862* (Stockholm, 1865), no pagination, see under 'Ostindiske Handeln'; Heckscher, '*Sveriges ekonomiska historia*, II, 2, pp. 693–5; Stavenow, *Sveriges historia*, vol. 9, *passim*.

[4] Swed. S. Arch., Kungl. Mai:ts Förordninger, 1759–61, Förordning ang. wisse utrikes waror så wäl lösgifwande ifrån förbud til införsel, som beläggande med mindre... afgifter, 21 September 1761.

[5] Lund, U.L., MSS Department, De la Gardieska Samlingen, historiska handlingar, Adolf Fredericks Arkiv, Oeconomica: jämförelse mellan Svenska Ostindiska kompaniet och utländska inrättningar af samma slag, år 1757.

[6] Axel Nielsen, *Dänische Wirtschaftsgeschichte* (Jena, 1933), p. 221.

[7] J. O. Bro-Jørgensen, *Industriens Historie i Danmark, Tiden 1730–1820* (Copenhagen, 1943), p. 104.

on the contrary, to foster a measure of free trade.[1] This was, though, the last respite given to foreign imports. A mercantilist policy favouring manufacture and protection intervened, and British goods were progressively excluded from Denmark, and later also from Norway.[2] Colonial produce was imported directly by the Danish Asiatic Company trading to China and India which, after its refounding in 1732, was partly owned by the Crown and given extensive privileges.[3] The Danish West India Company traded with the Danish possessions of St Croix, St John, and St Thomas in the Caribbean and, like its sister company, obtained privileges through the interest of the king and some of the most influential courtiers.[4] Its sugar-trade was fostered first by discriminatory duties on foreign produce,[5] and from 1750 onwards by outright prohibitions on the import of most grades of foreign sugar and of sugar products into Denmark and Norway.[6] British manufactures were driven out of the Danish–Norwegian market by a series of decrees from the 1730s to 1760. A sumptuary law of 1736 prohibited the wearing of articles and apparel which had been largely supplied by England,[7] and an expedient measure to encourage the wearing of Danish instead of English cloth was taken in the following year when a cut in the salaries of all civil and military officers was compensated for by a free issue of Danish cloth.[8] English salt, an important article of trade, was expressly excluded from Denmark and Norway in 1746 while its imports from other countries remained

[1] Dan. S. Arch., Rentekammeret, Sekretariatet: Toldforordning, 29 February 1732 [N.S.].

[2] Denmark and Norway were administered separately as regards trade, and commercial regulations specified which component, in part or whole, of the double kingdom was affected by them. On problems this gave rise to, see V. la Cour, *Mellem Brødre. Dansk–Norsk Problemer i det 18. Aarhundredes Helstat* (Birkerød, 1943), pp. 137ff.

[3] A. Olsen, *Danmark–Norge i det 18. Aarhundrede* (Copenhagen, 1936), pp. 21f.

[4] *Ibid.*

[5] Dan. S. Arch., Forordninger og Aabne Breve, Placat, 25 April 1735.

[6] P. P. Sveistrup and R. Willerslev. *Den Danske Sukkerhandels og Sukkerproduktions Historie* (Copenhagen, 1945), p. 41, citing edict referring to Denmark of 31 May 1750; also J. H. Schou (ed.), *Chronologisk Register over de Kongelige Forordninger og Aabne Breve som fra Aar 1670 till 1775 Aars Udgang ere udkomne* (Copenhagen, 1777), vol. 4, edicts referring to Norway of 12 January and 14 February 1751, 3 February and 18 February 1755.

[7] Bro-Jørgensen, *Industriens Historie*, p. 105, citing edict of 16 April 1736.

[8] B. M., Egerton MS 2695, Titley papers, official diary, no pagination, entry of 22 August 1737. The measure was held to have had some effect on British cloth imports.

7

unaffected;[1] glassware of all descriptions came to be excluded by 1760;[2] the import of tobacco was restricted by an order of the same year,[3] and Danish agricultural produce was given a monopoly position in southern Norway.[4] High duties further discouraged foreign grain and flour from entering northern Norway.[5] The most serious interference with legitimate British trade with Denmark was accomplished by duties which amounted to prohibitions, and by actual prohibitions, on all woollen goods, on linens, and cottons in the late 1730s and early 1740s.[6] These restrictions did not apply to Norway where a duty of 20% on prime cost, intended to be prohibitive, was only placed on all woollens in 1759, while a premium of 5% was given to merchants importing Danish textiles.[7] These numerous regulations[8] found their place in the Customs Roll of 1762[9] which marked the highest point in Danish mercantilist policy, from which no retreat was made for a decade.

British shipping was likewise discriminated against by Sweden and Denmark–Norway through the imposition of higher export duties on produce shipped in foreign bottoms, and through higher port charges. Sweden in 1722 and 1726 gave preferential treatment to her own ships carrying goods from their native harbours,[10] and

[1] Dan. S. Arch., Rentekammeret, Secretariatet, Placat of 23 August 1746. An earlier prohibition on the import of English salt into Denmark is referred to in this edict.

[2] Dan. S. Arch., *ibid.*, Placat of 26 March 1760.

[3] Dan. S. Arch., *ibid.*, Placat of 31 December 1760.

[4] Southern, or søndenfjeldske, Norway comprised in the eighteenth century the region to the south of Dovre and east of the Langenfjelde, with the Naze as the western border. The remaining part of Norway was styled Northern, or nordenfjeldske Norway. Customs regulations for these two regions were often different. See M. Vahl and G. Hatt, *Jorden og Menneskeliv* (Copenhagen, 1927), vol. 4, pp. 521.

[5] Dan. S. Arch., Rentekammeret, Sekretariatet, edicts relating to grain and flour in the years 1732, 1735 and 1744; and Generaltoldkammeret, Sekretariatet, edicts of 1762.

[6] Dan. S. Arch., Forordninger og Aabne Breve, edicts of 17 November 1739 and 10 November 1741 which were reiterated by the edict of 19 December 1753.

[7] *Ibid.*, edict of 18 May 1759 and Placat of 12 October 1759.

[8] No connected account appears to have yet been given of the customs regulations for Denmark and Norway in the earlier eighteenth century which therefore had to be assembled from the various sources given above. For the period after 1760, see Aa. Rasch, *Dansk Toldpolitik 1760–1797* (Aarhus, 1955), *passim*.

[9] Dan. S. Arch., Generaltoldkammeret, Sekretariatet, Toldforordning of 17 May 1762.

[10] Heckscher, *Sveriges ekonomiska historia*, II, 2, p. 670.

8

laid moreover a special duty on bar-iron exported in foreign ships.[1] Denmark–Norway had taken similar action in the preceding century when substantially higher port charges were imposed on foreign ships,[2] and earlier privileges given to British merchants were withdrawn and higher export duties placed on cargoes sent by foreign ships.[3]

British regulations affecting trade with the Scandinavian powers were few, although protests and threats of reprisals against Danish and Swedish treaty infractions were many. Import duties on iron, the principal Swedish produce, had been imposed for the first time in 1679 and were raised in 1694[4] without, however, appearing to have had any effect on the volume of imports.[5] A more indirect method was used to lessen English dependence on Swedish tar by an Act encouraging the production of naval stores in the American colonies.[6] The development of alternative sources of supply of produce imported from Scandinavia had been urged as early as 1697 by the Commissioners of Trade.[7] Their report was only acted upon after the Stockholm Tar Company had made the terms of trade too unattractive, and the danger of depending for essential naval stores on a power that might interrupt supplies became too obvious.[8] This danger was again recognised when a crisis in Anglo-Swedish affairs led in 1717 to an interruption of iron imports from Sweden, and a consequent agitation by merchants and manufacturers to find new sources of supply became very strong.[9] The newly-opened mines and forges of Russia were able to furnish an increasing amount of iron whose import was facilitated by the Anglo-Russian

[1] Heckscher, *Sveriges ekonomiska historia*, II, 2, p. 671.
[2] J. A. S. Schmidt (ed.), *Rescripter, Resolutioner og Collegial-Breve for Kongeriget Norge* (Christiana, 1847), vol. I, p. 23, edict of 16 April 1672.
[3] *Ibid.*, p. 45, edict of 10 May 1688 and p. 45, note 1, abstract of later regulations.
[4] T. S. Ashton, *Iron and steel in the industrial revolution*, 2nd ed. (Manchester, 1951), p. 105.
[5] H. Scrivenor, *A comprehensive history of the iron trade* (London, 1841), pp. 325ff., tables I, III, V and VIII, showing the quantity of iron imported from foreign countries, 1711–55.
[6] 3 and 4 Anne c. 10.
[7] Chance, 'England and Sweden', p. 679.
[8] G. N. Clark, 'Neutral Commerce in the War of the Spanish Succession and the Treaty of Utrecht', *British Year Book of International Law, 1928*, p. 71.
[9] Ashton, *Iron and steel*, pp. 111f.

9

treaty of 1734 which helped to deflect trade from Sweden.[1] Direct retaliation against Swedish import-prohibitions by substituting colonial for continental iron was proposed in the following year by the British envoy in Stockholm to the Northern Secretary of State, Lord Harrington, who approved of this advice after it had been considered by the Commissioners of Trade.[2] The matter was discussed in parliament where a committee of the House of Commons examined the feasibility of encouraging colonial iron production and imports by waiving the import duties on American iron. Witnesses argued before the committee that retaliation against Swedish prohibitions on the entry of British merchandise could and should be taken,[3] but nothing was done for the time being. Yet another committee of investigation served, at least, the purpose of alarming the Swedish representative in London sufficiently to make him approach members of Parliament and the Secretary of State who, while speaking darkly of reprisals, gave him to understand that retaliatory measures were for the present quite unlikely.[4] In fact, they were not taken until 1750.[5] A Commons committee in that year recommended after it had considered British trade with Scandinavia that duties on colonial iron shipped directly to London should be lifted,[6] but as the duties on colonial pig-iron had been small, this measure could have little effect until the colonies produced more bar-iron on which the incidence of duties had fallen more heavily.

In the end, Britain did no more than continue her protests to Sweden over discrimination against British trade in general, and in particular over the higher export duties on Swedish iron shipped in non-Swedish vessels. Sweden blandly disregarded all such protests and Britain let it go at that, although she pointed out from time to time that she would be quite within her rights if she retaliated,

---

[1] D. Gerhard, *England und der Aufstieg Russlands* (Berlin, 1933), p. 16.

[2] J. F. Chance (ed.), *British Diplomatic Instructions, Sweden, 1727–1789* (London, 1928) (cit. *Diplomatic Instructions, Sweden II*), pp. 56f., Harrington to Finch, 16/27 September 1735.

[3] *J.H.C.*, vol. xxii (1737), evidence of John Bannister, p. 851; Captain Tomlinson, p. 852; W. Astell and Joseph Farmer, p. 853.

[4] Swed. S. Arch., Ämnesserier, Handel och Sjöfart, ser. ii, bundle 9, Wasenberg to Cantzly-Collegium, London 21 March 1738 [O.S.].   [5] Ashton, *Iron and steel*, p. 118.

[6] *J.H.C.*, vol. xxv, p. 979, report of 6 February 1749–50; and Acts, 23 Geo. II c. 29.

as Sweden was breaking the Anglo-Swedish treaty of 1661.[1] There
was really nothing Britain could do so long as she depended on
Swedish iron imports, and even the sharp increase in Russian iron
imports from the end of the Seven Years War onward did not
entirely free her from dependence on the special high grades of
Swedish bar-iron. By 1770 the increase in home production and
in Russian iron imports had become so large that Swedish imports
were of relatively slighter importance, but by that time British
industry needed all the iron it could get. To deprive industry
deliberately of any iron at all was unthinkable, and in any case,
government was not prepared to intervene in economic matters
unless it was driven to it. There was no group which could induce
the government to take action against Swedish imports: British
exporters to Sweden simply were not numerous enough to carry
sufficient weight, and their complaints were lost in government
correspondence.[2] Imports from Sweden therefore continued to
enter Britain freely, whereas many British goods were either prohibited outright from entering Sweden or were charged prohibitive
or heavy import duties.

Protests and threats of reprisals against Danish–Norwegian
restrictions and prohibitions on the import of British goods were
equally ineffective. Denmark–Norway's principal export to Britain
against which reprisals could in theory be taken was timber. The
import duties levied on it were low[3] as they were based on a moderate
rate that remained unaltered from the middle of the seventeenth
to the end of the eighteenth century.[4] In fact, Norwegian timber
like Swedish iron was indispensable: domestic and ship building
as well as industry could not do without it until an alternative
source of supply was found. Again, merchants and government
looked to the North American colonies for timber supplies to take
the place of imports from Norway, but the hoped-for massive

[1] *Diplomatic Instructions, Sweden II*, pp. 29f., Secretary of State to Finch [envoy to
Sweden], 23 June 1732 [O.S.]; pp. 31f., Secretary of State to Finch, 21 November
and 29 December 1732 [O.S.]; p. 28, Secretary of State to Finch, 9 May 1732 [O.S.];
and pp. 53f., Secretary of State to Finch, 6 June 1735 [O.S.].
[2] P.R.O., C.O. 389/30, Commissioners of Trade to Lord Holdernesse [Secretary of
State], 8 July 1756.
[3] *R.H.C.*, vol. 15, timber duties (1835), XIX, pp. 348ff., table B.
[4] Books of Rates, 12 Car. II c. 6, and 11 Geo. I c. 7. As also Act, 50 Geo. III c. 77.

shipments from North America did not materialise until later in the century. In the meantime, the famous Act of 1720[1] for the encouragement of the importation of naval stores from the colonies could have no greater effect on the timber-trade than two earlier Acts of the reign of Queen Anne[2] so long as duties on foreign timber remained low, as lifting the duties on colonial timber could not compensate for the high freight-rates from America.[3] Threats to raise the duties on timber in retaliation against Danish–Norwegian trade restrictions were, indeed, made. The British envoy at Copenhagen, Walter Titley,[4] recommended reprisals on Norwegian timber in 1737,[5] but the Board of Trade advised against it since no substitutes were obtainable from elsewhere.[6] Titley's warning that British trade would fare worse still if firm action was not taken against Danish treaty-infractions[7] proved correct, but diplomatic protests alone made no impression on Denmark.[8] Although Danish treaty-infringements did not lead to trade reprisals, they served as an excuse to deny Denmark most-favoured-nation treatment when it was claimed in 1744 in conformity with the Treaty of 1670 to allow the free carriage of enemy goods enjoyed by Holland under the provisions of her commercial treaty with England.[9] The heavy incidence of Danish prohibitions on British trade in particular, continued to exercise Titley, who complained about them again to no effect shortly before the Seven Years War,[10] and suggestions

[1] 8 Geo. I c. 12.

[2] 3 and 4 Anne c. 10, and 12 Anne c. 9

[3] *R.H.C.*, vol. 15, timber duties (1835), XIX, evidence of W. Parker, pp. 200f., and of H. Warburton, p. 339.

[4] Titley was envoy to Denmark–Norway from 1730 until his death in 1768, and was only assisted during the last years of his life by others. A short biography of Titley is given in *D.N.B.*, vol. 56, pp. 419f., and notes on his career in J. F. Chance (ed.), *British Diplomatic Instructions, Denmark 1689–1789* (London, 1926), [cit. *Diplomatic Instructions, Denmark*], p. 89.

[5] *Diplomatic Instructions, Denmark*, pp. 112ff., Harrington to Titley, 2 August and 14 October 1737 [O.S.].

[6] P.R.O., S.R. 44/129, Harrington to Board of Trade, 14 October 1737 (O.S.), and S.P. 75/137, Board of Trade to Harrington, 4 December 1737 [O.S.].

[7] P.R.O., S.P. 75/137, Board of Trade to Harrington (citing Titley), 17 December 1736 [O.S.].

[8] P.R.O., S.P. 75/137, Memorial of Board of Trade for transmission to Titley, 13 May 1737 [O.S.].

[9] P.R.O., S.P. 100/1, Board of Trade to Carteret, 20 September 1744 [O.S.].

[10] P.R.O., S.P. 75/96, Titley to Newcastle, 13 May and 26 May 1753.

of trade reprisals were made again after the War, echoing earlier advice which still had not been taken.[1] Danish–Norwegian, like Swedish goods, therefore entered Britain without undue hindrance and remained major articles of trade in sharp contrast to the diminishing importance of British merchandise in the Scandinavian market.

[1] P.R.O., O. 388/95, Cosby [minister-resident, assistant to Titley] to Pownal [Secretary, Board of Trade] 16 March 1765; and B.M., Egerton MS 2696, Gunning [minister-resident, assistant to Titley] to Conway [Secretary of State], 4 May 1767.

2 *The Organisation of Trade*

The range of Scandinavian exports through legitimate channels to Great Britain in the middle of the eighteenth century was very narrow. Norway supplied the British market with timber, some iron, small quantities of pitch and tar, and dried fish. Shipments of copper from Norway had ceased after an English company working mines near Bergen went out of operation,[1] but an occasional cargo was still obtained from Sweden which had earlier sent large quantities of copper to England.[2] Swedish exports to Britain were during the 1750s and 1760s very largely of bar-iron, while timber, and pitch and tar, played a lesser role. Imports from Denmark were insignificant, as the country had little to offer besides grain which was sent to Norway, and meat sold to the Continent. Some calf-skins and hides, entered in the customs ledgers as coming from Denmark–Norway,[3] were no doubt of Danish origin, and one may suppose that shipments of hemp and flax during the war years came from the Elbe region, or under coloured papers in Danish ships from the eastern Baltic.

The ports from which produce was shipped were few, as navigation along the broken Scandinavian coast was hazardous to sailing-ships, which had to rely on the services of pilots operating only from some harbours.[4] The northernmost ports open to

[1] W. Beawes, *Lex mercatoria rediviva*, 2nd ed. (London, 1761), p. 827. The company was the Charitable Corporation which was liquidated in the late 1730s. It had the lease of copper-mines at Aardahl, south of Bergen, and after shipping some cargoes to Newcastle in the early 1730s, suspended operations as unprofitable.

[2] H. Hamilton, *The English brass and copper industries to 1800* (London, 1926), pp. 57, 60, 276–7.

[3] The annual accounts of the inspector-general of custom and excise – the customs ledgers – preserved in P.R.O., Cust. 3 and Cust. 14, do not distinguish in the eighteenth century between Denmark and Norway which are listed as a single unit. Requests were made from time to time to separate the accounts for the two countries, but not complied with.

[4] The Norwegian pilotage system in particular was, of necessity, highly developed, and all ships entering or leaving harbour were under compulsion by an edict of 5 March

trade[1] were Trondheim and Bergen, neither of great importance in the trade with Britain. Trondheim exported some timber and fish to the Mediterranean mainly in Scottish bottoms,[2] and a rather insignificant direct trade with Scotland was also carried on. The town itself, moreover, was small and its commercial life underdeveloped. A contemporary trader found little more to say of it than that it possessed a fine cathedral, and exported some good quality deals.[3] While the commerce of Trondheim was dominated by Scottish shippers and merchants, that of Bergen remained throughout the century under the domination of the Dutch. Its trade in the middle of the century was with Holland, the Mediterranean, and the Baltic, exports to Britain in 1757 amounting only to 14,000 Kroner.[4] A number of Scottish ships were active in the Bergen trade, taking flour, grain, woollens and coal to the port, and returning with timber.[5] At least some English ships from the East Coast also went as far north as Bergen to take on cargoes of timber and tar.[6] By far the largest share of the English trade belonged to the southern ports serving the great timber region of Christiania and Christian-

---

1725 (Dan. S. Arch., Kongl. Forordninger) to employ a pilot. The system itself is described by Beawes, *Lex mercatoria*, pp. 829–32.

[1] The province of Finmarken beyond Trondheim in northern Norway was a prohibited area in which trade was only permitted under royal licence not obtainable for foreign imports and exports. See A. Raested, *La mer territoriale – études historiques et juridiques* (Paris, 1913), pp. 131f.

[2] E. Holm, *Danmark–Norges Historie under Frederik V, 1746–1766* (Copenhagen, 1898) vol. 3, pt 2, p. 264.

[3] A description of commercial life in Norway at the middle of the century was given by a Mr R. Norcliffe, of Hull, to W. Beawes who acknowledged the contribution (p. vi) to his work, cited above. The note on Trondheim is in Beawes, *Lex mercatoria*, p. 828.

[4] Holm, *Danmark–Norges Historie*, p. 259. The Krone (crown) stood at that time at five to the Pound at par. Cf. Beawes, *Lex mercatoria*, p. 828, that the Bergen trade had 'decay'd'.

[5] Norw. S. Arch., Bergen Toldbøger, 1756 I, entries 37 and 76, *Margrath and Arbroath* with coal; entries 950 and 1105, cargo of woollens and cottons; entries 56 and 123, *James and Catherine*, woollens and cottons. *Ibid.*, 1760 I, entries 23 and 43, *Good Intent*, cargo of Scots flour [oatmeal?]; entries 26 and 44, *Mitchel and Polly*, cargo of wheatmeal and oatmeal. *Ibid.*, 1763 I, entries 131 and 151, *Agnes and Jannet*, cargo of woollens. All these ships returned to Scotland with timber.

[6] Custom House, King's Lynn: tally books, timber tally for ship *John and Mary*, John Philips master, 1754; and timber tally for English ship, from North Bergen (the prefix was employed to distinguish between Bergen in Norway and Bergen-op-Zoom in the Netherlands) with timber and a few barrels of tar, 1749. The name of the ship and its master are illegible, but it is stated to be 'of Lynn'.

15

sand[1] in which the saw-milling resources of the country were concentrated.[2] Christiania, the present-day Oslo, was the largest exporter of timber and wood-products, shipping nearly exclusively to England,[3] while the trade of the next largest timber-port, Drammen, was shared with Holland.[4] The remaining southern ports, though, were dominated by Anglo-Norwegian commerce. Christiansand relied on England during the middle of the century to buy the timber specially milled in dimensions preferred in the English markets;[5] Tønsberg's saw-milling industry and timber-fleet was expanded during the Seven Years War in response to English demand;[6] Larvik traded mainly with London, and added iron to its exports in the late 1750s;[7] and the smaller ports of Fredrickshald, Porsgrund, Skien, Mandahl and others sought to cut their timber to suit English partiality for certain sizes.[8] The Danish–Norwegian government supported the commerce of several of these towns by allowing them bonding facilities to encourage overseas merchants to trade with them, and by 1750 the larger ports had been granted privileges that tended to attract increasing numbers of English shippers.[9]

Denmark, being prevented from taking most British exports, and having little to offer herself to England, was largely by-passed by British trade, though the passage of the Sound made Elsinore of some consequence to shipping. Every ship passing the Sound in either direction had to heave-to for a customs examination, and

[1] Contemporary place-names are used, eighteenth-century Christiania thus being the same city as the Kristiania of earlier this century, and the Oslo of to-day.

[2] J. Schreiner, 'Det nye sagbruk', in: A. Bugge and S. Steen (eds), *Norsk Kulturhistorie*, vol. 3 (Oslo, 1938), pp. 126f.

[3] E. Bull and V. Sønstevold, *Kristianias Historie* (Oslo, 1936), vol. 3, p. 262: Table of timber shipments for the years 1753 to 1766. The accounts show that nearly all timber from Christiania went to England, no difference to shipments being made by war.

[4] Schreiner, 'Det nye sagbruk', p. 131, and Holm, *Danmark–Norges Historie*, p. 260.

[5] S. Steen, *Kristiansands Historie, 1741–1814* (Oslo, 1941), p. 313.

[6] O. A. Johnsen, *Tønsbergs Historie*, vol. 2 (Oslo, 1934), pp. 470ff.

[7] O. A. Johnsen and others, *Larviks Historie*, vol. 1 (Kristiania, 1923), pp. 312–15, and table, p. 318.

[8] Beawes, *Lex mercatoria*, pp. 828f. Schreiner, 'Det nye sagbruk' pp. 129f., notes that the export of timber cut to sizes preferred by Dutch merchants was discouraged and in some areas the manufacture of such timber was prohibited.

[9] Hans Jensen, *Dansk–Norsk Vekselvirkning i det 18. Aarhundrede* (Copenhagen, 1936), pp. 59–62.

pay dues on its cargo according to a tariff rating the majority of merchandise. Goods not included in the tariff were charged at 1 % *ad valorem* to most-favoured nations, which included Great Britain.[1] Certain fees were paid to the customs officers and translators, to officers of the guard-ship, and to customs clerks, with further charges being levied by the harbour authorities, the total amounting to about twenty Rixdaler[2] beside the duties on merchandise. Disputes over charges were not infrequent, but merchants generally preferred to give in rather than face a long delay to their ships. One such dispute involving a British ship was referred by the English envoy, Titley, to the Danish government. It was over duties on unrated goods, and there is little doubt that the British shipper was in the right. In the end he paid up to prevent a greater loss through being laid-up for too long a time.[3] Duties, fees, and port charges had to be paid in Danish currency which could be bought from dealers at Elsinore who, for a premium, would see to the despatch of the shipment through the customs. Elsinore, having like the Norwegian ports bonding privileges, thus became an important exchange mart and commercial centre for the Baltic trade.[4]

Copenhagen, the larger city, had hardly any share in direct and legitimate British trade. Efforts by the Danish government to make it the principal centre for trade with the Baltic did not have a great effect on English commerce which by-passed the city. Only a few colliers arrived during the year to sail further into the Baltic for a return cargo to England,[5] and some ships called to unload leaf tobacco.[6]

[1] The regulations in force during the 1750s and 1760s are listed in T. A. de Marien, *Tableau des droits et usages de commerce relatifs au passage du Sund* (Copenhagen, 1776). The most-favoured nations at that time, apart from Great Britain, were the Netherlands, Sweden, France, Portugal, Naples and with the exception of some years, Spain. Other nations paid 1¼ % on unrated goods. The tariff is printed in full on pp. 30ff.

[2] *Ibid.*, pp. 66–72. The Rixdaler of Denmark was the equivalent of the Krone of Norway, and like it stood at five to the Pound at par.

[3] P.R.O., S.P. 75/98, Holdernesse to Titley, 25 January 1755, letter and appended memorial on transit dues, and *ibid.*, Titley to Holdernesse, 18 February and 5 April 1755. [4] Marien, *Tableau*, pp. 18f.

[5] J. Schovelin, *Fra den danske Handels Empire*, vol. I (Copenhagen, 1899), pp. 15–18, and cf. a despatch of Titley to Bute of 25 April 1761 (in P.R.O., S.P. 75/112) that Copenhagen was only used by colliers.

[6] P.R.O., S.P. 75/118, Cosby to Sandwich, 16 March 1765. Cosby, Titley's assistant, refers in his despatch to the trade of the previous years, and *ibid.*, S.P. 75/96, Titley to Newcastle, 26 May 1753.

The larger Swedish ports, Gothenburg and Stockholm, were in a different position from Copenhagen through their extensive iron-trade. The larger part of Stockholm's iron exports went to England in both Swedish and English ships, and Gothenburg shipped nearly all its iron to English ports.[1] Of the smaller towns, only Öregrund to the north of Stockholm played any role in Anglo-Swedish trade through the export of the finest grade iron from the mines in the district.[2]

The principal British centre for the Scandinavian trade was London, handling in the 1750s and 1760s about one-half of timber imports, and two-fifths of iron imports into England and Scotland.[3] Exports were distributed differently, London and the English and Scottish out-ports sharing the Danish–Norwegian market in about equal proportions, while the Swedish market was mainly supplied by the out-ports.[4] Of those, few, if any, East Coast ports can have failed to be engaged in the Scandinavian trade. Hull merchants dealt with Christiania, Moss and Frederickshald in Norway,[5] with the Swedish iron-ports,[6] and no doubt with other Norwegian ports, and Copenhagen, as well. The trade connection of King's Lynn with Norway has already been noted,[7] Sweden also contributing to the commerce of the port through direct iron shipments.[8] In a petition signed by the 'principal Traders to the Baltick' appear the names of merchants from several East Coast ports – though none from Hull and King's Lynn – from Aberdeen and Dundee, and from Bristol, Leeds and Liverpool.[9] Many of the names are

[1] M. G. Jars, *Voyages métallurgiques* (Paris, 1774), vol. I, p. 157.

[2] *J.H.C.*, vol. XXII, report of committee on manufacture of iron, evidence of A. Spooner, p. 854; and Jars, *Voyages, loc. cit.*

[3] See appendix 1, Figs 2 and 3, and appendix 2, Figs 6 and 7.

[4] See chapter 6.

[5] Nor. S. Arch., Personalia nr 38. a. 2, Thomas Fearnley, Kopibok, ff. 4–8, and 33f.

[6] A. Gatty, *Sheffield past and present*, (Sheffield, 1873), p. 215, and Ashton, *Iron and steel*, p. 246. Both note the strong position of Hull in the Swedish iron-trade.

[7] See above, p. 15, n. 6.

[8] Custom House, King's Lynn: tally books, iron tally, ship *'Lynn'*, Henry Hood master, with iron from Stockholm. The date is illegible, but evidence points to the 1750s.

[9] P.R.O., C.O. 388/54, ff. 29–30, petition in favour of granting the British consul at Elsinore a fee on ships passing the Sound, London 14 March 1766. Further evidence on the trade of Bristol and Liverpool with Norway is found in tables of timber shipments from Larvik, printed in Johnsen, *Larviks Historie*, p. 318. Such shipments

known also in the Norway trade, and the Swedish iron-trade. Liverpool in particular was a favoured West Coast centre of the trade with Scandinavia as the salt-works in its neighbourhood furnished return cargoes for ships bringing timber and iron.[1] The many British ports serving the Scandinavian trade suffered in one respect, though, when compared with ports in Denmark, Norway, and Sweden. Merchants in the latter were able to put most British imports into bonded warehouses and thereby escape payments of duty on re-exportation, or defer customs payment on goods for home consumption until bond was broken. No such facilities existed in British ports for Scandinavian merchandise until the beginning of the nineteenth century, but this inconvenience does not appear to have deterred importers.[2]

Government showed some concern over the Anglo-Scandinavian trade when giving instructions to envoys to report on trade conditions, to assist commerce and to safeguard the rights of merchants of their own nation. Walter Titley at Copenhagen[3] took these duties seriously enough, and even went so far as to present the king of Denmark and his court with barrels of the best salt herrings to obtain their patronage for the newly opened British herring fisheries. The king was appreciative enough of the gift, though Titley's enterprise must have struck him rather as the equivalent of carrying coals to Newcastle.[4] Needless to say, herring did not become an article of export to Denmark as Titley had hoped, since the Danish catch alone was more than sufficient for her requirements. There is no further record of Titley's attempting to promote British exports by such direct means, but he remained active in protesting

were, however, exceptional, most cargoes being consigned to London and the East Coast.

[1] *J.H.C.*, vol. xxv, pp. 1034f., report on petition of merchants in the salt-trade, 7 March 1749–50 [O.S.], evidence of John Hardman of Liverpool.

[2] W. Vaughan, *Tracts of docks and commerce* (London, 1839), pp. 31 and 36.

[3] *Diplomatic Instructions, Denmark*, pp. 89f., instructions to Titley; and p. 5, general instructions. To these was added a standing order of 1715 to report annually to the Board of Trade. The order was in fact not acted on again until 1765.

[4] P.R.O., S.P. 75/94, Titley to Newcastle, 4 May 1751 [N.S.], and enclosure; and *ibid.*, 24 July 1751 [N.S.]. Titley's concern over establishing a market for British herring in Denmark which exported some herring herself, would show him to have been rather naive in commercial affairs, an impression borne out by other instances.

against infringements of treaty stipulations granting British merchandise free access to the Danish–Norwegian market,[1] and in interceding for merchants in difficulties with the authorities.[2] Titley was rather hampered, though, in his well-meant efforts to further British trade, by his conception of an envoy's proper position which did not allow him to make acquaintances among the merchant class.[3] Lacking any first-hand knowledge of commerce, and unwilling to meet people on whose experience he could have drawn, Titley may not have been the best person to smooth the way for British trade by negotiation with Danish ministers, or through advice to his government.

England had appointed no envoy to Sweden between the recall of Colonel Guy Dickens in 1748, and the appointment of Sir John Goodricke in 1758.[4] Goodricke's early career is something of a mystery. He is not mentioned in the *Dictionary of National Biography*, and has found no biographer. Some light on his career before he was appointed to the Swedish legation has been thrown by a letter he wrote from The Hague in 1757 to an acquaintance in London, asking him to speak on his behalf to Pitt: 'You are able to inform him that, having been appointed His Majesty's Resident Minister in Brussels in the year 1750, I came over to this country to instruct myself in the affairs of the Barrier and of the Trade to the Austrian

[1] P.R.O., S.P. 75/96, Titley to Newcastle, 12 May 1753, advising that he had been able to prevent the imposition of further import-prohibitions on British produce into Norway. *Ibid.*, S.P. 75/109, Titley to Holdernesse, 29 March and 8 April 1760, ineffectual protests over import-prohibition on glass which had been a valuable export article.

[2] Dan. S. Arch., T.K.U.A., Engl. A. II, 30, Titley to Bernstorff, 25 April 1755, and Bernstorff to Titley, undated draft reply, unsuccessful attempt by Titley to have taxes on a British merchant in Copenhagen remitted. P.R.O., S.P. 75/98, Titley to Holdernesse, 5 April 1755, report on intercession on behalf of British shipper in difficulties over Sound payments. *Ibid.*, S.P. 75/100, Titley to Holdernesse, 17 February 1756, intercession on behalf of British merchant at Elsinore who had gone bankrupt.

[3] P.R.O., S.P. 75/114, Grenville to Titley, 5 October 1762, asking that every courtesy be shown to an English merchant in Copenhagen. By reply of 23 October 1762, Titley advised Grenville that he had not thought it in keeping with his position as envoy to know members of the merchant community.

[4] Notes on the official career of Guy Dickens and Goodricke are in *Diplomatic Instructions, Sweden II*, pp. 89, 129 and 133. The appointment of Robert Campbell as minister-resident in 1757 was conditional on his credentials being accepted at the Swedish court. They were not, and he was therefore never minister-resident.

Netherlands; that this Employment was taken from me by a Dark Intrigue.' Goodricke went on to say that he had obtained no other appointment even after Newcastle in 1752 had asked him to remain in Holland and confer with the Dutch ministers on 'the Barrier etc.' He had stayed at The Hague for two years without salary although the British envoy, Colonel Yorke, had been sympathetic and helpful, and now wanted him to be appointed secretary to the legation.[1] Goodricke, so it appears, had some experience as a diplomat unlike his intended predecessor, Colonel Robert Campbell, whose mission to Stockholm in 1757 was a complete fiasco and ended in his being told to return home. Goodricke also had the unusual distinction for a diplomat of the time of having made a particular study of commercial affairs. The government was sufficiently impressed by him to appoint him to the potentially quite important Swedish post. When Goodricke, however, reached Copenhagen on his way to Stockholm, he was informed by the Swedish envoy to Denmark that he would not be allowed to enter Sweden. He therefore spent the remaining war years in Copenhagen on instructions from the government while retaining his commission as minister-resident to the court at Stockholm. His interest in commercial matters was great, and he set himself to meeting merchants and transmitting their views on trade to London. But, having no official position in Denmark and being cut off from Sweden, Goodricke could do little for them, particularly as he was on bad terms with Titley.[2] He was reduced to writing despatches on trade, of which, it would appear, little notice was taken.[3]

Sweden herself retained in London until 1758 a secretary of legation, Arnold Wynantz, as chargé d'affaires.[4] He had connections

---

[1] P.R.O., Chatham papers, 30/8, vol. 33, letter of 25 January 1757 to G. F. Lane.

[2] P.R.O., S.P. 75/106, Titley to Holderness, 13 November 1759. Titley asked the Northern Secretary in this despatch that either Goodricke with whom he could not get on should be removed from Copenhagen, or that Titley himself should be allowed to retire.

[3] A series of these despatches is in P.R.O., S.P. 75/115, Goodricke to Halifax, 26 February, 8 March, 30 July and 23 August 1763, dealing with herring fisheries, the coal, leather and iron trades, shipping, and smuggling. None received any acknowledgment, and there is no record of these despatches having been passed on to the Board of Trade.

[4] Wynantz, like Goodricke, has not found his way into reference works. He himself listed his appointments in a letter asking for a higher salary, showing that he had

in the commercial world through a relative of the same name who was a considerable London merchant,[1] and had dealings with a Swedish house of iron-importers and financiers in the City.[2] Wynantz reported regularly on trade directly to those Swedish government departments which would have been most interested in his information, and exerted himself to prevent any obstacle being put into the way of the iron-trade.[3] Wynantz was not alone in acting on behalf of Swedish merchants in England. Greater services may have been given them by a political refugee from Sweden, Christoffer Springer, who had earlier worked in Stockholm in the British interest.[4] He became a pensioner of Newcastle's after finding his way to London in 1754[5] and, much to Wynantz's annoyance, was on friendly terms with English merchants and cabinet ministers who, Wynantz suspected, took greater notice of Springer's intercessions than of his own.[6] Springer kept in touch with merchants in Sweden,[7] was visited by them when they travelled in England,[8] and is reputed to have acted as the spokesman of the

been employed in government service since youth: Swed. S. Arch., Diplomatica, Anglica I, Wynantz to Kanslipresidenten, 13 April 1756.

[1] Francis Wynantz was a signatory to a petition of Baltic merchants, in P.R.O., C.O. 388/54, f. 30; and see Heckscher, *Sveriges ekonomiska historia*, II, 1, p. 402.

[2] Swed. S. Arch., Diplomatica, Anglica I, Brev. till W. från Kanslikollegium o. a. ämbetsverk, Kommerskollegium to Wynantz, 9 July 1753; and *ibid.*, Wynantz's koncept, volume for year 1757, undated draft replies acknowledging commercial information given by the firm of Spalding and Brander.

[3] *Ibid.*, Diplomatica, Anglica I, Wynantz to Kanslikollegium, which gives a long series of despatches retailing his efforts to prevent any discrimination against Swedish iron during the parliamentary debates on the iron-trade in 1756 and 1757. See despatches of 11 and 25 February and 23 November 1756; 4, 18 and 25 March, 5 and 22 April and 3 May 1757.

[4] The events leading to Springer's flight from Stockholm are given in E. R. Adair, *The Exterritoriality of ambassadors in the sixteenth and seventeenth centuries* (London, 1929, p. 225).

[5] Payments to Springer from the secret service funds are listed in Sir Lewis Namier, *The structure of politics at the accession of George III* (London, 1929), vol. 2, pp. 537ff.

[6] Swed. S. Arch., Diplomatica, Anglica I, Wynantz to Kanslipresidenten, 1 July 1757. Wynantz was particularly chagrined over the influence which he attributed to Springer over ministers.

[7] *Ibid.*, Kanslipresidenten to Wynantz, 27 May 1757. Complaints are made in this letter that Springer corresponded with Stockholm, and was taking too great a part in trade matters in London.

[8] The popularity enjoyed by Springer among Swedish merchants in London is noted in S. Rydberg, *Svenska studieresor till England under frihetstiden* (Uppsala, 1951), pp. 98f. and *passim*.

Swedish colony in London in the absence of an official representative after Wynantz's recall in 1758.[1]

Of the two successive Danish envoys to England during the mid-century, the first, Count Rantzau, who stayed in London from 1754 until 1757, took little interest in commercial affairs. After his recall at the request of Holdernesse, with whom Rantzau had quarrelled, Danish trade was given every assistance by Count Bothmer who took Rantzau's place. Bothmer got on well with members of the cabinet, and was able to persuade Newcastle on more than one occasion to have proceedings dropped against Danish–Norwegian shippers transgressing English customs regulations.[2] He used every means to acquire a knowledge of the Anglo-Danish trade, even taking on to the legation staff a young merchant who had made a special study of it, to act as a commercial secretary.[3] Bothmer's own acquaintances among Danish merchants in London, and English merchants in the Danish–Norwegian trade, were many. The Danish-born financier and writer on economic subjects, Nicholas Magens, was a confidant and helped Bothmer to allay fears on the bourse over Danish credit.[4] An English merchant, Nicholas Tuite, whose interests were in the West Indian and Mediterranean trade as well as in the sugar-trade with Denmark, advised Bothmer on ways to advance the legitimate and the smug-

---

[1] This information is given in the biographical note on Springer in *Biographisk lexicon öfver namnkunnige svenska män*, vol. 15, pp. 199f.

[2] Reporting on the case of a Norwegian ship in which tea was discovered by customs officers, Bothmer remarked that he would see Newcastle about obtaining the release of the vessel. Newcastle had often obliged in the past in similar cases. Dan. S. Arch., T.K.U.A., Engl. B, 110, Bothmer to Bernstorff, 16 September 1760.

[3] Bothmer explained in private letter to Bernstorff that he could not find the time to give all the trade intelligence which he thought necessary, and would therefore employ an experienced man recommended to him by a Danish merchant to gather commercial news affecting Denmark and Norway. In Dan. S. Arch., T.K.U.A., Engl. B, 109, 29 December 1758.

[4] Arrangements with Magens to co-operate with Bothmer are recorded in a despatch of 1759 in Dan. S. Arch., T.K.U.A., Engl. B, 109, 17 April 1959. The prominent position of Magens in financial affairs is noted by Namier, *Structure of politics*, vol. 1, pp. 67, 69, 235 n. 3, 235 and 237. Namier was mistaken in believing that Magens was of Dutch or German origin. A deed by which he arranged for a scholarship for a boy from his native Danish village is in Dan. S. Arch., T.K.U.A., Engl. C, 264, under date of 30 April 1751, together with a dry note by Bernstorff that too many boys were already being sent to university, and the money could be spent to better purpose. Several works by Magens used in this book are cited in the bibliography.

gling trade of the Danish colonies with England,[1] and the firm of Cottin & Co. kept him informed on likely openings for Danish shipping in English ports.[2] Such sources of information enabled Bothmer to make detailed proposals for extending Anglo-Danish commercial relations, which appear to have been acted upon. One of these proposals was that Danish merchants should buy English cloth for export to the Levant where English trade was in decline due to the Seven Years War, and another was a detailed exposition of the working of the exchange course between Copenhagen and London, with suggestions on its improvement.[3]

Anglo-Scandinavian commercial relations were further affected by the illegal activities of members of the Swedish and Danish legations. Industry in Scandinavia was anxious to obtain the services of English craftsmen, whose skill and knowledge of trade secrets was to help in building or improving manufactures intended to make the Scandinavian countries at least independent of British imports. Laws against the 'enticing' of workers out of the country were disregarded, many were induced to take work overseas, and others were kidnapped. It was no accident that the importation of glass into Norway was prohibited within a few years of numbers of English glass-workers settling there with the encouragement of the Danish government.[4]

Envoys were meant to be assisted by consuls in promoting trade and in safeguarding the rights of their nationals, particularly seamen and merchants. There were, however, few consuls at the time, and those few were generally appointed in the outports. Bernstorff, for

[1] Relations between Bothmer and Tuite (this is the signature he came to use, earlier ones being Tweed and Tuit), and Tuite's activities can be followed from documents and letters in Dan. S. Arch., T.K.U.A., Engl. B, 107, Bothmer to Bernstorff, 2 December 1757; *ibid.*, 110, Bothmer to Bernstorff, 7 November 1760; *ibid.*, Engl. A. II, 30, Tuite to Isselin & Co. of Copenhagen, 1 June 1759; and *ibid.*, Danske Kancelli, Indlaeg til Vestindiske Sager, memorial of Tuite dated Copenhagen 12 July 1754 with appended letter of Commerce Collegium to Count Holstein, 23 August 1754.
[2] Despatch in *ibid.*, T.K.U.A., Engl. B, 113, Bothmer to Bernstorff, 21 December 1764.
[3] Dan. S. Arch., T.K.U.A., Engl. B, 112, Bothmer to Bernstorff, 26 April 1763, and 109, Bothmer to Bernstorff, 13 July 1759. For the probable effect of Bothmer's suggestions, see below, ch. 7, pp. 128–9.
[4] See appendix 5 for a description of the traffic in skilled craftsmen.

382.0942   K415w

c. 1

example, when being petitioned by a Danish merchant for a
consulship in London, thought it unnecessary for a consul to be
stationed in a capital where an envoy was already expected to be
looking after commercial affairs.[1] A few years later Bernstorff did
appoint a consul in London, but that consul happened to be a very
prominent London financier and merchant who could be of service
to Denmark–Norway in a number of ways.[2] Britain was equally
sparing in her appointment of consuls in Scandinavia until late in
the century, but the importance of the Sound to British shipping
made an exception and had early led to the stationing of a consul at
Elsinore. Titley especially wrote a memorial on the consulship
at Elsinore, stating that 'the Commerce of Great Britain in the
Baltick could very hardly, if at all, be carried on, without the
assistance of some such Publick Officer, as the King's Consul at
Elsenore; who not only watches over that Trade and asserts the
Rights and Privileges obtained by Treaty for His Majesty's Subjects,
but, in order to facilitate the Passage of the ships bound upwards
[into the Baltic], is Himself engaged to the Danish Custom-House
for the payment of the Sound-Duty on Their Behalf'.[3] On the
death of consul Tigh in 1752, Titley therefore asked that his place
be filled immediately, and recommended for the post an English
merchant, Nicholas Fenwick, who, unlike his brother and partner
in their Elsinore firm, was unmarried and therefore 'free (and I hope
will remain so) from all Connections, that might possibly biass
Him in the Execution of that Office'.[4] Fenwick was duly appointed,
and later also employed by the Russia Company to send it lists of all
ships passing the Sound.[5] Masters of British ships were expected
to call on Fenwick with their passports or other papers, and ask his

---

[1] Dan. S. Arch., T.K.U.A., Engl. B, 106, Rantzau to Bernstorff, 1 June 1756.

[2] See below, pp. 29–30.

[3] P.R.O., S.P. 75/96, memorial dated 21 February 1753. Titley, incidentally, was
mistaken in believing, as it would seem, that only a British consul could clear British
ships. Masters were in fact free to make their own arrangements for clearance through
the Sound.

[4] P.R.O., S.P. 75/96, Titley to Newcastle, 25 January 1752 [N.S.]. Titley also mentioned
that Fenwick had assisted Tigh for several years.

[5] Cambridge U.L., Russia Company, Minutes, 1756–78, p. 32, entry of 21 February
1758, and see B.M., Egerton MS. 2694, Fenwick to Titley, 14 July 1754 on Fenwick's
connection with the Russia Company.

25

assistance when necessary.[1] It was understood that for a customary commission, the consul would clear vessels of his nation through the Sound and stand surety for the payment of Sound duties when they were deferred until the return voyage. Fenwick, although he kept his appointment till the 1780s, soon turned out to be unsuitable for the consulship. He went bankrupt, the Sound authorities refused at one time to accept his bond for the payment of duties on ships cleared by him, he quarrelled with the governor of Elsinore who would no longer assist after that quarrel in helping Fenwick to apprehend absconding sailors, and it can have come as no surprise that masters of British ships preferred getting clearance from the French consul, a source of much complaint by Fenwick who pointed out both his loss of income and the dangers to British shipping in war through the French obtaining useful intelligence.[2] Although Fenwick's assistance to shippers in the Swedish trade can only have been slight, he was of some help to merchants by keeping the Admiralty informed on convoys and on the movements of Gothenburg-based French privateers during the Seven Years War.[3]

The only other British consul in Scandinavia at the time was at Bergen. His appointment, the first in Norway, had also been made on the recommendation of Titley despite the objections of Norway merchants who saw no point in having a British consul where their trade was small, and who also feared that consulage fees would be asked of them.[4] In the event, the consul appointed,

[1] Commission to Fenwick dated 19 February 1752, in P.R.O., F.O. 90/9, ff. 30–3. The customary procedure for clearing ships at the Sound is given in S.P. 75/114, Titley to Bute, 22 May 1762 and enclosed letter of Bernstorff to Titley, 4 May 1762.

[2] P.R.O., S.P. 75/100, Titley to Holdernesse, 17 February 1756, reporting Fenwick's bankruptcy and refusal of Sound authorities to accept his bond. *Ibid.*, S.P. 44/139, Titley to Bute, 4 August 1761, and appended papers, referring to difficulties over deserting sailors. Dan. S. Arch., T.K.U.A., Engl. A. II, 30, Titley to Bernstorff, 27 August 1763, dealing with renewed payment difficulties. P.R.O., S.P. 75/98, Titley to Holdernesse, 10 June 1755 and S.P. 75/114, Titley to Bute 22 May 1762, reporting Fenwick's complaints that the French consul and others were clearing British ships.

[3] P.R.O., Ad. 1/3833, Fenwick to Cleveland (Secretary, Admiralty), 12 June and 3 July 1756; Ad. 1/3834, as above, 21 June 1757, 24 October and 9 December 1758; Ad. 1/3835, as above, 8 September, 30 June and 11 August 1759. These are intelligence reports on privateers, convoys, and movements of Danish ships suspected of carrying contraband.

[4] For his commission, dated 9 November 1744, see P.R.O., F.O. 90/8. Reference to his appointment on Titley's recommendation is in *ibid.*, S.P. 44/129, Carteret to

Alexander Wallace, a prominent Norwegian-born merchant of
Scottish parentage and education, proved to be of the greatest
assistance to shipping during the Seven Years War. He looked
after crews from British vessels which had been taken prize and
brought into Norwegian harbours, advanced them money to prevent
them from signing-on in foreign ships, and eventually sent them
back to England.[1] He also interceded for the release of the ships
themselves, reported their capture, gave assistance to British warships off the Norwegian coast, and, with the help of deputies in other
ports, kept the Admiralty very fully informed on French privateers.[2]

There was no British consul in Sweden, nor a Swedish in England,
until later in the century.[3] Denmark, however, gave during the
mid-century several consular commissions to merchants in England,
the Channel Islands, and Scotland. The first to be appointed was
one Bernard Falck in 1750, son of a retired Danish naval officer at
Falmouth. He stated in his application for a consulship that he
was a Danish citizen, had once assisted a ship-wrecked Danish
vessel in the Channel, stressed the services to the Crown by his
father, and added that he could be of help in victualling Danish
West Indiamen and obtaining cargoes for them. The Danish board
of trade advised at the time against his appointment as there was
hardly any Danish traffic through the Channel, but the West India
Company supported it, and it was pointed out that the son of a
distinguished officer ought to be provided for. The increase in
Danish shipping during the Seven Years War to the West Indies
and the Mediterranean, and also to the English West Coast, may
have subsequently justified a consular office at Falmouth. In any
case, Falck's commission was extended in 1763 to the Bristol area.[4]

Board of Trade, 14 September 1744 [O.S.]. Advice of merchants on consul in Bergen
ibid., S.P. 95/133, Board of Trade to Chesterfield, 11 December 1746 [O.S.].
[1] A biographical note on Wallace is in W. H. Christie, *Genealogiske Optegnelser om
Slaegten Christie i Norge 1650–1890* (Bergen, 1909), p. 16. Wallace's services to
British sailors may be inferred from his accounts for payment of expenses in P.R.O.,
S.P. 75/137, Wallace to Suffolk, 27 August 1776, and appended papers.
[2] His activities are detailed in P.R.O., S.P. 109/72, Wallace to Bute, 2 June 1761;
S.P. 75/112, memorial to Bute, 5 May 1761; Ad. 1/3834, Wallace to Cleveland,
21 September 1757; Ad. 1/3836, as above, 1 September, 13 June and 5 May 1761.
[3] But see K. Samuelsson, *De stora köpinanshusen i Stockholm, 1730–1815*, (Stockholm,
1951), p.47, on earlier Swedish consular activities in London.
[4] Dan. S. Arch., T.K.U.A., Engl. A. II, 31 *b*, Commertz-Collegium to Count Schulin,
Copenhagen, 28 February 1750, application of Falck with endorsements by various

Despite all his efforts to be appointed, Falck seems never to have been formally accepted as consul by the British customs or other authorities. Neither he himself nor the Danish envoy in London at any time sought an approbation of his patent or appointment from one of the Secretaries of State, and that had become necessary by the mid-century before a foreign consul was accepted and confirmed in what few privileges he had. He may simply have been quite content to collect consulage fees from any Danish–Norwegian ships which ran into harbours in his consular area, relying for his authority merely on his Danish commission. It is always possible, though, that the Falmouth and later also Bristol customs authorities knew nothing of such recent regulations as approbations for consuls and allowed Falck his largely nominal privileges while Falck in turn saw no reason to bother a Secretary of State when it seemed unnecessary. The usual lack of communication and co-ordination between government departments in London and provincial offices makes this a quite likely explanation. Falck also seems not to have troubled himself with reports to Copenhagen, and little can therefore be gathered about his activities.

More is known of Isaac Dobrée, appointed consul for the Channel Islands in 1753.[1] He was described as the principal merchant on Guernsey,[2] where he would have been in the best position to watch over the fortunes of Danish and Norwegian ships carrying tea and other East India goods from the Copenhagen sales, to be run from the Channel Islands into England.[3] Dobrée was soon in trouble with the governor of Guernsey who refused to have dealings with him when he attempted to represent the interests of Danish ship-masters, on the grounds that a native of the island, and therefore a British subject, could not be consul for a foreign nation. The

hands, and attached papers from other departments and the West India Company. *Ibid.*, same to same, 20 May 1750, report on Danish shipping in the Channel. *Ibid.*, commission dated 6 June 1750, and re-commissions of 16 and 26 December 1763.

[1] The patent of commission in Dan. S. Arch., T.K.U.A., Engl. C, 274, dated 5 November 1753, is made out for a consulship at Jersey, but elsewhere Dobrée who lived in Guernsey, is referred to as consul for the latter island. His commission no doubt included the other islands as well.

[2] Dan. S. Arch. T.K.U.A., Engl. C, 274, Case by A. Hulme-Campbell on the legal position of Dobrée as consul, dated 26 February 1755.

[3] See below, ch. 7, on the smuggling trade.

matter was referred for legal opinion which held that the law of England had nothing to say on the subject.[1] The silence of the law did not protect Dobrée against the governor and customs officials about whose 'persecution' of him he complained until his death in 1763.[2] He had no successor.

London did not have a Danish Consul until 1759 when a well-known Anglo-Dutch financier, Henry Muylman,[3] was appointed to the position after some competition from other London merchants.[4] Muylman was prominent in the Baltic trade, held one of the four consulships of the Russia Company and was a member of its committee advising the Admiralty on convoys.[5] His instructions on appointment as Danish consul were very comprehensive. He was to report every month on conditions of trade, and was allowed to employ vice-consuls to assist him. All Danish–Norwegian ship-masters coming into London were to present their public papers to him within twenty-four hours of arrival, give a full account of their voyage, and an entry of this advice was to be made into his official ledgers, the consular fee paid by shipmasters to be £1. Disputes between captain and crew, or any Danish subjects, were to come before him, his judgment being legally binding. He should, however, not use his consular office to force anyone to trade with him, and shippers were free to use as agents whom-ever they chose.[6] Muylman had offered to act as consul without

[1] Dan. S. Arch., T.K.U.A., Engl. C, 274, Case by A. Hulme-Campbell, 26 February 1755, and opinion of Geo. Hay, Doctors Commons, 27 February 1755.

[2] *Ibid.*, Dobrée to Rantzau, Guernsey, 21 April 1757; *ibid.*, Engl. C, 264, Bernstorff to Rantzau, 15 March 1757, retailing in detail Dobrée's complaints, asking for redress, and for recognition of consular office by Secretary of State; and Engl. B, 112, Bothmer to Bernstorff, 15 March 1763 on complaints earlier received, and advice on Dobrée's death.

[3] A biographical note on Muylman is given by Namier, *Structure of Politics*, pp. 69f.

[4] Dan. S. Arch., T.K.U.A., Engl. B, 106, Rantzau to Bernstorff, 1 June 1756, reporting on applications for a consulship. Rantzau advised that only a very circum-spect man should be appointed as a consul could too easily make extra work for an envoy by getting into scrapes with the authorities.

[5] Cambridge U.L., Russia Company, Minutes 1756–78, p. 34, election of Henry Muylman into consulship, 1 March 1758, and pp. 37 and 61–2, elections to convoy committee, 1 March 1758 and 1 March 1759. Muylman was one of the signatories to a petition of the 'principal' Baltic traders, in P.R.O., C.O. 388/54, petition of 14 March 1766.

[6] Dan. S. Arch., T.K.U.A., Engl. C, 274, copy of instructions, dated 4 May 59. Muylman's commission is approved and entered in P.R.O., F.O. 90/9, ff. 63–4. The commission is dated at Copenhagen 27 April 1759.

salary,[1] apparently hoping that some business would come his way through his office. He obtained indeed shortly after his appointment the London agency of at least two large Danish firms which had previously dealt with another merchant,[2] but complaints about over-charging lost him the new connections.[3] Muylman resigned as consul in 1764,[4] to be succeeded by a Danish official specially sent from Copenhagen.[5] Whether Muylman did fulfil any of the duties listed in his instructions is a matter for conjecture as his ledgers, if ever they were kept, cannot be found.[6] He certainly was in touch with the Danish envoy, acted as agent and banker for Danish firms, and may have settled cases of dispute between master and crew, though it is unlikely that fellow-merchants of Danish nationality referred disputes among themselves to Muylman. Yet, whatever his official activities, the presence of a consul having official standing, would have had some disciplinary effect and thereby have led to the lessening of possible friction in a port.

Finally, Copenhagen gave on the petition of Norwegian timber-merchants, a consular commission to Christian Mulderup, who had been sent to Scotland to act as the agent of shippers from Christiansand.[7] The request of a commission for their agent was most likely prompted by the knowledge that a consul was em-

[1] Dan. S. Arch., T.K.U.A., Engl. A. II, 31*b*, Bothmer to Bernstorff, 9 April 1759.
[2] *Ibid.*, Engl. B, 109, Bothmer to Bernstorff, 16 October 1759, reporting Muylman, having been charged by the houses of Borré & Fenger, and Wilder, to clear their shipments and handle cases of disputed prize goods, was charging higher commissions than the previous agent of the firms; and *ibid.*, Engl. C, 266, Bernstorff to Bothmer, 15 September 1759 with appended notes, gives more on the affair.
[3] *Ibid.*, Engl. B, 109, Bothmer to Bernstorff, 6 November 1759, that Bothmer had spoken to Muylman who was unrepentant. Enclosed copies of letters from Muylman to Bothmer, and Muylman to Borré & Fenger.
[4] *Ibid.*, Engl. A. II, 31*b*, draft of dismissal at Muylman's own request, 29 June 1764.
[5] The commission of this consul, von Passow, is entered in P.R.O., F.O. 90/10, under dates of 29 June 1764 and 31 October 1764 (approbation).
[6] Danish archivists do not know of their existence, and agree that it is improbable that they ever existed as no regular correspondence, entry-books, or the like from part-time consuls have yet come to light.
[7] Dan. S. Arch., T.K.U.A., Engl. A. II, 316, Commertz-Collegium to Bernstorff, Copenhagen, 8 January 1763, on the request for a commission, and approval; *ibid.*, 17 January 1763, draft commission; *ibid.*, Commertz-Collegium to Bernstorff, 29 March 1763, approving of request that the north of England above Flamborough Head should be included in the consul's jurisdiction, and *ibid.*, new commission dated 23 April 1763. Mulderup's commission and approbation are entered in P.R.O., F.O. 90/8, under date 12 April 1763.

powered to settle disputes between master and crew, and it may also have been thought that a consulship would be an indication to customs authorities and clients of Mulderup's respectability.

Danish–Norwegian and Swedish merchants living in England enjoyed substantially the same rights as merchants of British nationality, suffered from no particular restrictions on their trade in England itself or with their native countries,[1] and obtained justice on equal terms with British subjects. They found it therefore unnecessary to combine into any organisation, such as a factory, to protect their interests against a foreign authority. It was the tendency for Swedish merchants in London[2] to trade with Sweden and to act as agents in England for firms in Stockholm and Gothenburg. One prominent Swedish house in London, Spalding & Brander, kept in close touch with merchants from Sweden travelling to London, assisted their affairs, and acted as agents for firms in Stockholm as well as being financial agents for the Swedish government.[3] Another large firm of the mid-century, Anders & Carl Lindegren, shared with Spalding & Brander a large part of the Swedish commission business in London, and also had bills drawn on them by the Swedish government.[4] The Board of Trade recog-

---

[1] Foreign merchants in England were at the sole disadvantage to English merchants of being charged higher duties when importing some commodities on their own account. See, for example, P.R.O., T. 70/1205, f.A.41, 'Duties payable on some commodities into England', undated, mid-eighteenth century: the duty on Swedish iron in English ships on English account was £2 1s. 6d. and on foreign account £2 3s. 3¾d., less than 5% difference. When imported in foreign ships, the difference was less than 4%. Yet it was still a discrimination against foreigners and would explain why they took out papers of naturalisation as shown by *J.H.C.*, vol. xxv, p. 909, Bill to naturalise Charles Lindegren [a Swedish merchant in London], dated 4 December 1749 [O.S.] and *ibid.*, vol. xxvii, p. 335, Bill to naturalise Jens Pederson [a Norwegian timber-merchant in London], dated 11 December 1755.

[2] No Swedish or Danish–Norwegian merchants can be traced in the out-ports during the mid-century, apart from the Danish consuls in Falmouth and Scotland already noted.

[3] Swed. S. Arch., Diplomatica, Anglica I, Brev till W. från Kanslikollegium o. a. ämbetsverk, Kommerskollegium to Wynantz, 9 July 1753; see also Samuelsson, *De stora köpmanshusen*, p. 47; and Rydberg, *Svenska Studieresor*, pp. 87–91, and *passim*.

[4] Swed. S. Arch., Diplomatica, Anglica I, Brev till W. från Kanslikollegium o. a. ämbetsverk, Krigskollegium to Wynantz, 23 July 1755; *ibid.*, Wynantz' Brev till Kanslikollegium, Wynantz to Kanslikollegium, 15 October 1756, and 20 September 1757; Samuelsson, *De stora köpmanshusen*, pp. 46 and 50; Rydberg, *Svenska studieresor*, pp. 90f., and *passim*. See also B.M., Egerton MS 2694, ff. 272–4, for financial connection of the Lindegrens with the important Stockholm house of C. & C. Grill.

nised their standing in the Swedish trade when calling on both firms in 1765 to give advice on a projected treaty with Sweden.[1] Smaller Swedish merchants in London, like Johan Spieker[2] and Henry Uhthoff,[3] were also active on behalf of principals in Sweden. That they were not necessarily restricting themselves to trade with Sweden is shown by membership of the Russia Company of, for example, Uhthoff.[4] The only advantage of membership could be found when importing from the eastern Baltic, and trade with Russia may therefore be assumed.

The trade of Danish–Norwegian merchants in London presents the same pattern. The most prominent of them, Johan Collet, was a commission agent for timber-merchants in Norway among whom his own family were well represented. On his death in 1759 the business, reputed to have been the largest and financially most influential timber-firm in London, passed to a Dane, Claus Heide, who continued to deal with Norway,[5] and also took on commissions for Danish shippers to the West Indies.[6] Jens Petersen or Pederson, a Norwegian naturalised in England, shared with Collet and Heide the bulk of the Norway timber-trade to London.[7]

To gain better connections in the trade, an English house might send an agent to represent it in Scandinavia. This was done by the Hull firm of Haworth & Stephenson whose agent, Thomas Fearnley, settled in Norway in 1753 and also travelled on occasion for his principals in Sweden. Fearnley established himself by 1759 in

[1] B.M., Add. MS 14035, f. 250, draft letter of Board of Trade, 5 June 1765, to be sent to six merchants noted in the margin.

[2] W. R. Meade: 'Thomas Dunn och Johan Spieker – två engelsk–findländska köpmän', *Finsk Tidskrift*, vol. 149 (January 1951), reprint, pp. 5 ff.; and Rydberg, *Svenska studieresor*, p. 90.

[3] Dan. S. Arch., T.K.U.A., Engl. B, 110, Bothmer to Bernstorff, 25 August 1761, sending advice on Uhthoff; and P.R.O., Court of Bankruptcy, Order Books, B 1/39, ff. 190 *et seq.*, bankruptcy proceedings against Uhthoff.

[4] Cambridge U.L., Russia Company, Minutes, 1734–56, f. 447.

[5] Nor. S. Arch., ser. localia, Larvik, Underdanigst Rapport...angaaende den Norske Traehandel til London, signed F. L. Fabricius, dated London, 6 February 1759, f. 8. See appendix 4 for the complete document in translation. Also, *Norsk Biografisk Leksikon*, vol. 3, pp. 82 ff., s.v. 'Collet'.

[6] P.R.O., S.P. 75/105, memorial by Bothmer on Danish ships which were taken prize, 7 February 1759.

[7] See appendix 4, p. 196.

The Organisation of Trade

Christiania as an independent merchant, exporting timber to England and importing cloth and other English goods.[1] In another instance, an English trader at Drammen corresponded with a Wiltshire cloth-manufacturer, buying his woollens and commissioning him to make up shipments of other merchandise, while selling timber through a Norwegian agent in London.[2]

Nicholas Fenwick's activities as agent for British shipping at the Sound were complemented in Denmark by John and David Brown, Scottish immigrants who had settled in Copenhagen where they imported coal and cloth, and became leading financiers with close English connections.[3]

British merchants in Sweden were no exception to the general rule that merchants settled abroad tended to trade substantially, if not exclusively, with their native country. Their trade was to some extent confined by an edict of 1724 ordering foreigners to import only the produce of their own country, and laying restrictions on foreign shipping.[4] These disabilities ceased, though, with naturalisation which could be obtained after a short residence. Nevertheless, British houses led by merchants long naturalised, traded practically exclusively with England. The largest Stockholm iron-exporters were the partners Jennings and Finlay, both naturalised and ennobled for their services to Sweden.[5] Of their total business, 90% was with England,[6] which the partners visited from time to time to

[1] Nor. S. Arch., ser. Personalia, nr 38, a. 2, Thomas Fearnley, *passim*.

[2] *Ibid.*, ser. Privatarkiver, nr 65, Lauritz Smith, Kopibok 1755–66, accounts with Samuel & Thomas Fludyer of London, 1737–55, and letters to Fludyer of 20 June 1755 and 3 May 1757. See also Namier, *Structure of politics*, vol. 1, p. 157, on the Fludyers who were London financiers and had a cloth-manufactory in Wiltshire. Lauritz [or Lars] Smith's business was carried on after his death by his widow who continued to employ Jens Petersen as her London timber-agent. See appendix 4, p. 196.

[3] P.R.O., S.P. 75/100, Titley to Holdernesse, 17 February 1756, report on John Brown who had applied for the consulship at Elsinore on Fenwick's bankruptcy, and enclosed letter by Brown. Also, *Dansk Biografisk Leksikon*, vol. 4, pp. 191ff., s.v. 'Brown'.

[4] R. G. Modée (ed.), *Utdrag utu alle...publique handlingar* (Stockholm, 1742), vol. 1, p. 575, edict of 10 November 1724, and p. 645, explanatory placat of 26 February 1726.

[5] *Svenska män och kvinnor* (Stockholm, 1942–55), vol. 4, p. 593, s.v. 'Jennings', and vol. 2, p. 518, s.v. 'Finlay'. See also on the Finlay family G. A. Sinclair, 'The Scottish Trader in Sweden', *Scottish Historical Review*, vol. 25, pp. 293f.

[6] Samuelsson, *De stora köpmanshusen*, p. 74 and *passim*.

make trade arrangements.[1] The next largest iron-shippers, the Scottish firm of Tottie in Stockholm,[2] also shipped very largely to England.[3]

English merchants in London and the out-ports had not the same inducement through family or other personal connections to trade with one particular country to the virtual exclusion of others. Yet, with the exception of financiers in the trade,[4] they also specialised very largely in commerce with Scandinavia, rarely venturing further than the eastern Baltic for Russian iron and naval stores. The supply of these materials from America except of tar, was as yet of little consequence, and a potential trade with the colonies attracted few merchants with established connections in Europe. A Norwegian observer of the London iron- and timber-market in the late 1750s who claimed to have met all the Norway merchants and timber dealers, reported only one as having shown an interest in the North American trade.[5] The argument of the time that colonial resources should be developed to the mutual advantage of England and the colonies had its attractions for theorists, and for ironware-manufacturers and timber-users hoping a lowering of prices, but left Baltic and Scandinavia merchants quite unimpressed.

The extinction of the Eastland Company's privileges in the trade with Denmark–Norway and Sweden in the preceding century had broken a formal association of merchants to Scandinavia which was not replaced. Informal associations of importers of Swedish

[1] Finlay was in England in 1750 to receive the freedom of the Russia Company: see Cambridge U.L., Russia Company, minutes, 1734–56, f. 446. Jennings came to London in 1760 to negotiate terms for iron shipments: see P.R.O., S.P. 95/103, 'Wilkinson' [Baron Gedda, a British agent in Stockholm], report of 28 April 1760, and S.P. 75/108, Goodricke to Holdernesse, 10 May 1760. For other visits to England see Rydberg, *Svenska studieresor, passim*.

[2] H. Rosman and A. Munthe, *Släkten Arfwedson: Bilder ut Stockholms Handelshistoria* (Stockholm, 1945), pp. 203ff., gives extensive notes on the personal and business affairs of the Tottie family.

[3] Samuelsson, *De stora köpmanshusen*, pp. 26, 74, 219 and *passim*. Other British merchants noted in Stockholm during the mid-century are Maister and Worster. Their trade was also with England.

[4] See below, ch. 6.

[5] See appendix 4, pp. 196f. This merchant, James Norman, remained in the Norway trade. Members of his family later settled in Norway, and the firm of Norman became by the end of the century the greatest Anglo-Norwegian timber-business in Christiania and London.

iron, and of Norwegian timber continued to exist, and made themselves effectively felt. Evidence from the 1730s shows that English iron-merchants combined to force Swedish exporters to lower their prices, and were successful in their common effort. The Swedish chargé d'affaires who reported on the incident, referred to the close association of iron-merchants,[1] and all the evidence points to such trade and industrial associations continuing to exist in later decades. One may assume that when John Jennings, the leading iron-exporter of Stockholm, came to England in 1760 to negotiate for better prices,[2] his proposals were considered by a group, and not by individual importers. Similarly, London timber-merchants may be shown to have been in close contact with each other. Considering the price of Norwegian timber too high, they informed exporters in 1754 that they would not place orders until it came down. The Norwegians persisted in their demands, and London merchants in consequence sent only a few ships to Norway.[3] Imports into London of deals, the most commonly used timber, dropped that year to 10,000 Hundred from 14,000 in 1753, to recover again to 13,500 in 1755.[4]

Norwegian timber-merchants, like their English correspondents, were in consultation with each other to regulate conditions of trade. A shortage of timber in England in the late 1740s led exporters, particularly from Christiania and Drammen, to raise their prices which were subsequently maintained at a higher level by general agreements of shippers from the principal ports.[5] The leading Swedish iron-merchants also were associated since 1747 through the Iron Bureau (*Jernkontoret*) which by the strictest control over output from mines and works adjusted supplies for the export market to likely demand, with a view to obtaining maximum prices.[6]

---

[1] Swed. S. Arch., Ämnesserier, Handel och Sjöfart, ser. II, Handlingar rörande Utrikeshandel, nr 9, Wasenberg to Cantsly-Collegium, London, 21 March 1738[O.S.].

[2] See preceding page, n. 1.

[3] Nor. S. Arch., Personalia, nr 38, a. 2, Fearnley, ff. 55–73, letters of Fearnley to Haworth & Stephenson [Hull]. Christiania, 9 and 16 March and 8 July 1754.

[4] The figures, rounded off to the nearest 500, are from P.R.O., Cust. 3/53–5, imports from Denmark–Norway to London.

[5] See appendix 4, pp. 194–5.

[6] The functions of the Iron Bureau are described by Heckscher, *Sveriges ekonomiska historia*, II, 1, pp. 501ff. All the leading exporters, as well as smaller ones, were members of the Bureau and subject to its discipline through their ownership or

A 'confederacy' of mine-owners and iron-merchants had already earlier been reported by Guy Dickens.[1]

Combination in some form or other was then usually resorted to by merchants to further their interests as importers or exporters.

The Seven Years War did little to modify the general order of Anglo-Scandinavian trade except through its effect on the organisation of shipping. French privateers in the North Sea did their best to capture English ships bound for Scandinavia or other ports, though they did not interfere with Danish–Norwegian and Swedish ships carrying their countries' own produce, so long as it was not contraband. The threat to shipping led to the inauguration of convoys as far as the Sound. The Baltic itself had been declared neutral in a Danish–Swedish convention[2] and was therefore safe for English ships, as Denmark and Sweden were determined to enforce the article relating to the Baltic.[3] Denmark further reasserted in 1756 and 1757 as neutral a four-sea-mile-wide belt along the Danish–Norwegian North Sea coast,[4] and later included by agreement with Sweden the Cattegat within the area in which no hostilities were to be permitted.[5] The Swedish North Sea coast was safeguarded by similar edicts of 1756 and 1758.[6] British war-

holdings in mines and iron works. See also Samuelsson, *De stora köpmanshusen*, pp. 25f. and 99ff. on the interests of Finlay & Jennings, the Totties, Worster, and Maister in iron-mines and works.

[1] P.R.O., S.P. 44/129, Carteret to Board of Trade, 20 April 1744.
[2] The text of the convention, signed on 12 July 1756, is in P.R.O., S.P. 75/101, bound in under date.
[3] The operative article was the third, disclaiming incidentally reprisals in the Baltic against injuries to Danish-Swedish shipping by the belligerents: 'haec tamen Navigatio Baltico in Mari non est suscipienda, utpote quod tutum, estam belli, quam effectuum ejus omnium permanebit immune'.
[4] H. S. K. Kent, 'The Historical Origins of the Three-Mile Limit', *American Journal of International Law*, vol. 48 (1954), 546f. See also Schmidt (ed.), *Rescripter*, vol. 1, pp. 423 and 439, edicts of 7 May 1756 and 13 May 1757.
[5] This Danish-Swedish declaration is in P.R.O., Ad. 1/3825, Fenwick to Cleveland, 11 August 1759. Its effect was none too great as Titley had to complain at Copenhagen about French privateers continuing to be active in the area. Denmark sent a squadron against them which returned, so it was claimed, without having seen a privateer. Titley commented drily in his despatch that the Danes could not have looked very closely. In P.R.O., S.P. 75/106, Titley to Holdernesse, 15 September 1759.
[6] The first edict is bound in under date of 8 March 1756 in P.R.O., Ad. 1/3833, and the second is cited by P. C. Jessup, *Law of territorial waters and maritime jurisdiction* (New York, 1927), pp. 35-7. See also Kent, 'The Three-Mile Limit', *loc. cit.*

ships occasionally patrolled off the Norwegian coast to protect shipping outside these limits as no convoys were assembled except to and from Elsinore.[1] The Sound convoys were arranged for during the sailing season from May till November by the Admiralty in consultation with the Russia Company,[2] and news of their sailing was posted at Lloyd's Coffee-house.[3] The protection of convoys and patrols was not complete, and vessels to and from Scandinavia were taken by privateers.[4] The danger deterred many British ships from staying in the trade, which came to be served largely by Danish–Norwegian and Swedish vessels.[5] The restrictions which both privateers and convoys put on the movements of British ships remaining in the trade were serious. Of vessels to and from the Sound, some at least preferred to run for it rather than be delayed by convoys,[6] and one can only conclude for certain that British shipping was put to great inconvenience and worked under a great disadvantage compared with vessels from the Scandinavian countries.

The most pronounced effect of war on the organisation of Anglo-Scandinavian trade was in fact on shipping. There was

[1] Activities of British warships off Norway are referred to in S.P. 75/106, Titley to Holdernesse, 15 September 1759; and S.P. 110/85, Jenkinson [Secretary, Admiralty] to Captain Stewart, 16 April 1762.

[2] Cambridge U.L., Russia Company, Minutes, 1756–78, ff. 19 *et seq.*, Memorial of Russia Co. to Admiralty, 15 April 1757; *ibid.*, ff. 50 *et seq.*, letters on convoys; *ibid.*, ff. 61–2, election of Russia Co.'s convoy committee to advise Admiralty.

[3] Dan. S. Arch., T.K.U.A., Engl. B, 105, Henneken [secretary of legation in London] to Bernstorff, 19 August 1755.

[4] P.R.O., Ad. 1/3834, Fenwick to Cleveland, 25 June 1757; *ibid.*, Wallace to Cleveland, 21 September 1757; 1 September and 13 June 1761, and others.

[5] See, for the changing proportion of British and Scandinavian ships, appendixes, figs 2, 3, 6 and 7. Some British ships may have been transferred during the war to Scandinavian owners. There is, however, no evidence for it, but some against it, as a French Admiralty order of 1744 which still remained in force during the 1750s and 1760s declared that British-built ships were to be good prize. Scandinavian owners would therefore have been reluctant to buy British vessels. The implications of the French order are noted in J. S. Worm-Müller (ed.), *Den norske sjöfarts historie*, vol. I (Kristiania, 1923), pp. 514f. I discussed the point with Professor O. A. Johnsen in Oslo and was assured that no direct evidence of the transfer of British vessels to Norwegian ownership has been found for the Seven Years War period.

[6] P.R.O., S.P. 75/112, Titley to Bute, 25 April 1761. Titley reported that 'a great number' of colliers had arrived at Copenhagen without convoy. *Ibid.*, Ad. 1/3834, Fenwick to Cleveland, 25 June 1757, reporting that 'many' ships would not sail in convoy because of the great delay. *Ibid.*, Ad. 1/3834, same to same, 9 December 1758, that some thirty out of sixty ships waiting at Elsinore for convoy-escort had run for it.

a very marked deflection of shipping from London to the out-ports. An explanation for it has been given very neatly in title and text by the anonymous author of 'An Essay on the Increase and Decline of Trade in London and the Out-Ports wherein is shown that... all the merchants in the Out-Ports are not clandestine Dealers, and licensed Smugglers, as hath in too general Terms been asserted'.[1] After this revealing title, the author continued his argument on page 31 in the text of the pamphlet that '*all* the Merchants in the Out-Ports do not deserve the odious names of Clandestine Dealers and Licensed Smugglers...If therefore the Out-Ports have *gained* upon London...this ought not to be attributed universally to fraudulent and clandestine Dealings, but, in many of those Ports, to more just and honest Causes [such as] the *Advantages* which several of those Ports enjoyed from their *Situation*, during the late *War*, wherein their ships were not so much exposed to the Enemy, as those were which sailed from London.' This explanation was published in 1749 after the War of the Austrian Succession, but was equally valid after the Seven Years War. The loss of shipping to London was balanced by the increase in shipping to the out-ports, and the out-ports continued to gain a greater relative share of the trade with Scandinavia after the war. For the rest, war brought little change. Envoys and consuls were, with the exception of Wynantz, left undisturbed to do what they could for the commerce of their countries, and actually increased their efforts. War had brought home to all of them the importance of trade, and the increasing amount of economic information in the despatches of envoys as well as the increasing number of consular appointments after the Seven Years War show that this heightened interest in economic affairs was a lasting one. As for the merchants, they carried on as usual, adding perhaps privateering to their ventures, or bringing more ingenuity to their smuggling activities, but above all seeing to it that war diminished neither the volume nor the diversity of the Scandinavia trade.

[1] London, 1749.

3 *The Timber-Trade*

British commercial relations with Denmark–Norway were dominated by the timber-trade in which England had the main share, to the virtual exclusion of Scotland which participated in it only through freighting for the English importer.[1] Scottish imports of Norwegian timber were a fraction of the supplies that reached England, amounting to less than a twentieth in the case of deals which by themselves constituted half the timber shipments to Great Britain, and to even smaller amounts in the case of other types of plank, of masts, and of baulks.[2]

The average annual imports into England of all Danish–Norwegian commodities during the ten-year period 1755 to 1764 were rated at £78,000[3] of which more than four-fifths were accounted for by timber coming from the Norwegian forests, with the possible exception of a few loads from the Elbe valley.[4] Norway was not the only country with extensive timber-stands supplying the British market. The eastern Baltic, that is, the timber regions east of the river Oder, furnished great masts, oak, the valuable Baltic spruce deals used in ship-building, large quantities of barrel-staves, fir baulks, and some fir, or ordinary, deals. Shipments from the

[1] For an account of the timber-trade throughout the century, see H. S. K. Kent, 'The Anglo-Norwegian Timber Trade in the Eighteenth Century', *Economic History Review*, 2nd series, vol. 8 (1956), 62–74.

[2] The average annual imports of deals into England for the period 1755 to 1764 were 25,000 Hundred, and only 1,200 Hundred into Scotland. During the whole ten-year period, Scotland imported only a few dozen masts, and equally small numbers of baulks and planks. Scottish imports are entered in detail in the customs ledgers for Scotland, P.R.O., Cust. 14/1 *a* and 1 *b*, 1755–64.

[3] Annual imports for the years 1755 to 1764, both inclusive, were entered in the customs ledgers for England, P.R.O., Cust. 3/55–64, as having been £74,000; £83,000; £70,000; £85,000; £87,000; £58,500; £78,500; £70,500; £89,000; and £85,000, each figure being rounded off to the nearest 500.

[4] See above, p. 3, for Danish exports to England from the Elbe region. No evidence of timber shipments from the Elbe has been found, but the possibility cannot be excluded as the upper reaches of the river are in a forest region.

American colonies of oak and pine were still small, and of little consequence until later in the century.[1] Fir timber in small quantities was also obtained from the White Sea area, and oak from Germany and from Holland which drew on the Rhenish forests. The supplies from all these sources hardly affected the Norway trade through which England obtained most of her sawn timber and smaller masts.

Sweden was as yet of no importance as a timber-exporter to England. Only the better grades of plank were generally acceptable on the British market, and the Swedish product could not compete with the Norwegian, as saw-milling technique was further advanced in Norway than in Sweden,[2] reflecting on the quality of plank. Sweden had, moreover, lost her best-developed saw-milling areas to Russia through cessions in 1721 and 1743,[3] and the wood cut in the remaining accessible forests had the reputation in England of being unfit for better work.[4] When supplies of satisfactory timber were available, delivery was uncertain, and the Admiralty found during the Seven Years War that it could not obtain Swedish timber which had been contracted for.[5] Norway, favoured by proximity, remained therefore the largest supplier of the most commonly used woods, redwood and whitewood.

Redwood, formerly known in the East Coast ports as red deal,

[1] The American colonies supplied some oak, and fir and pine logs, as well as masts. The first shipments of deals, that is, sawn timber, did not reach England until the mid-1750s, the quantities being very small. See P.R.O., Cust. 3/50–65, and Cust. 14/1 *a* and 1 *b*, for records of timber imports. Further details on colonial shipments of deals are given in *R.H.C.*, vol. 15, timber duties (1835), XIX, pp. 353ff., evidence of H. Warburton on imports in the 1750s and 1760s.

[2] A comparison of accounts of Swedish saw-milling given by Heckscher, *Sveriges ekonomiska historia*, II, 1, pp. 343f., with descriptions of Norwegian practice given by J. Schreiner, 'Det nye sagbruk', pp. 120ff., shows that the thin steel saw-blade which alone gave smoothly-cut planks was introduced into Norway from Holland in the 1710s, and into Sweden not until the late 1730s or early 1740s. Heckscher notes (p. 344) that the installation of thin-bladed saws led to greater exports to England.

[3] Heckscher, *Sveriges ekonomiska historia*, II, 1, p. 346.

[4] *R.H.C.*, vol. 15, timber duties (1835), XIX, pp. 364f., evidence of H. Warburton that Gothenburg deals were 'fit for the rough purposes, both in and out of doors, on account of their durability: but they are not fit for fine joiners' work'. And also, that they were too rigid, knotty, and inclined to warp, and therefore commanded a lower price than Christiania deals.

[5] *R.H.C.*, 1st series, vol. 3 (1771–3), report on supply of naval timber, 1771, p. 17, that 'Offers had been made from Sweden, but the Person who had undertaken to bring the Supply did not perform it'.

and in London and elsewhere as yellow deal,[1] is the timber of the Scots Fir, *pinus sylvestris*. It is more resistant to decay, and thus has a wider range of use than whitewood, *picea excelsa* or the Common Spruce, styled white deal in the timber-trade. Redwood and whitewood were imported both as sawn and as whole timber, the latter being shipped in three main states of manufacture. 'Die-square timber' was generally four- to ten-inches sided, hewn perfectly square, and could be used without further work being expended on it in building construction. 'Flat timber' had the same uses,[2] and, as the name implies, was rectangular in section, hewn to exact measurement, and cut into lengths as required. The third, 'common timber', was the cheapest and generally of white-wood. It was roughly octagonally sided to save shipping-space, and served much as pit-props. The total quantity imported annually remained fairly steady around 20,000 Loads of 50 cubic feet.[3] The average cost per Load landed in England was in the vicinity of £1,[4] and was rising during the war due to higher freight-rates.[5]

Imports of 'timber' or 'fir timber' accounted during the period 1755 to 1763 for about one-sixth at real value of total imports. A far more important class of wood imported was deals, defined by customs regulations as sawn boards up to 3¼ inches in thickness,

---

[1] This regional idiosyncrasy has persisted to the present day, the standard term redwood only being introduced during the last war.

[2] The uses in the eighteenth century of the various sizes of 'timber' and of sawn planks are listed in E. Chambers' *Cyclopaedia*, 1st ed. (London, 1738), vol. 2, s.v. 'Timber', and *R.H.C.*, vol. 15, timber duties (1835), XIX, pp. 50, 55, 91f., 200f., and 364ff.

[3] See appendix 1, Fig. 4.

[4] 'Timber' was rated during the eighteenth century in the customs ledgers, England, P.R.O., Cust. 3, at 14s. to 16s. the load. The rating dated from 1696 when the English series of ledgers commenced, and appears to have been based on then ruling prices, an average for the various grades being struck. The rating in the Scottish series, P.R.O., Cust. 14, was different. The Scottish series commenced in 1755, and all commodities appear to have been rated at prices ruling at that time, 'timber' being rated at 18s. the load. Evidence from other sources suggests that this was on the conservative side for redwood, but a correct assessment of the price for whitewood. (See *R.H.C.*, vol. 15, timber duties (1835), XIX, pp. 403ff., appendix 40.) The inference may be drawn that the 'timber' imported into Scotland was mainly white-wood. See also S. Kjaerheim, 'Norwegian Timber Exports in the Eighteenth Century. A Comparison of Port Books and Private Accounts', *Scandinavian Economic History Review*, vol. 5, no 2 (1957).

[5] See below, p. 193.

from 7 inches to 11 inches in width, and from 8 to 20 feet in length. Boards of narrower width but otherwise same dimensions were styled 'battens', and paid lower duties, and those of a width above 11 inches belonged to the category of 'planks' for which the highest duties were charged.[1] Merchants employed a greater variety of terms, differentiating between grades of quality in deals, and subdividing their dimensions more widely.[2] Norway produced only a negligible quantity of planks, and of them only a few reached England. Battens, though extensively milled in Norway, were not very acceptable on the English market, and the quantity shipped was therefore small.[3]

Duties on deals, as on all other sawn timber, were levied not on cubic measurement, but on the Hundred of 120 pieces irrespective of quality or variations in size. It would therefore have been of advantage to merchants to import the heaviest deals of the highest quality, but in practice this was not possible. The then available, slow-growing Norwegian timber rarely gave deals above 12 to 14 feet long, and the favoured redwood was not as freely obtainable as the lower-quality whitewood.[4] The thickness of deals imported depended on available supplies, and on the prevailing rates of duty and English labour costs. When duties were considered reasonable, as during the middle of the century,[5] and labour costs were high,

[1] Customs regulations and duties on timber are set out in S. Baldwin, *A survey of the British customs* (London, 1770), pt 1, pp. 66ff.

[2] See appendix 4, pp. 191ff.

[3] The quantity of battens imported between 1750 and 1770 was fairly steady at 4,000 Hundred annually. See P.R.O., Cust. 3/50–70, and Cust. 14/1 *a* and 1 *b*.

[4] Thomas Fearnley, the English agent in Norway of a Hull firm, was always anxious to obtain redwood only, which had a better sale in England. See his letters in Nor. S. Arch., Personalia, 38. a. 2., Fearnley [to be cited below as Fearnley papers] to Mr Stromboe, a Norwegian timber merchant, f. 12, dated Frederickshald 10 March 1753; to Haworth & Stephenson of Hull [Fearnley's principals], f. 15, dated Frederickshald 16 July 1757 (*sic* – the date should be 1753); to Stromboe, f. 21, Frederickshald 21 August 1753; and others. English merchants also preferred to obtain the longest possible lengths, but there again, the supply was not equal to the demand: note for example Fearnley to Waddington [an English importer], f. 27, Frederickshald 13 September 1753: 'I had a Lr. from Mr Stromboe of Xtiania, . . . With Assurance of his Utmost endeavours in Providing the desir'd qty. of Long Deals altho' the most in demand from all Parts.'

[5] *R.H.C.*, vol. 15, timber duties (1835), XIX, evidence of H. Warburton, that duties were then considered nominal. Warburton submitted accounts of his firm dating back to the 1750s.

orders were placed for $\frac{1}{2}$-inch deals suitable for walls and pannelling, $1\frac{1}{4}$-inch deals for flooring, and $2\frac{1}{2}$ inches for general joinery work. Heavier deals were 'split', that is, handsawn into thinner boards for particular uses.[1] These might be found in merchantship-building for which red deals were largely required.[2] The Royal Navy also experimented during the Seven Years War with 'fir', that is, redwood-built frigates, as oak, the usual building-material for the hull, was in short supply. The building of all-redwood warships was, however, not continued with as their length of service was short, and costs too high,[3] but Norway red deals were regularly used by the Navy as deckplanking.[4]

The less durable white deals were not suited for any outdoor work, and were mainly used in cheap furniture manufacture, as mining-timber, and in box-making. Their low cost, in which the incidence of duties was felt more heavily than in red deals, may have led to their being imported in the heaviest sizes to be resawn in England.

The only remaining category of timber obtained from Norway in substantial amounts was masts. Few 'great' masts, that is, masts of a diameter above 12 inches, came from the Norwegian forests, but 'middle' and 'small' masts of respectively 8 to 12, and 6 to 8 inches diameter, were obtained in larger quantities than from any other source, to be used in naval construction, and in industry and trade for derricks and hoists. The numbers imported remained

[1] See appendix 4, pp. 191f.

[2] B.M., Add. MS. 38387, ff. 84–5, 'Foreign Articles used in building, and fitting a ship of Eight Hundred Ton'. The specifications called for 200 loads of 'Norway Firr [red] Deals', apart from Norway masts. See also *R.H.C.* (1820), vol. 3, foreign trade, appendix on the timber-trade, p. 14, evidence of E. Solly: That Norway timber had in the past been used extensively in merchantship-building, particularly in ports like Sunderland, Newcastle and Whitby. See also Johan Schreiner, 'Et problem i norsk trelasthandel', *Historisk Tidsskrift* (Oslo), 43 (1964), on the milling of thin boards.

[3] *R.H.C.*, 1st series, vol. 3 (1771–3), report on supply of naval timber, 6 May 1771, p. 17: 'That in the Course of the last year, the Navy have used Fir in the Construction of Ships of 18 Guns, by way of Experiment, and in Order to gain Time; but they do not think it answers, on Account of its Want of Durability; and likewise is more expensive, as the Merchants will not undertake to build a Fir Ship at the same Price they will an Oak Ship'.

[4] R. G. Albion, *Forests and Sea Power – the Timber Problem of the Royal Navy, 1652–1862* (Harvard, 1926), pp. 26–7.

fairly steady between 1750 and 1770 at 2,000–3,000 each of middle and small masts annually, with some fluctuations due to the war's effect on shipping. These figures compared with a few hundred up to a thousand from the East Country and Russia together, and a few hundred annually from the American colonies. Sweden supplied hardly any masts, the numbers never exceeding a few dozen per year.[1] The dependence of the ship-building industry on Norway may be gauged from the specifications of an 800 ton ship which called for 17 New England and Riga masts of from 3 to 7 feet circumference, that is, middle and great masts of approximately 11 to 24 inches diameter, and for 49 'Norway masts' of 1 foot 6 inches to 3 feet circumference,[2] the smaller masts presumably to be used as booms or spars.

How great the dependence of other industries and the domestic building trade on Norwegian timber was, cannot be accurately assessed as no certain quantitative estimate of home supplies is available. Complaints about the deforestation of the English countryside had been frequent since at least Elizabethan days, but it would be rash to argue in the absence of reliable statistics that the growth of manufacture and population was alone responsible for outstripping native supplies for building and industrial uses.[3] The greater suitability of Norwegian wood for building and other purposes,[4] its cheapness due to greater resources and easier accessi-

[1] See appendix 1, table 1.
[2] B.M., Add. MS 38387, ff. 84–5.
[3] The increase in the merchant fleet and the Royal Navy was held responsible for the need to import ship's timber as native supplies were no longer sufficient. See *R.H.C.*, vol. 3 (1771–3), report on supply of naval timber, 6 May 1771, pp. 15f., that imports were imperative because of the large building of merchant- and East Indiamen. As to the Royal Navy, its numbers had been greatly increased in 1745, and 'at the Opening of the War in 1755 the Number and Size still increased; in 1756 the Size of the Ships was considerably increased; insomuch that Seventy Gun Ships, which formerly were about 1,300 Ton, now are increased to 74 Guns and 1,600 Ton; that during the last War there were 50 or 60 ships of the Line built, the least of them carrying 60 Guns.'
  The numbers of East Indiamen built in England in the years 1759 to 1763, both inclusive, are printed in the same report, appendix 5, p. 35. They were 29 ships of over 600 tons.
[4] The reputation which Norway deals enjoyed in the building trade may be noted from later evidence given before the Committee on Timber Duties, *R.H.C.*, vol. 15 (1835), XIX: evidence of William Parker, a former timber-merchant and builder, that houses built by him of Norway timber lasted twice as long without repair as

bility, and the saving in manufacture by mechanical sawing with water-power while handsawing remained the standard English practice – these considerations must all have played their part in the demand for the Norwegian product. The availability of sufficient shipping to bring it to England was assured despite war, and it may well have been found more advantageous to transport such a bulky commodity by water to the English coasts rather than obtain it from inland forests by long road haulage. The Navy, at least, found by the mid-century that supplies of large logs were nearly exhausted within such a distance from the sea as made transport to the dockyards by road or water economical.[1]

The customs accounts of masts imported into England may be assumed to be fairly reliable as masts were entered by number, and their shape made them too prominent and awkward for smuggling. The figures given for timber declared by the Load are more open to suspicion, but can hardly fail to show over a number of years the trends in the import of wood from various sources. It is clear from the customs entries that Norway was during the mid-century the largest supplier of both middle and small masts, and of timber rated by the Load, that is, 'die-square', 'flat' and 'common' timber. There is some difficulty in interpreting the accounts of imports of sawn timber rated by the Hundred, and not by cubic content. Bearing in mind that Norway deals were generally 10 to 14 feet long, and Baltic and White Sea deals 14 to 20 feet, a comparison of import figures modified to allow for differing sizes, still shows that Norway was the largest source of sawn timber, leaving the Baltic, Sweden, and the colonies well behind.[2]

Apart from deals, battens, masts, and 'fir timber', Norway exported to England small quantities of staves, poles, firewood,

others built of colonial timber (pp. 91f.); evidence of George Baker, builder engaged on the British Museum and the National Gallery, that Norway timber was the best (p. 217); and evidence of John Armstrong, carpenter and builder, to the same effect (pp. 220f.). There was no dissenting opinion.

[1] *R.H.C.*, vol. 3 (1771–3), pp. 15f., deposition by naval board witnesses that all 'their Purveyors and Timber Merchants agree, that the large Timber near the Sea Coast, that is to say, within such Distance that the Land and Water Carriage does not exceed 38/- a load, is nearly exhausted'. See also *R.H.C.*, vol. 15 (1835), XIX, pp. 348ff., that the freight per load, counting the Hundred deals at five loads, stood in 1770–1 at about 10*s*. Christiania to London.

[2] See below, appendix 1.

and, according to customs accounts, also some oak. Entries of oak shipments raise the question of fraud and smuggling as its export from Denmark–Norway was prohibited since the seventeenth century. Some oak may have been smuggled aboard English ships which could not be searched after loading,[1] but the records show that oak was nearly always carried in Danish–Norwegian ships, the amounts increasing during the War up to 1,000 Loads annually.[2] It may be assumed that such cargoes did not originate in Norway, but came from the Baltic under coloured papers. Such fraudulent practices are known to have occurred, and in one instance a whole fleet was involved in carrying timber with false invoices. The *Gentleman's Magazine* reported in 1753 that 'Fourteen Danish [sic] ships, laden with wood, have actually been seized at Liverpool; the reason whereof was because it was of the growth of Livonia, and Danish ships act contrary to treaty [i.e., article 7 of the treaty of 1670 which is cited above, p. 3] when they bring other wood into England than the product of their own country.'[3] Accounts of the incident were sent to Copenhagen by the Danish–Norwegian envoy at London, Rosenkrantz, who mentioned in his despatch that the ships had been loaded at Riga with pine-plank consigned to one Thomas Blackburne of Liverpool.[4] Rosenkrantz appealed to Newcastle on instructions from his court for the release of ships and cargoes, adding that salt and tobacco had already been loaded in exchange for the timber. Trade in Baltic timber by Danish–Norwegian shippers, he told Newcastle, had been carried on regularly without molestation for the past 20 years. Newcastle, however, could not intervene this time, and the cargoes, valued at £7,000, were forfeited.[5] This case was not an isolated one. Two more Danish–Norwegian ships were seized the following year in Scotland for carrying Baltic timber under coloured

[1] See above, p. 3. Treaty of 1670, article 9.
[2] P.R.O., Cust. 3/50–70. The entries for some years are given in 'feet', i.e. cubic feet, and have been converted into Loads.
[3] *Gentleman's Magazine*, vol. 23, issue of 31 August 1753, p. 390. It was customary to refer to Norwegian as 'Danish' ships.
[4] A Blackburne of Liverpool, and another of Leeds, signed in 1766 a petition of the 'principal traders to the Baltick'. P.R.O., C.O. 388/54, ff. 29–30.
[5] Dan. S. Arch., T.K.U.A., Engl. B, 103, nos. 212 and 213 with enclosures, and no 271. *Ibid.*, Engl. C, 260, no 95.

papers,[1] and a German ship was believed to have been guilty of the same offence,[2] the various seizures indicating that this evasion of the Navigation Acts was not uncommon.

Not only Baltic, but also some Swedish timber reached England ostensibly as Norwegian produce. It was floated across the frontier to sawmills mainly in the Frederickshald district, and shipped from there.[3] The extent of this traffic was considerable enough to attract the attention of the Danish–Norwegian government which objected to foreign timber being bought on Norwegian account, and attempted to stop this drain of money by an edict in 1745.[4] The attempt was unsuccessful as some years later arrangements were still being made for Swedish timber to be shipped from Norway.[5]

The amount of Swedish and Baltic timber which reached England by this way and came to be entered in the customs accounts as Norwegian produce, cannot be assessed. One may assume, though, that it was not very large as Norway herself had sufficient produce to ship from her own forests, and over-entries on that head credited to Norway were, most likely, more than balanced by under-entries due to straight-out smuggling of Norwegian timber into England. It was, indeed, believed that timber could not be smuggled and was therefore a convenient commodity on which duties might be levied without fear of evasion of payment,[6] but the evidence is against that contemporary view. Thomas Fearnley, the English timber-shipper settled at Christiania, wrote in 1753 to the yard foreman, John Holland, of the Hull timber-merchants Haworth & Stephenson, that he 'shod be glad You wod Consign me a Capt. to Smugle heartily, I'll engage to furnish him with Goods from hence...mind & Clear this Early in the Spring, for depend upon it I'll give you Satisfaction with Norway Deals next year.'[7] Holland,

---

[1] Dan. S. Arch., T.K.U.A., Engl. B, 103, no 229; *ibid.*, Engl. B, 104, no 260 and unnumbered despatch of 12 July 1754; *ibid.*, Engl. C, 260, instructions of 5 February and 19 June 1754.

[2] P.R.O., Court of Exchequer, Rolls, Mich. Term 1753, Middlesex, E 159/600, judgment on John Dixon.

[3] Schreiner, 'Det nye sagbruk', p. 131.

[4] Schmidt (ed.) *Rescripter*, vol. 1, p. 313, rescript of 23 April 1745.

[5] Nor. S. Arch., Fearnley papers, f. 116, letter of 20 April 1766.

[6] *R.H.C.*, vol. 15, timber duties (1835), XIX, p. 358.

[7] Nor. S. Arch., Fearnley papers, f. 33, letter of 20 November 1753.

who was active enough to become an independent importer, would no doubt have taken the hint. Methods of smuggling were noted at about that time by the factor of a large Norwegian landowner who had been sent to London to study means of increasing shipments to England from his employer's sawmills and iron-works. Smuggling timber into London, he reported,[1] was difficult as the customs officers were too knowledgeable. It was therefore better to try it in smaller ports where it could easily be arranged to the mutual satisfaction of shipper and purchaser. The prospective buyer boarded the vessel before she entered harbour and, without being able to inspect the cargo closely, made his purchase on the evidence of the bill of lading. The shipper could therefore within reason assign to the timber better grades than it merited. The deal was concluded on the understanding that part of the cargo would be landed secretly, and duty was then only paid on the rest which was openly unloaded at the wharf in order, presumably, that the purchaser could account for having Norwegian timber in his possession. His saving in duty more than recompensed him for being overcharged for the cargo, and both parties were satisfied.

A further addition to the quantity of Norwegian timber entering England without being recorded in the customs accounts was due to the war policy[2] of bringing up shipments consigned to France or, later, Spain. Such cargoes were not condemned, but to deny their use to the enemy, were bought for the royal dockyards.[3] Diplomatic correspondence on this practice suggests that the quantities affected were considerable,[4] and other correspondence between the Secretaries of State and the Admiralty on complaints from shippers shows further that Norwegian timber-merchants did not intend to lose any money by this forcible diversion of part of their trade.[5] The prices they put on their cargoes were invariably very high.

[1] See appendix 4, p. 193.   [2] See below, pp. 138f.   [3] Acts, 19 Geo. II c. 36.
[4] Dan. S. Arch., T.K.U.A., Engl. B, 109, despatches and appended memoranda of 13 July, 3 August and 28 February 1759.
[5] P.R.O., Ad. 1/4124, letter and enclosure of 30 January 1761; *ibid.*, Ad. 1/4125, letters and enclosures of 20 May, 25 June, 20 and 31 August 1762, and 11 May 1763. The complaints by shippers were about the Admiralty refusing to meet their bills, to which the Admiralty replied that freight charges and timber prices had deliberately been overstated. The Secretaries of State in turn asked that the bills be met to avoid unpleasantness.

The organisation of the timber supplies which reached England by legitimate or illicit means was largely determined by the Norwegian pattern of landownership. The greater part of the forests was owned by small proprietors or communes producing only a few parcels of timber each, and therefore unable to ship directly to the English market without the help of middlemen who assembled stocks at the ports. These middlemen, the Norwegian timber-merchants, in turn dealt with the English importers who rarely had direct correspondence with prime owners able to make up complete cargoes from their own resources.[1] The Norwegian shippers, either timber-merchants or, exceptionally, large land-owners like the Count of Laurvig, had to gain the confidence of their English correspondents in their honesty when fulfilling orders, as no bracking, that is, the grading and stamping of timber by officials, was undertaken in Norway.[2] English timber-merchants tended therefore to place their orders with the better-established Norwegian houses,[3] or to send their own agents to Norway to assemble cargoes.

The direct placing of orders with Norwegian houses led to what was known as the contract system,[4] which operated in favour of the shipper, who bore few risks under it. Contracts for delivery of timber were given by English timber-merchants generally at the beginning of the sailing season in April or May after they had been informed by Norwegian houses of the ruling prices for the year. These prices were agreed upon between themselves by the Norwegian shippers,[5] and were based on advice they had received

[1] Schreiner, 'Det nye sagbruk', p. 131. Schreiner notes that exporters handling the produce of larger estates were generally still dependent on additional supplies from peasant-holdings.

[2] Shipments of unsatisfactory goods could lead to the shipper losing his English customers. One such instance is the subject of complaint by Fearnley in a letter dated Frederickshald, 4 May 1766, in Nor. S. Arch., Fearnley papers, f. 122.

[3] The same few names occur in the Fearnley papers time after time as shippers: Ancher (or Anker), Leuch, Zacharison, Elieson, Vogt, and others.

[4] This was described in great detail by Fabricius whose manuscript report on the timber trade is given in translation as appendix 4. Fabricius' report is confirmed and amplified by the Fearnley papers, cited above. Fearnley, who had gone to Norway as agent of an English firm, made himself independent and became a timber-shipper whose correspondence with English clients illuminates the problems of shipper and importer.

[5] See above, p. 35.

from agents in England on the state of the market and likely demand, on the availability of the various grades of timber in Norway, and on the rate of exchange. The price thus arrived at was quoted f.a.s., that is, free alongside ship. All charges had to be borne by the importer, who chartered Norwegian or English vessels to carry the cargoes ordered and paid the insurances, handling charges, and customs dues both in Norway and England. A fee of customarily 2 to $2\frac{1}{2}\%$ of the total cost was lastly credited to the shipper for his services in assembling and despatching the timber. Prime foreign cost, including export duties of around 20% *ad valorem*,[1] amounted to about two-thirds of total landed cost for a good grade of wood, and to less than half for a poorer quality on which the incidence of freight and import duties fell more heavily.[2] Prime foreign cost remained remarkably steady despite the Seven Years War,[3] as did import duties, fluctuations in the total landed price being due to higher freight charges during the War which rose to nearly double the pre-War level.[4] Freights fell again after the War,[5] but their share in the total landed cost of better-quality wood was not large enough to affect the retail price, which continued at a steady level.[6]

So soon as a cargo which had been contracted for with a Norwegian shipper had been loaded, a bill of exchange was drawn on the purchaser, or, on occasion, part of the amount due might be drawn

---

[1] There is no basis for the statement in V. La Cour, *Mellem Brødre*, p. 66, that a rise in export duties adversely affected timber exports to England by the middle of the century.

[2] See appendix 1, table 3.

[3] See appendix 1, table 2.

[4] See appendix 4, p. 193. 'The rate from Laurvig [Larvik] which used to be 15/- to 17/- has risen since the beginning of the war to an average of £1. 8. 0. Freights are higher from Drammen and Christiania where...loading is more difficult and takes longer.' It may be noted that the distance to the latter ports is longer, and navigation in Oslo Fjord difficult.

[5] Freights from Christiania to London for the Hundred deals of dimensions $12' \times 9'' \times 2\frac{1}{2}''$ stood in 1763 at £2 4s. 8d.; in 1765 at £2 3s. 7d.; and in 1767 at £1 17s. 1d, See *R.H.C.*, vol. 15 (1835), XIX, pp. 348ff.

[6] Retail prices for whole and split deals, wainscot boards and oak laths supplied by two sources to Greenwich Hospital are tabulated in Sir W. Beveridge, *Prices and Wages in England* (London, 1939), vol. 1, pp. 296f., and notes on supply, pp. 282ff. Between 1730 and 1765, prices fluctuated between 1.17s. to 1.25s. for whole deals; between 0.67s. to 0.75s. for split deals; between 3.50s. to 3.75s. for wainscots (which were practically wholly imported from Holland); and between 2.25s. to 2.75s. for oak laths (imported mainly from the Baltic).

by bill when the order was placed.[1] The bill was customarily at two months sight,[2] and for preference payable at London rather than in the out-ports.[3] The rate of exchange on England was unfavourable, ranging from 2% to 4% or 5% when payable at London, with generally an added ¼% on the out-ports.[4] A more favourable rate of exchange with foreign centres would on occasion lead to bills being drawn on them rather than on England. Fearnley, for example, arranged through a Hull firm for credits to be made available with J. A. Crop & Co. of Amsterdam to be drawn on when it should be of advantage, and he used the account for thirty-days bills.[5]

The English timber-merchants – the yard-keepers – who had to meet these bills required considerable capital. Credits to Norway might have to be advanced for a considerable time to maintain satisfactory relations with Norwegian shippers;[6] sawn timber was

---

[1] Nor. S. Arch., Fearnley papers, f. 146, letter to Edw. Smyth, dated Fredericshald 8 July 1766: '[It] being Customary here to pay for deals As soon as the Ship is dispatch^d. Sometimes ½ the Amo^t, is advanced long before the Ship appears.'
  See also appendix 4, p. 189, that payment is 'generally made by bills sent to Norway, otherwise a bill is drawn so soon as the loading is completed'.

[2] Copies of protested bills on England, nearly all at two months sight, are entered in Sjaelland Arch., Notarialprotocoller, 1755–1759, ff. 153, 171, 314, and 394.

[3] Nor. S. Arch., Fearnley papers, f. 184, letter to Holland & Co. [of Hull], dated Fredericshald 15 September 1766: 'Next post shall Make free to Value upon you ...pble. in Londo as bills pble. in Hull are not so Negotiable & by Some Rejected.' *Ibid.*, f. 62, to Jens Korn [of Copenhagen], dated Christiania 4 May 1754: 'English bills drawn According to Custom from hence at 2 Months Sight direct upon Lond. or if they Should be drawn upon Hull Pble. in Lond.'

[4] See appendix 4, p. 194: 'Up till now [1759], the difference in value between Danish [Norwegian] and English money has not been above 3%, English money being of less value in Norway than in England.' Information on higher exchange rates, and on added rates for the outports, is in Nor. S. Arch., Fearnley papers, f. 29, letter to [Haworth & Stephenson of Hull], dated Christiania 13 October 1753, asking that the Hull firm open an account with a London banker on whom Fearnley could draw rather than on Hull to save the firm the added exchange; also ff. 68–9, letter to same, Christiania, 13 June 1754, giving information that exchange rate fluctuated between 3% and 5%.

[5] Nor. S. Arch., Fearnley papers, f. 49, letter to J. A. Crop & Co., dated Christiania 19 January 1754, and f. 57, bill payable at Amsterdam, dated Christiania 16 March 1754.

[6] Nor. S. Arch., Fearnley papers, ff. 42–3, letter to [Haworth & Stephenson], Christiania 6 December 1753, that Norwegian timber-merchants require credit as there is a long interval between their purchasing logs, having them sawn and finally shipping them. *Ibid.*, ff. 25–6, letter to G. Stromboe [of Frederickstad], Fredericshald 11 September 1753, reply to request by Norwegian timber-merchant to draw during

meant to be seasoned for at least eighteen months in the merchant's yard before retailing to prevent it from splitting;[1] and, further, the lack of bonding-docks demanded capital to meet customs payments well before sales could be made. This pressure on the resources of importers led to the gradual disappearance of the contract system under which the merchant–importer had to meet direct payments to the shipper, and its supersession by the agency system.

The agency system[2] was well established by the middle of the century in London, but has not been met with in the out-ports before 1763 when the Christiansand shippers appointed their own agent for Scotland and Northern England.[3] The most prominent London timber-agents during the mid-century were Norwegians of whom Collet, Heide, and Petersen have already been instanced, and one or two Englishmen.[4] Their function was to finance the trade without normally engaging in the sale of timber on their own account. For the customary agent's fee of 2% to $2\frac{1}{2}$% of the total cost of the cargo, the agent advised his principals in Norway of likely demand for timber, found a purchaser, arranged insurance on the cargo in his own name for an additional fee of $\frac{1}{4}$ to $\frac{1}{2}$% of the sum assured,[5] took delivery of the shipment on arrival and directed it to the purchaser's yard. His main function was, though, to advance credit to his principals, or obtain it for them. Credits were given not only to shippers who consigned their cargoes to him, but also to Norwegian merchants who merely used his services to effect insurance. Fearnley, who shipped directly on contract to the out-ports, used the London agent Claus Heide only to arrange insurance, but was nevertheless given advances by Heide,

the winter for several hundred pounds on a Hull firm of importers as London and Yarmouth merchants customarily gave this facility. From further letters, ff. 29–30 and 41–2, it appears that credits were advanced as requested.

[1] *R.H.C.*, vol. 15, timber duties (1835), XIX, p. 342. It is of interest that a timber-merchant whom I questioned on this point assured me that eighteen months of seasoning is a measure of perfection often laid claim to and rarely attained.

[2] Fabricius reported on it, as on the contract system, in detail. His observations are in appendix 4, pp. 189ff.

[3] See above, pp. 31f.

[4] See above, p. 32, and also appendix 4, pp. 196f.

[5] Insurance of Norwegian timber in the eighteenth century is exhaustively treated by K. Lorange, *Forsikringsvesenets historie i Norge* (Oslo, 1935), pp. 24–35.

who acted as his banker.[1] Credits were also extended to purchasers who normally paid half the amount due for a cargo in four-months bills, one extra month being allowed for unloading, and the balance in cash. Although the agent did not guarantee payment to his principals,[2] he attempted for the sake of his own reputation to find purchasers of such financial standing that their bills could be discounted at $\frac{1}{2}\%$ the month.[3] During the last years of the Seven Years War, the scarcity of money led to credits being demanded by the purchaser for two years or longer, bills on occasion being drawn for such time,[4] and the agent was then called upon to advance money both to shipper and purchaser so that trade could continue.[5] Finally, when an agent could not find a purchaser for a cargo consigned to him, he obliged by arranging for the storing of the shipment in a merchant's yard, advancing customs duties and rent for storage, and disposing of the timber when opportunity offered. His principals were allowed in the meantime to draw on him as if the cargo had already been sold.[6]

Not every Norwegian shipper employed an agent, or received contracts for supply. Cargoes of timber were then sent to English ports on speculation, particularly during the later years of the War. Prices for such shipments were often depressed; the English merchant knew that a sale had to be made, as the loss to the shipper would be even greater if the timber were taken further afield, or returned to Norway.[7] English merchants who preferred neither to deal through an agent nor to give direct contracts, might send their own representative to Norway to assemble cargoes and to

---

[1] Nor. S. Arch., Fearnley papers, ff. 129–30, 139, 166, 181, 203–5, letters to Heide and others, Frederickshald, 8 and 29 June, 11 August, 14 September and 16 November 1766.

[2] The emergence of *del credere* agents who guaranteed payment for an additional fee was a later development in the timber-trade.

[3] See appendix 4, p. 189.

[4] A. Olsen, *Danmark–Norge*, p. 56, citing a Norwegian timber-merchant's correspondence.

[5] See appendix 4, p. 194, that extension of credit by Collet at the end of the War of the Austrian Succession, when the same conditions applied, led to the price of timber being maintained.

[6] Lorange, *Forsikringsvesenets historie*, p. 30; and also *R.H.C.*, vol. 15, timber duties (1855), XIX, pp. 341f.

[7] La Cour, *Mellem Brødre*, p. 146, notes such instances.

arrange for at least part of their payment through barter of English goods. The activities of one such representative, Thomas Fearnley, have already been noted extensively, and not the least of them was to act as an unofficial bracker in his firm's interest and thus assure it of timber of a satisfactory quality.[1]

London, in which the principal financiers of the timber-trade were active, was predominant during the mid-century as a centre of the trade, about half of all shipments to England being directed to the capital.[2] The War led to a greater share of shipments going to the out-ports as it was safer making direct shipments from Norway[3] rather than transhipping at London into coasters which distributed timber principally to the West Coast ports.[4] An extension of credit facilities in the provincial centres may be an added explanation for the more even distribution of shipments to England. The London merchants, who had already lost some of their pre-eminence in the 1740s, fought hard to retain their position. The Danish–Norwegian envoy to England, reporting in 1753 the arrest of a fleet of ships at Liverpool for clandestinely carrying Baltic timber,[5] gave his opinion that the seizure had been due to the jealousy of London merchants who had shipped much timber to the West Coast. To hinder the rise of rivals, they had asked their agents in the Baltic to watch the loading of ships to the out-ports. On receiving information that Danish–Norwegian ships were taking on timber at Riga for Liverpool, the customs were told of it and provided with copies of Riga brack-marks from which the provenance of the timber could be proved. The ships would have been safe, the envoy concluded, if they had come into London.[6]

Shipping which brought timber to England was unevenly

---

[1] Nor. S. Arch., Fearnley papers, f. 14, letter to [Haworth & Stephenson of Hull], 16 March 1753: Fearnley, writing to his principals, hopes that a cargo just despatched 'may meet your Approbation having used my utmost Endeavours to see the same well Wreaked'.

[2] See appendix 1, Figs 2 and 3.

[3] See above, p. 38.

[4] The London port books for the eighteenth century were destroyed by fire with the exception of one which has no record of coastwise shipping. Some evidence exists, however, in the records of other ports which have been described by T. S. Willan, *The English coasting trade* (Manchester, 1938), *passim*, but particularly pp. 121ff.

[5] See above, p. 46.

[6] Dan. S. Arch., T.K.U.A., Engl. B, 103, despatch of 10 August 1753.

divided between British and Norwegian bottoms with a preponderance of English vessels in the immediate pre-War years. The War altered the proportions of British and foreign ships in the trade.[1] A sudden diminution in the number of English, accompanied by a steep rise in the number of Norwegian ship-voyages in 1755 which cannot be wholly accounted for by increased imports, suggests despite the lack of direct evidence[2] that at least some British ships were sold to Norway on the outbreak of hostilities through fear of privateering which would commence on a declaration of war. The Norwegian merchant fleet continued to increase rapidly,[3] and by the end of 1756 practically all the timber carried to London, and the greater part of shipments to the out-ports, was in Norwegian bottoms. Until the end of 1762, few British ships were left in the trade, but so soon as hostilities ceased, Norwegian vessels were increasingly displaced by British ships which, however, did not regain their earlier preponderance. The rise in the number of British ship-voyages was slow in the case of London, and startlingly sudden to the out-ports: this is the impression given by the quantities of timber shipped, according to the customs accounts, in British and foreign ships. These accounts must however not be taken as exact evidence of the proportion of British and foreign tonnage engaged in the trade. Such evidence could only be obtained if one knew the number of voyages per season by every ship in the trade, and this we do not know and have no means of finding out with any certainty. Quantities of timber carried must therefore be taken only as an indication of the number of ships employed. It is even possible that the disproportion of Norwegian to English ships after the War was more marked than figures of shipments suggest. This possibility is given some added weight by the complaints of Norwegian ship's masters about the slow turn-around of Norwegian

[1] See appendix 1, Figs 2 to 4.
[2] See above, p. 37, n. 5.
[3] Holm, *Danmark–Norges historie*, vol. 3, pt 2, p. 262. The increase between 1746 and 1766 was by one half of total tonnage. It is suggested by O. A. Johnsen, *Tønsbergs Historie*, vol. 2 (Oslo, 1934), p. 475, that most of the increase occurred during the Seven Years War.

Another author, Magnus Jensen, *Norges Historie fra 1660 till Våre Dager* (Oslo, 1949), vol. 2, p. 154, states that the hold which England and also Holland had on Norwegian shipping was only broken by the Seven Years War.

ships in Norwegian ports as compared with English ships, which were loaded so quickly that they could make two voyages to one by a Norwegian ship. The reason for such preferential treatment in port, so the complaints went, was due to English ships paying cash for their cargoes.[1] The distribution of shipments between London and the out-ports irrespective of the nationality of the ships had already been affected by the War in favour of the out-ports. At the end of the War, it was fairly evenly balanced, with London gradually losing its earlier pre-eminence in the timber-trade.

As far as one can judge from the loads carried,[2] the ships in the trade were generally of between 100 to 300 tons. A typical load of a timber-ship from Norway is instanced in a book of instructions for customs officers, and it would appear that such a load was carried by a ship of 300 tons.[3] Shipments by Fearnley indicate that vessels of from 200 to 300 tons[4] were usual, and this is borne out further by timber tallies, kept on discharge in England.[5] Scottish ships trading to Bergen and returning with timber were generally smaller, and at times of less than 100 tons.[6] The number of voyages a ship could make in a season varied between three and six, depending not only on the weather, but also on the turn-around in port. The timber tallies at the Custom House, King's Lynn, show that unloading was in every case completed in less than a week, and usually in three days. The period of one month

---

[1] Dan. S. Arch., T.K.U.A., Engl. B, 114, consular report of 9 July 1965.

[2] It was quite unusual for a ship's tonnage to be stated, but one may assume that, roughly, one load of timber went to the ton. See *R.H.C.*, vol. 15, timber duties (1835), XIX, p. 361: 'The Henriette was registered 269 tons; and usually brought a cargo of about 300 loads of timber, converting wainscot logs, deals, half-deals or lathwood, into loads of timber, according to the customary rules of the shipping trade.'

These rules have not been preserved in present-day practice, but calculations based on the most commonly imported sizes of deals show that one Hundred of deals equalled approximately five loads, with battens and half-deals in proportion.

[3] Baldwin, *The British Customs*, pt 2, p. 72.

[4] Norw. S. Arch., Fearnley papers, bills of lading, ff. 35-7, and accounts of shipments, ff. 55, 93 and 131.

[5] Custom House, King's Lynn: Ship *Providence* from Crokery [Kragerö]: *John and Mary* from North Bergen; ship from North Bergen, name indecipherable, 1749. Another ship, however, the *John and Rachel* from Frederickshald, was nearer 400 tons.

[6] See above, p. 15, n. 5. The tonnage of these ships is stated in the Bergen port books as they were measured for an assessment of port dues.

customarily allowed for unloading and payment was merely an extension of credit. It is evident from Thomas Fearnley's correspondence that the voyage across the North Sea took generally less than a fortnight, several days of it often being spent beating into port, and that loading was completed in a few days.

English ships in the trade were rarely owned by the importer, but chartered for the single voyage or the season, while Norwegian vessels more often belonged to the shipper.[1] Return cargoes to Norway were usually made up by the English timber-merchants who normally did not deal in timber only, but also in other commodities. Haworth & Stephenson, the Hull importers with whom Fearnley was connected, shipped large quantities of cloth and ironmongery, lead, leather, flour, grain, and cheese for sale to Norwegian retailers, or in barter against timber.[2] The trade of this firm was not restricted to Norway, nor its imports to timber. Naval stores and iron were obtained by it from Russia[3] – one of the partners, if not both, was a freeman of the Russia Company[4] – and cloth, lead, and ironmongery were shipped to Holland[5] probably in exchange for oak boards.[6] John Rigg, a London timber-agent, owned 'a large cloth manufactory from which he sent much to Norway'.[7] John Holland, of Hull, with whom Fearnley had arranged to smuggle timber,[8] supplied Fearnley with a variety of goods in barter.[9] Marshall, a Newcastle timber-merchant, shipped coal to

[1] *R.H.C.*, vol. 15 (1835), XIX, p. 363, evidence of H. Warburton on former practice. Also, Nor. S. Arch., Fearnley papers, ff. 15, 119, 120, 151 *et passim*.

[2] Nor. S. Arch., Fearnley papers, ff. 4–5, Fearnley to [Haworth & Stephenson], Frederickstadt, 14 May 1753; *ibid.*, f. 8, same to same, Christiania, 27 June 1753; *ibid.*, f. 19, same to same, Frederickshald, 19 August 1753; *ibid.*, f. 28, Fearnley to John Stacy [who had supplied Haworth & Stephenson with overpriced goods], Frederickshald, 13 September 1753; *ibid.*, ff. 84–5, Fearnley to [Haworth & Stephenson] Christiania, 28 September 1754; and others.

[3] P.R.O. Exchequer Papers, King's Remembrancer, port books, Hull [cited below as port books, Hull], E. 190/366, b. 7, entries 407, 418 and 428.

[4] Cambridge U.L., Russia Company, Minutes, 1734–56, f. 434, admission of Benjamin Haworth of Hull, 21 February 1749–50.

[5] P.R.O., port books, Hull, E. 190/368, b. 5, entry 119.

[6] *Ibid.*, E. 190/366, b. 7, entry 446: Part-cargo of wainscot-boards for Benj. Haworth & Co. Wainscot-boards were nearly exclusively imported from Holland.

[7] See appendix 4, p. 196.

[8] See above, p. 47.

[9] Norw. S. Arch., Fearnley papers, ff. 76–7, Fearnley to Holland, Christiania, 19 July 1754; and *ibid.*, f. 206, same to same, Frederickshald, 16 November 1766.

Norway and received timber in exchange.[1] The masters of several Scottish ships calling at Bergen told the customs officers there that they would unload only if they obtained timber for their cargoes, otherwise they would continue down the coast until they found the opportunity for an exchange.[2] Such exchange was not uncommon and actually referred to as barter, Fearnley advising Haworth & Stephenson that he had 'disposed of 2 ps. of Cloth in Barter for Battins, Uffers and some other Goods'.[3] While barter persisted, the timber-trade was thus connected directly with the export of British merchandise.

[1] *Ibid.*, ff. 14–16, Fearnley to [Haworth & Stephenson], Frederickstadt, 14 May 1753.
[2] Norw. S. Arch., Bergen Toldbøger, 1760, I, entries 23 and 43; 25 and 52; 26 and 44; 27 and 53; 28 and 86; 29 and 76; 31 and 55; 32 and 78; 38 and 90. The first entry relates to arrival, the second to clearance. Nine ships came in within a few days, carrying mainly flour and salt. Salt, although a prohibited import, could be landed by special licence [see below, pp. 98f.]. The master of each one of these ships, none of which exceeded 100 tons, gave the same account to the customs officers on arrival. Every ship was cleared within a week, the masters then stating that they were taking on a return cargo of timber.
[3] Nor. S. Arch., f. 7, letter dated Frederickshald, 10 June 1753. Other barter arrangements are noted throughout Fearnley's correspondence with various timber-firms.

4 *The Iron-Trade*

The course and the volume of the iron-trade across the North Sea was affected to no greater degree than the timber-trade by the outbreak of the Seven Years War. The Swedish mines and forges continued to supply the greater part of the total amount of bar-iron shipped to British ports from Europe and from America even after Sweden in 1757 had joined her old ally France in the field against Prussia while prudently avoiding open hostilities against England. If for no other reason, Sweden could not afford to break with England, which was by far her most important customer, taking well over half of her bar-iron exports which in themselves accounted for three-quarters of her total outward trade.[1] English merchants and manufacturers were equally interested in preventing any interruption of their dealings with Sweden on whom the English metal industries depended for at least half of their bar-iron requirements. Efforts to lessen this dependence on a power whose political and also commercial hostility had been a constant threat to British industry since the early years of the century, remained largely unsuccessful. Hopes had been raised from time to time that the American colonies might produce more iron for shipment to the mother country, but American exports stayed disappointingly small despite every inducement held out by the government in London. Spain, which had in the past been prominent in the iron-trade with England, had long since become of little consequence as the growing demand outstripped her ability or wish to ship more than the 1,000 or 2,000 tons annually that were by the mid-century

---

[1] Heckscher, *Sveriges Ekonomiska Historia*, II, 2, p. 652, and *ibid.*, appendix, p. 30, table 15. This table shows that in the five-year period 1751–5, England bought 53·3% of Swedish bar-iron production; in the period 1756–60 the percentage was 57·1, and 55·3 for the years 1761–5. The next highest export figures were around 9% for the Netherlands. The Hansa Towns, Portugal and Spain, and France came next with around 5% each, the figure for France falling during the war while that for Portugal and Spain rose.

a mere fraction of English imports. The latest-comer among the iron-exporters to England, Russia, alone seemed likely to challenge Swedish preponderance in the English market. From a few tons at the beginning of the century, Russian exports had grown into the thousands to be second to Sweden's, and were continuing to increase.[1] For the time being, however, Swedish predominance in the iron export trade was unassailable both for the quantity shipped and for the quality of her iron, which placed the first grade beyond competition, and the second on a par with the best of other imported or English bar-iron.

English ironware- and steel-manufacturers had good reason to be apprehensive about their dependence on bar-iron supplies from foreign countries which might at any time prohibit exports to England as had once been done by Sweden earlier in the century. The resulting shortage of bar-iron which crippled the iron-working industry until Swedish supplies were again restored showed only too disturbingly how far short the output of English forges fell from meeting demand.[2] The shortage of charcoal which had already in the preceding century been so troublesome, was the main reason for the failure of the English forgemasters to work up sufficient bars for the smith and the steel converter. Charcoal was indispensable in iron-working until later in the eighteenth century when the wider introduction of mineral fuel and of new techniques into the foundry and the forge allowed British iron production to expand rapidly. Until then, however, charcoal was needed to produce pig-iron of a good enough quality for fining into bars, for the fining process itself, and again for the conversion of the bar into steel. The limit of English bar-iron production while charcoal remained irreplaceable was by contemporary estimates reached at probably 18,000, and possibly 20,000 tons annually.[3] These quanti-

[1] Iron imports from Russia into England during the century are noted by D. Gerhard, *England und der Aufstieg Russlands* (Berlin, 1933), pp. 51–2; and by D. K. Reading, *The Anglo-Russian Commercial Treaty of 1734* (Yale University Press, 1938), pp. 33ff. Imports in single years are listed occasionally in D. McPherson, *Annals of Commerce, Manufactures, Fisheries and Navigation* (4 vols., London, 1805).

[2] Ashton, *Iron and Steel*, pp. 111–12, gives the best short description of the incident and its consequences.

[3] *Ibid.*, appendix 2, pp. 235ff., summarises statistics on the supply of iron in England in the early eighteenth century. See also K. G. Hildebrand, 'Foreign Markets for

ties were not nearly enough to satisfy the needs of the iron-working industry. Imports were imperative and were rather wistfully looked for from the American colonies where ore had been found, and timber for charcoal was abundant. Despite much agitation to persuade the colonists to increase their iron production for the mother country by making exports worth their while through a remission of import duties into England, nothing effective was done until 1750 to encourage colonial iron imports. There was a likelihood in that year of Sweden and Russia going to war against each other, and iron supplies from either country seemed to be endangered. Colonial iron imports, it was hoped, might help to save the manufacturing industries, and the long discussed remission of import duties on colonial iron shipped directly to London was at last decided on.[1] It was fortunate for English industry that the storm in the Baltic blew over without affecting Swedish and Russian iron shipments, as the hoped-for increase of colonial supplies failed to follow the waiving of the import duties.[2] A further effort in 1757[3] to stimulate colonial bar-iron supplies by opening all ports to them besides London, which had so far alone been privileged to receive them directly, was no more successful than earlier efforts to raise the quantity of iron sent to England by the colonists. The Swedish government was not to know this, and was worried over the effect which new legislation on the iron trade might have on its own iron exports. Wynantz wrote from London so early as the end of 1756 to the president of the Swedish Chancellery (Kanslipresidenten), Höpken, that he had heard of a move by the London iron-merchants to press in the next parliamentary session for the free importation of American bar-iron into all ports. Early in the next year, 1757, he reported on a petition to Parliament by the Bristol merchants for the free importation of American bar-iron on the grounds that imports from Sweden and Russia drained the country of specie. In further reports he wrote of meetings which had been held in London by representatives of mine-owners and iron-masters who were not quite certain whether to support the iron-

Swedish Iron in the Eighteenth Century', *Scandinavian Economic History Review*, 6, no 1 (1958).   [1] Acts, 23 Geo. II c. 29.
[2] See appendix 2, Fig. 5.   [3] 30 Geo. II c. 16.

merchants or not, and who eventually decided that colonial iron imports were not in their interest, as colonial iron would be in direct competition with their own grades of iron. They therefore resolved, Wynantz reported, to sidetrack the whole matter in Parliament by having it referred to a committee, and thus disposing of it for good and ever. They were unsuccessful, though, and the House of Commons decided by a vote of seventy-eight to seventy-three that the proposal to open all ports to colonial bar-iron should be debated, and by a further vote of eighty to forty that the Bill should be brought in. It passed its third reading, after a long debate, on a division of ninety-three against forty-six votes. Wynantz assured Höpken that he would do all he could by working through well-placed friends and acquaintances to prevent further legislation aimed at freeing colonial bar-iron from paying duties in the out-ports. In any case, duties continued to be paid in the out-ports, while importation into London had been free since 1750. Höpken was not to be reassured, and in great agitation wrote to Wynantz that he foresaw the ruin of the Swedish iron industry by colonial imports, and ordered Wynantz to redouble his efforts to stop any further agitation for the import or the use of colonial iron to replace Swedish.[1]

Höpken need not have been alarmed. Shipments of bar-iron from the colonies did not rise from their insignificant pre-war total of a few hundred tons annually,[2] nor pig-iron from 2,000 to 3,000 tons until well into the 1760s.[3] Colonial iron, therefore, played no part in satisfying the extensive English demand for imports which had to be obtained from European countries.

Europe was scoured for the essential supplies which supported

[1] Swed. S. Arch., Diplomatica, Anglica 1, Wynantz' Brev till Kanslipresidenten, 1747–58, despatches of 23 November 1756, 11 and 25 February, 18 and 25 March, 22 April and 3 May 1757. *Ibid.*, Anglica 1, Brev till Wynantz från Kanslipresidenten och kanslitjaenstemän, section d, 1757–8, Höpken to Wynantz, 27 June 1757.

[2] See appendix 2, Fig. 5.

[3] Pig-iron was the first product of the ore which had been smelted with mineral coal for foundry work, or with charcoal when the pig-iron was to be fined into bar-iron. It sold for less than a third of the price of bar-iron and importation was therefore not economic unless pig-iron could be used for ballast. The American colonies were practically the only exporters of pig-iron to England. The quantities annually imported into England are listed in P.R.O., Cust. 3/50–70 for the years 1750–70, while in Cust. 14/1 *a* and 1 *b* are the imports into Scotland for the period 1755–70.

the great iron-working industry, and there was hardly an iron-producing or trading country that did not send its quota. Small quantities of pig-iron, scrap-, and occasionally bar-iron came from Holland, from Germany, and from the East Country ports, amounting in all to no more than a few hundred tons.[1] Larger shipments of bar-iron were obtained from Spain,[2] and a contemporary noted that the 1,000 or 2,000 tons annually imported were peculiarly suitable for anchor manufacture because of the Spanish iron's special properties.[3] A few hundred more tons of bar-iron were shipped to England from the Norwegian ports,[4] to bring up the total from all the countries so far mentioned to no more than 3,000 tons. That figure was far surpassed in the mid-century by imports with which Russia was credited. Russian shipments of bar-iron to England as entered in the customs ledgers had risen spectacularly from an odd sample at the beginning of the century to a recorded 15,000 tons in 1750,[5] a year in which imports were heavy because, no doubt, of their threatened interruption by a possible Baltic war. Such large export figures from Russia were not sustained in the next years. They dropped sharply in 1751 to 5,000 tons, rose again in 1755 to 10,000 tons at the threat of the Seven Years War, returned to the pre-War level of around 5,000 tons for the years 1756–8, and from then on rose quickly to approach the figures for Swedish bar-iron exports to England which were finally surpassed after the War. Until then, supplies from Sweden accounted never for less than one-half, and in some years for as much as three-quarters of foreign bar-iron imports which were generally in the vicinity of 30,000 tons annually.[6] On an average, customs records credit Sweden with near two-thirds of all bar-iron

[1] Statistics on iron imports from these countries are to be found in the series of documents cited in the above footnote. The East Country was the region between the river Oder in Silesia, and the Gulf of Finland. The designation East Country did not appear in the Scottish customs ledgers, where imports and exports from that region were separately entered under Prussia, Poland, and Livonia.

[2] See appendix 2, Fig. 5.

[3] See appendix 4, pt 2, p. 198 and footnote 2. Also, Beveridge, *Prices and Wages*, p. 658.

[4] Notes on the export of iron from Norway will be found in appendix 4, pt 2. The quantities are listed in P.R.O., Cust. 3/50–70, and Cust. 14/1 *a* and 1 *b*.

[5] For this and later statements on shipments from Russia, see appendix 2, Fig. 5.

[6] See appendix 1, Fig. 4.

shipments to England during the years 1755–63, or, to put it another way, with the same quantity as the estimated output of British forges. The Swedish forges were then at least of equal importance to the British in the supply of bar-iron to the metal industry if the customs accounts are accepted without further question. That, however, cannot be done.

Doubts about the accuracy of the English customs accounts relating to iron shipments from Sweden occur so soon as they are compared with Swedish export figures. These show that iron exports to Great Britain, i.e. England, Scotland, and Ireland, were consistently noted as being 25% to 40% higher than the corresponding figures for imports in the customs accounts for England only.[1] What little bar-iron was imported into Scotland came mainly from Sweden, and was then hardly ever recorded in the Scottish customs accounts as being more than 2% or 3% of the figures in the English customs ledgers;[2] there is no reason to suppose that Irish imports differed greatly from the Scottish.[3] The discrepancy between the records of exports from Sweden, and of imports into Great Britain is then still large. It may be narrowed by making allowance for iron bought by English merchants and shipped on their account to other countries without bond being broken in an English port,[4] but there is no way of telling what quantities were involved. Similar uncertainties are met with when one comes to consider that most elusive of all transactions, smuggling. All that can be said about smuggling of Swedish bar-iron into England or Scotland is, that contemporaries believed it to

[1] E. F. Heckscher, 'Un grand chapitre de l'histoire du fer: le monopole suédois', *Annales d'histoire économique et sociale*, 4, nos 14 and 15 (Paris, 1932).

[2] Imports of bar-iron into Scotland before the commencement of the Scottish series of customs ledgers, are listed by Scrivenor, *A Comprehensive History of the Iron Trade* (London, 1841), appendix, table 10, pp. 341–2. It is noteworthy that before and after the Seven Years War imports were practically exclusively in Scottish vessels, and during the war mainly in Swedish. See for this P.R.O., Cust. 14/1*a* and 1*b*.

[3] Imports of bar-iron into Ireland during the years 1771–3, and 1781–3 are listed in [Adam Anderson], *Historical and Chronological Deduction of the Origin of Commerce* (London, 1789), vol. 4, p. 527. The editors of volume 4 of this work state that imports had been increasing, and stood at *c*. 4,000 tons in 1783.

[4] That this happened may be deduced from the correspondence of an English iron-merchant, Richard Blount, which has been preserved in fragment in the Swedish State Archives, ser. Enskilda Samlinger, Arkivfragment, Arkivbildare: Kommerseråd Frans Jennings Correspondence.

have been prevalent. Samuel Garbett, the well-known eighteenth-century ironmaster who with his partner Roebuck was a self-appointed guardian of fair-trading practices, bombarded government offices with allegations against his rivals, declaring the while virtuously that he would continue to meet their unfair competition without stooping to smuggling 'though he has works by the sea-side, and in a convenient place'.[1] Straightout smuggling by running iron bars ashore from ships lying out to sea, or by spiriting them past tide- and land-waiters when unloading under their supervision, cannot have been too difficult. Bars of iron weighed on the average less than 40 pounds which, translated into size, did not make them very conspicuous when thousands were checked out of the hold. Finally, and most telling, there is evidence in the customs ledgers themselves that more Swedish iron reached England than is indicated by the entries headed as imports from Sweden.

Shipments of bar-iron from Russia, the East Country, and Denmark–Norway were almost invariably described in the customs ledgers as consisting of 'native' and of 'Swedish' iron. In the case of shipments from Denmark–Norway, the reason for this apparently confusing description is not far to seek. Merchants in Norway bought Swedish iron or accepted it in exchange for re-export only as Norway, herself an iron-producer, allowed the import of Swedish iron for no other purpose.[2] Such purchases for re-export may have been purely speculative or, as likely, a sound move to obtain a paying bottom ballast for timber cargoes in a country that had little iron for export. Possible differences in cost between direct shipment and re-export could be disregarded, as freight rates for iron were lower when it was shipped in small quantities with a main cargo relatively as light and as buoyant as timber, rather than

[1] Calendar of Home Office Papers, pp. 637–8, entry 2064, Garbett to Burke (secretary to General Conway, Secretary of State), 14 December 1765. For further correspondence of Garbett with government departments, see *ibid.*, p. 620, entry 2,000, and P.R.O., S.P. 44/141, Burke to Garbett, 12 December 1765 and Garbett to Burke, 14 December 1765 for complete text of letter of that date in the Calendar. See also appendix 5, below, for Garbett's and Roebuck's efforts to prevent the emigration of English iron-workers. Garbett and Roebuck figure prominently in Ashton, *Iron and Steel*.

[2] Jensen, *Dansk-Norsk Vekselvirkning*, pp. 59–60 and 62, cites Danish-Norwegian legislation on that subject.

making up a dangerously heavy and unwieldy load that could have strained a hull to the limit. Purchases of Swedish iron for re-export by merchants in Russia and the East Country may also have been made, though there is no direct evidence of it and it would appear somewhat unlikely as the distances were greater, and iron abundant in Russia herself. One can only look to the probable for àn explanation of Swedish bar-iron turning up in England under the guise of imports from the eastern Baltic, and an examination of custom-house procedure shows how that may have come about.

On arrival in port, the master of a ship gave to the clerks in the Long Room of the custom house the information they needed for striking the duties and for compiling eventually the statistical tables which were to appear every year in the customs ledgers.[1] One copy of this declaration was sent to the inspector-general's office, which was responsible for compiling the large folio ledgers showing the nation's trade with other countries during the past year. Each colony or foreign country had its separate section listing the goods that had entered into the trade, their quantity, estimated value, and whether they had been carried in British or foreign vessels. The bills of entry from which information for the tables in the ledgers was extracted gave among other details the ports of lading, and the place from which the vessel had come, which for a British ship trading to the Baltic was beyond reasonable doubt the port farthest from England. The location of this port determined which foreign country was eventually credited in the annual ledgers with having sent the entire cargo. A cargo taken on in Sweden and at St Petersburg or Riga would therefore enter the statistics of imports as having originated in Russia or the East Country. The ledgers unfortunately did not specify, except in a rare instance, the proportions of Swedish to other iron when there was a mixed cargo. There are two such instances, the only ones that have been found, in the entries relating to the English out-ports in the years 1761

---

[1] Custom-house procedure is described in great detail by E. E. Hoon, *The organisation of the English custom system, 1696–1786* (London and New York, 1938), *passim* and particularly chapter 4. See also G. N. Clark, *Guide to English commercial statistics 1696–1782* (London, 1938), pp. 1–32 in which an analysis of statistics is given, and of the methods employed in compiling them.

and 1763.[1] Of 3,998 tons of bar-iron credited to imports from Russia in 1761, 3,904 tons are separately listed as Swedish, while, however, 12,446 which reached London appear in the entry for that port in the usual form of Russian and Swedish iron. In the same year, too, 196 tons of bar-iron out of a total of 205 from the East Country are specifically listed as Swedish, the remaining 9 tons appearing in the column of imports carried by foreign ships. The entries for 1763 are similar.[2] Evidence from two years cannot, of course, give any valid indication of the share of Swedish iron in the statistics of imports from Russia and the East Country, but it serves to show that in at least two particular years no less than a quarter of bar-iron imports credited to other sources was actually Swedish. The total Swedish share in foreign bar-iron shipped to England must then have been rather larger than is shown by the English official statistics of the time, and to have surpassed to some extent the contribution made by British forges to supplies for the metal-working industry.[3]

Not all Swedish bar-iron imported into England was used in industry. Some was re-exported without having been worked up, to Africa, to the Caribbean and North American colonies, and to India. The quantities recorded annually in the customs accounts were never large, and rarely reached 500 tons, of which a quarter went to New England, Virginia and Maryland, an amount little less than total colonial shipments to England.[4] Some 20,000 tons per year of Swedish iron then still remained in England where the demand for it was intense because of its properties and its finish. Two grades were imported. The first or '*oregrund*' made from the ore of the famous Dannemora mines had no real rival although an odd sample of colonial iron was at times claimed to be as good. Only from *oregrund* could the finest quality steel be manufactured, and this grade had the additional advantage over any possible colonial competition of being a standard product. The mark of

[1] P.R.O., Cust. 3/61 and 63, tables of imports from Russia. The figures for 1763 show total imports from Russia of 13,630 tons of bar-iron of which 3,832 tons are noted as having been Swedish, and the remainder 'Russian and Swedish'.
[2] *Ibid.*, tables of imports from East Country.
[3] See also appendix 4, pp. 199 f., for Swedish iron being shipped from Norway.
[4] P.R.O, Cust. 3/50–70, tables of exports, London and out-ports.

War and Trade in Northern Seas

the Dannemora forgemasters was a guarantee to the purchaser that he was receiving iron of the very highest quality whose properties were constant, a distinct boon when it came to converting bars into steel.[1] *Oregrund* accounted for about 15% of imports from Sweden, or some 3,000 or even 4,000 tons.[2] A Hull merchant, Joseph Sykes, is reputed to have become at a later date the sole importer of it, but tantalisingly little has so far been found out about his or any other iron-importer's dealings.[3]

The second grade or 'ordinary Swedish' equalled in quality the best grades of any other bar-iron on the English market, and was therefore in direct competition with first grade or 'best tough' English bars. It could be converted into steel good enough for edge tools, or be worked into high-quality iron implements. Ordinary Swedish was, however, considered harder iron than best tough, needing more labour and more fuel in working up. The consequently higher working costs of ordinary Swedish bars were reflected in its price, which was slightly lower than that of the corresponding English grade.[4] Unlike *oregrund*, ordinary Swedish was not a stan-

[1] The properties of *oregrund* bars are very fully described by Jars, *Voyages*, vol. 1, pp. 120 and 157. On its uses see Ashton, *Iron and Steel*, p. 238 and *passim*. Claims for colonial iron to approach the best Swedish in quality were made e.g. in 1737 in evidence presented to a parliamentary committee of inquiry into iron manufacture, while other evidence before the same committee claimed it to be no better than second-grade Swedish iron, or inferior to any Swedish iron. The evidence given to the committee is in *J.H.C.*, vol. XXII, pp. 850ff.

[2] Heckscher, *Sveriges ekonomiska historia*, II, 2, appendix, p. 30, table 15, legend, and *ibid.*, II, 1, pp. 401 and 405. Also, Jars, *Voyages*, vol. 1, p. 157.

[3] Sykes is something of a mystery-man. He is known through fragments of correspondence to have carried on a large trade, but little else has been found out about him. On his trade and family connections, see the introduction by Professor Hayek to his edition of Henry Thornton's *Enquiry into the Nature and Effects of the Paper Credit of Great Britain* (London, 1939), p. 28 and *passim*. Professor Ashton mentions Sykes on pp. 57 and 246 of his *Iron and Steel*, and some biographical data are in W. A. Gunnell (ed.), *Sketches of Hull Celebrities* (Hull, 1876), p. 395. I have found documentary evidence of his trading activities in P.R.O., S.P. 95/133, Denison (London agent or attorney of Sykes) to Earl of Holdernesse, London, 11 September 1759, on iron shipment by Sykes and others which had been taken by Prussian privateer; and *ibid.*, petition by Sykes and others, dated Hull, 12 September 1759, for release of another iron cargo; and *ibid.*, affidavit by N. F. Facks, master of a Swedish ship (n.d., n.p., Portsmouth, January 1760) that he had discharged yet a third iron cargo for Sykes at Hull in November 1759.

[4] The uses and properties of ordinary Swedish iron are given in detail in *J.H.C.*, vol. XXII, p. 854, evidence of Abraham Spooner before Committee of the House.

68

dard product, and pulls from the mines which shipped from Stockholm were regarded as being better than those from some of the West Coast mines whose port of shipment was Gothenburg. The small amount of Swedish iron, presumably from West Coast mines, which reached England via Norway had no better reputation than Norwegian bars, which were regarded as being too hard, often cold-short, and so magnetic that shipwrights feared to use them in their work as they were believed to affect the compass.[1] Shipments of iron from Gothenburg, however, were only about one-quarter of those from the Swedish East Coast ports, and the quantity of poorer iron from Sweden cannot therefore have been large.[2]

Both grades of Swedish iron were imported in a wide range of sizes and shapes. An observer noted in 1758 that round, flat, and square bars reached the London market, and he meticulously wrote down their specifications.[3] Round bars ranged in diameter from $\frac{3}{4}$ to $1\frac{1}{2}$ inches; the smallest square bars measured $\frac{3}{4}$ inch in section, progressing by $\frac{1}{2}$ inch to 2 inches in section; flat bars or plates came in 21 distinct widths between 1 and 7 inches, each width being available in 4 thicknesses of $\frac{3}{8}$ to $\frac{3}{4}$ inch. Moreover, the finish of the bars was the finest of any he had seen.

Among such a selection of sizes were at least some that could be used by the consumer without having to pass through an English smithy. One London merchant specifically asked his Stockholm correspondent to include in a shipment 'tyer Iron 9 foot exact long $2\frac{1}{2}$, $2\frac{3}{4}$ & 3 inch broad, $\frac{5}{8}$, $\frac{3}{4}$ & $\frac{7}{8}$ inch thick',[4] clearly no longer bar but rather manufactured iron which was liable to much heavier

---

[1] See below, appendix 4, pt 2.

[2] An analysis of the Sound Toll Registers for the years 1750 to 1760 showed that before the war on an average some 8,000 to 9,000 tons of bar-iron passed the Sound for England in English ships, and another 3,000 to 4,000 in Swedish ships. During the war years most of the iron was carried in Swedish ships. Deducting the total amount carried through the Sound from imports recorded in the customs ledgers gives roughly a proportion of 3 to 1 for shipments from Swedish East and West Coast ports. See N. Bang and K. Korst, *Tabeller over Skibsfart og Varetransport gennem Øresund 1661–1783*, vol. 2, pt 2, *Tabeller om Varetransporten 1721–1760* (Copenhagen, 1945), pp. 521–761.

[3] See below, appendix 4, pt 2.

[4] Swed. S. Arch., ser. Enskilda Samlinger, Arkivfragment, Arkivbildare, Jennings correspondence: R. Blount to F. Jennings, London, 22 June 1744.

import duty,[1] and yet there is no record of manufactured iron from Sweden having passed through the customs in the middle decades of the century except in one instance. Samuel Garbett was responsible for that single entry. He had made himself the spokesman of whatever English forgemasters or iron-manufacturers were concerned over the practice of Swedish exporters serving English iron-merchants too well at the expense of English industry, and asked the government to class flat bars, i.e. plates, as manufactured iron. The commissioners of customs refused to act unless he and Roebuck agreed to bear the legal costs if it should come to a court action. Garbett was willing, and two consignments of Swedish iron plates were accordingly stopped at London, for which the importers paid the higher duty chargeable on wrought ware without going to court. Next, a consignment was intercepted at Hull, but there the importers were prepared to raise 'a common purse' and test the unwonted zeal of the customs authorities in court. To Garbett's chagrin, 'The trial...[was] by some unintelligible means, dropped', no ruling was obtained on a revision of duty assessments, and Swedish bars indistinguishable from manufactured iron continued to enter the country at the lower rate of duty.[2]

This fixed duty was in no way a deterrent to the import of Swedish bar-iron. It stood at £2 1s. 6d. a ton when the iron was imported by English merchants in English ships, at a few shillings higher for foreign merchants or vessels, and at a maximum of £2 12s. 7d. when imported by foreign merchants in foreign ships.[3] Sweden herself also charged export duties of £3 12s. 6d. a ton which were increased in 1756 for iron carried in non-Swedish ships.[4] Despite these surcharges on the prime cost, Swedish iron easily held its own in the English market in competition with native iron and increasing imports of Russian iron, as its production costs

[1] The duty on manufactured or 'wrought' iron was 47% higher than on bar-iron, i.e. an extra £1 10s. 0d. Calendar of Home Office Papers, 1760–5, p. 2064, entry 637.

[2] *Ibid.*, p. 620, entry 2000, Garbett to Burke, 9 November 1765, and p. 2064, entry 637, same to same, 14 December 1765.

[3] These charges are listed in P.R.O., T. 70/1205, f. 41, 'Duties payable on some commodities imported into England' (No date, *c.* 1750). cf. Ashton, *Iron and Steel*, that the duty was invariably £2 1s. 6d. The duty on a ton of steel was, incidentally, close on £10 which explains why foreign steel was hardly imported.

[4] Heckscher, *Sveriges Ekonomiska Historia*, II, 2, p. 671.

were very low. The anonymous author of a tract of the period, 'The Interest of Great Britain supplying herself with Iron',[1] gives the cost of Swedish bar-iron at the forge as £4 5s. 0d. the ton; transport and handling charges advanced prime cost at port to £9–£10, which included the Swedish export duty of c. £3 12s. 6d. The prime cost of Russian iron was held to be a quarter of that for Swedish iron-bar, and therefore made it competitive on the British market although it had to be transported overland for long distances before it reached its port of shipment, St Petersburg. Cost at the forge in England was at the time estimated at £15–£16. Swedish and Russian bar-iron could therefore undersell English iron, particularly as 'the freight from the Baltick [was] lieing the merchant in no more than what it will cost the British maker to carry his iron but twenty miles by land-carriage'. The lower production costs in Sweden, the author of the tract concluded, were due to lower land values and labour costs which were about a quarter of those in England. There is little doubt that Swedish iron could have been sold in England for less if it had not been for the deliberate policy of the Swedish ironmasters to keep prices as high as possible without pricing their product out of the market. They were encouraged in this policy by the Swedish government primarily through the creation in 1747 of the Iron Bureau (*Jernkontoret*) which had as one of its main tasks the allocation of credits to the Swedish iron industry.[2] Instead of having to sell for want of ready money when demand for iron was slack and prices therefore low, the Iron Bureau, which was under the control of the ironmasters themselves, arranged State Bank loans on the security of iron up to seven-eighths of its current value. Unlike the Norwegian timber industry which depended at least in part on credit from England, the Swedish iron industry could rely on internal credit and was therefore able to regulate sales, and through them prices, more easily. The next step in the regulation of prices for Swedish iron – and, it must be

[1] Cited by A. Fell, *The early Iron Industry of Furness and District* (Ulverston, 1908), pp. 308–9.
[2] The background to the institution of the Iron Bureau is fully discussed by A. W. Essén, in his *Johan Liljencrantz som handelspolitiker – Studier i Sveriges handelspolitik 1773–1786* (Lund, 1928), pp. 46ff. On the Iron Bureau, see Stavenow, *Sveriges Historia*, vol. 9, p. 285, and Rosman and Munthe, *Släkten Arfwedson*, p. 177.

remembered, that this meant very largely prices in the English market – was taken through restriction of output ordered by a decree of 1753. No new forge was to be erected nor the production of existing ones increased, and this prohibition remained substantially in force till near the end of the century.[1] The monopolistic policy of the Swedish ironmasters was in the short run highly successful. Demand for iron in England outstripped supply and prices rose steadily. One sharp increase coincided with the restrictive measures introduced in Sweden, the next with the outbreak of war in 1755–6, and another occurred at its height in 1759–60.[2] The profits made by Swedish iron-merchants who often owned the mines and forges, were large. Whereas the percentage difference between price at the forge and export price had been 56·4% in 1756, it had risen to 129·5% in 1761, from which high point it declined again to 96·8% at the end of the War. The absolute increase in export prices over the period of the War was equally spectacular, starting in 1756 with 56 copper dalers per ship-pound, to end at 102–4 dalers in 1763.[3]

Higher export prices were not the only factor making for price increases in England. Freight rates also went up during the War as in the case of the timber-trade, and so did insurance charges. The shortage of money experienced in England later in the War would most likely also have had its effect on prices through greater

[1] Heckscher, 'Un grand chapitre de l'histoire du fer: le monopole suédois', *Annales d'histoire économique et sociale*, 4, no 15 (1932), pp. 231–2. There was no known intention to stimulate manufacture by this regulation. The intention of the decree was to regulate export prices, and Ashton, in *Iron and Steel*, p. 120, has been misled by his source into reading more into it. The effectiveness of the decree is shown by the increase in iron prices which followed it.

[2] Heckscher, *Sveriges Ekonomiska Historia*, II, I, pp. 415 and 430, table I and text; also Ashton, *Iron and Steel*, pp. 131–2. Heckscher has made too much in his text, though, of the increase in export prices, as he has left entirely out of account the depreciation of the Swedish currency. By a report of mid-1758, the Swedish copper daler (dkm.), which was the unit of exchange, had fallen from 36 to the Pound Sterling at par, to 55–56 dalers to the Pound. There is no information, however, of the rate of exchange in successive preceding years, and no certain evidence when parity last ruled. The state of the Swedish economy in the immediate pre-war years suggests that the exchange was then much closer to parity. The report on Swedish finance here cited is in P.R.O., S.P. 75/104, Goodricke to Holdernesse, 25 July 1758. See also below, p. 75, n. 1.

[3] Heckscher, *Sveriges Ekonomiska Historia*, II, I, tables I and 2, p. 430.

length of credit being given by the importer to the retailer or consumer.[1]

The importer, indeed, filled a twofold demand. He made not only iron but also credit available to the consumer, whereas the Swedish exporter expected to be paid on delivery for any order placed with him. The importer could therefore not be done without so long as consumers needed credit, and even the largest do not seem to have been able to manage without it. Benjamin Huntsman, a leading steel converter, regularly bought his Swedish bar-iron supplies through a middleman rather than ordering them directly from Sweden.[2] Sheffield was said to have been 'entirely supplied with steel irons [from Sweden] by some half-dozen houses at Hull, which gave long credit – even twelve months or more. This credit was capital to our town, especially to the makers of steel, saws, and files...so long as credit was needed at Hull, it was given with an open hand.'[3] The importer himself drove the hardest bargain he could with his Swedish correspondents, placing his order in great detail for a variety of different-sized bars, arranging for it to be shipped only when the exchange rate was favourable and prices within a certain range, and expecting the exporter without further commission payments to charter ships when this had not been done already in England.[4] The Swedish exporter, in turn, besides filling orders for specific deliveries, dealt with agents in England to whom consignments might be sent for disposal. The London houses best-known in the mid-century as agents for principals in Sweden were Spalding and Brander, and the brothers Lindegren, Swedes themselves who had become naturalised in England.[5]

[1] See below, appendix 4, pt 2. It may be noted that the insurance market was already at that time international, Swedish merchants acting so early as the 1730s as agents in Sweden for London houses. See on Baltic and North Sea insurance in the eighteenth century, T. Söderberg, *Försäkringsväsendets historia i Sverige intill Karl Johanstiden* (Stockholm, 1935), *passim*, particularly pp. 181ff. Premiums from Stockholm were $\frac{1}{2}$% higher for English West Coast than East Coast ports.

[2] Ashton, *Iron and Steel*, p. 246.   [3] Gatty, *Sheffield*, p. 215.

[4] Swed. S. Arch., Enskilda Handlinger, Arkivfragment, Arkivbildare, correspondence of Jennings and Blount.

[5] See above, p. 31. No records of these houses have come to light except fragments of correspondence. Mr G. S. Lindgren, M.P., has kindly made enquiries for documents of the family but was unable to trace any.

Merchants handling iron on either side of the North Sea were not exclusively or even principally committed to the iron-trade only. The greatest Stockholm houses in the iron-trade had dealings in, so it seems, anything that might have shown a profit.[1] A substantial London importer of Swedish bar-iron, Richard Blount, also placed orders for tar and timber, and showed a somewhat suspicious interest in the Gothenburg tea-market from which smugglers to England were supplied.[2] Thomas Fearnley, who has been met with in the Norwegian timber-trade, also traded in iron which he shipped to England from both Norway and Sweden. When commissioned by a Hull firm to load a ship in a small Swedish port with timber, Fearnley tried as well to persuade Swedish acquaintances to consign 30 or 40 tons of iron with it and, when no iron was to be had near the port, travelled to Gothenburg to buy it there. English merchants who sent him cloths or leather for sale on commission in Norway, asked on occasion to have the proceeds remitted in Swedish iron, and in other instances English goods were directly bartered for Swedish iron and also steel which, however, amounted to no more than a few tons in a year.[3]

Barter deals were of course only feasible when small quantities were involved, and in larger transactions and undoubtedly in the majority of smaller ones, payment was made in cash and by bills of exchange drawn by the exporter either directly on his customer or agent, or by arrangement on a banker in London or abroad. The earlier-mentioned London merchant, Richard Blount, for example, advised a Swedish correspondent to draw on a house in Amsterdam, while the Hull firms with which Fearnley dealt had bankers in London, as was usual for merchants in the out-ports.[4] Since Sweden obtained most of her imports from France and also Holland, it was convenient for Swedish merchants to draw on Continental

---

[1] Samuelsson, *De stora köpmanshusen, passim*, particularly ch. 3.
[2] 'Their [Gothenburg merchants] sales of Tea I believe will be low as our Ships cannot carry on the Smuggling Trade from Gothenburg as they used to do in time of Peace.' R. Blount to F. Jennings of Stockholm, London 29 May 1744, in Jennings correspondence of Swed. S. Arch., Enskilda Samlinger, Arkivfragment, Arkivbildare.
[3] Nor. S. Arch., Fearnley papers, ff. 37, 69, 79, 116, 121, 123–4, 164, 171–8, 250–1 *et al.*
[4] See for a general discussion also K. Samuelsson, 'International Payments and Credit Movements by the Swedish Merchant-Houses, 1730–1815', *Scandinavian Economic History Review*, 3, no 1 (1955).

houses, but the rapid rise of the English money market in the mid-century may well have made London the principal clearing centre for bills from Sweden by the time of the Seven Years War. It is at least suggestive that the leading Swedish financier of the day looked to London and not Holland or Hamburg for loans when Swedish government finances were in the doldrums towards the end of the War.

The first indications of what was in the wind came in the despatches of Goodricke who reported from Copenhagen that the principal Swedish iron-merchant, mine-owner, and financier of the day, Jennings, had called on him on his way to England where he intended to make long-term arrangements for Swedish iron exports. Swedish finances were very shaky, Goodricke had found out, and the State Bank was believed to have sponsored Jennings' mission. The bank's bills were discounted by 30% to 40% for specie, but it had large securities in iron pledges through its connection with the Iron Bureau. Jennings, so Goodricke believed, intended to negotiate the Bank's iron pledges for gold and silver.[1] This despatch was corroborated by a report from a Swedish spy in British service at the Court of Stockholm, one Baron Gedda, who used the code name of 'Wilkinson'.[2] The sharp increase that year in shipments from Sweden would indicate that Jennings had some success.[3] Two years later, Goodricke reported that Jennings and his partner Finlay had undertaken to lend the government 'a large sum' and had sent an agent to England to raise it there at $6\frac{1}{2}$% interest.[4] And, to round off this record of Jennings' enterprise, when Swedish houses were threatened with bankruptcy during the great financial crisis of 1763, Goodricke reported that they were depending on London to pull them through as 'Our Merchants are the only ones able to make any advances at present, and our Country the only one from which Sweden receives any Ballance in Money'. As matters stood, Goodricke reported, Jennings alone was confidently expected to weather the storm since his English corre-

[1] P.R.O., S.P. 75/108, Goodricke to Holdernesse, 10 May 1760.
[2] S.P. 95/103, Wilkinson's report to London, Stockholm 28 April 1760.
[3] See below, appendix 2, Fig. 5.
[4] S.P. 75/113, Goodricke to Bute, 13 February 1762.

spondents could give him a large enough loan.[1] Whether loans were made by English to Swedish houses is not known as no records appear to have been preserved, but Jennings at least justified Goodricke's confidence in him and survived the crisis.

Once a bill was drawn in Sweden, it could be exchanged for ready money by selling it at a discount to importers who had to make payments abroad, or to government agencies for remittance to diplomatic agents. It was customary to draw for the full amount of the invoice when iron had been shipped on order, and for the greater part of the estimated value of the cargo when it was sent on consignment to agents. The agent remitted the balance due, less his commission, when the shipment entrusted to him for disposal had finally been sold.[2]

London was not only a financial centre of the Anglo-Swedish iron-trade. It was also the most important single market for iron, taking a good two-fifths of recorded shipments from Sweden before and during the War.[3] Small quantities were re-exported, others were distributed to the royal dockyards and to private yards working on government contracts, and the rest was used locally in manufacture, as there were no substantial English iron-producing areas within economic distance of London.[4] Distribution of Swedish iron for use by the Royal Navy had an importance quite out of proportion to the amount imported. Swedish iron alone was allowed in the construction of ships for the Royal Navy as it had proved itself well suited and the Admiralty would take no risks with any other. This ruling remained in force until the end of the century, although samples of bar-iron worked up from colonial ore had indeed been tested at a royal dockyard through the initiative – spurred possibly

[1] P.R.O., S.P. 75/115, Goodricke to Halifax, Stockholm 3 and 13 September 1763.
[2] Copies of bills of exchange are plentiful, and their circulation can be followed in detail from their endorsements. For examples see Swed. S. Arch., Diplomatica, Anglica I, Brev till A. Wynantz från Kanslikollegium och andra ämbetsverk, sect. Statskontoret och Räntekammaren, 1748–58; and also, P.R.O., S.P. 95/106, ff. 161 *et seq.* Some financial practices in the iron-trade are discussed in E. F. Söderlund, *Swedish Timber Exports 1850–1950* (Stockholm, 1952), pp. 85–6.
[3] See below, appendix 2, Fig. 6.
[4] Re-exports from London were practically entirely to India, and from the out-ports to Africa and America. See also below, appendix 4, pt 2, on the placing of government contracts for Swedish bar-iron, and Ashton, *Iron and Steel*, appendix C, pp. 239ff., on local distribution.

76

by national sentiment – of an English ironmaster, and had been declared as good as any Swedish. The results of the tests were submitted to a parliamentary committee in 1737, only to be flatly contradicted by evidence given by a number of independent iron-masters. Their attitude was made quite clear at a parliamentary enquiry into the iron-trade in 1750. The ironmasters and mine-owners of 'Sheffield, Gloucester, and the County of York' then stated that the position of Swedish iron in the English market would not be affected by increased imports of colonial iron which could not replace Swedish, but could certainly replace English iron and would therefore ruin the English iron industry.[1] It may well have been in the back of their minds that once duties on colonial iron had been entirely lifted, it would be hard to reinstate them if colonial iron should come into the country in any quantity and be a menace to the English iron industry, whereas it would be much easier to raise already existing duties on Swedish iron and make it non-competitive. Agitation to raise the duties on Swedish iron was indeed loud by 1765 when the iron-trade was once again the subject of parliamentary debate, and a Bill was to be introduced to raise the duty by £2. Nothing came of it as the government was just then negotiating a treaty with Sweden.[2] On a further attempt to introduce a similar Bill into Parliament, matters were so arranged that the session was prorogued before any action could be taken. Sandwich, the Northern Secretary, intended to take full credit for it and instructed Goodricke that 'You will make the most Merit you can, of a Plan of this Sort having been dropt', but Goodricke was not to make promises for the future in case the government wanted to increase the duties at a later date.[3]

Of the out-ports, Hull and Newcastle were most important in the trade. A contemporary also mentioned Bristol and Liverpool, but these were identified more closely with the products of the foundry than of the smithy and forge. What was needed locally was sent from these import centres to the nearby inland manufacturing

[1] *J.H.C.*, vol. XXII, pp. 850–1, and *ibid.*, vol. XXV, pp. 1019 and 1021.
[2] P.R.O., C.O. 391/72, entries of 1, 2 and 25 April 1765; *ibid.*, C.O. 389/31, Lords Commissioners of Trade and Plantations to Secretary of Treasury, 26 April 1765; *ibid.*, S.P. 95/107, Goodricke to Sandwich, Stockholm, 9 July 1765, secret.
[3] P.R.O., S.P. 95/106, Sandwich to Goodricke, 24 May 1765.

towns where tens of thousands of workers depended on the regular supply of Swedish bars.[1]

The ships which carried these supplies to the English market had before the War been mostly British, a rather surprising fact at first sight as the outward voyage had generally to be made in ballast.[2] Sweden admitted by the mid-century few English goods, and would not allow foreign ships to trade coastwise which might in part have recouped the owner or charterer for his loss on half the voyage.[3] The explanation appears to be that the smaller English ships were more suitable in the trade than the ships of greater tonnage favoured by Swedish owners, and their cargoes easier to insure. Richard Blount was quite upset when his Stockholm correspondent Francis Jennings sent him a cargo of bar-iron in a Swedish ship, and he wrote to Jennings that 'I must tell you I would have given one Shilling per last more freight for one half the Burthen, as such large foreign Ships run great hazards upon our coasts', and made his own arrangements for the next shipment.[4] Blount was one of the larger men in the trade, buying whole cargoes in one transaction. The smaller merchants made up a cargo between them, and more often than not ships loaded small parcels of iron and of timber consigned by half-a-dozen exporters to their different customers in a port. Thoughtfully, Swedish exporters generally included in their shipments a few barrels of French brandy which, needless to say, did not find their way into the statistics of imports.[5]

The Seven Years War changed the pattern of shipping in that Swedish-registered ships came to ¦be much more engaged in it. Iron was not a contraband of war and could therefore be carried without hindrance in neutral ships, whereas English ships had to

---

[1] See appendix 4, pt 2.

[2] See below, appendix 2, Figs 5 and 6. The greater number of British ships passing the Sound into the Baltic were in ballast, and many ships trading to Gothenburg had only a nominal cargo.

[3] See above, p. 5.

[4] Swed. S. Arch., Enskilda Handlinger, Arkivfragment, Arkivbildare, Jennings Correspondence, Blount to Jennings, London, 17 August 1744.

[5] Gothenburg Provincial Archives (Landsarkivet i Göteborg), City accounts and port books (Göteborgs Stads Räkenskap Böker m. d. Verificationer), 1725, 1750, 1775. The entries show that British ships to Gothenburg were almost invariably of less than 100 tons, and most generally nearer 50.

run the gauntlet of French privateers in the North Sea and particularly in the approaches to the Sound. Sweden had opened her West Coast harbours to them,[1] and the formidable Captain Thurot who was later to land with a force in Ireland, actually used Gothenburg as his base. Convoys had been organised from and to the Sound, and cruisers made independent sweeps in the North Sea, but the dangers were still great and many prizes fell to the French.[2] It is small wonder that ships flying the English flag left half the trade to their Swedish rivals until the end of the War, when they returned to it in as great numbers as before.[3]

With the exception of the changed distribution of shipping, the iron-trade between England and Sweden during the War showed few outward signs of strain. But a strain there was. The Russian forges were producing increasing quantities of a good quality bar-iron for export to England,[4] and the falling-off of recorded imports from Sweden after the War might well have happened earlier if it had not been for the exceptional demands during it. Sweden had taken the opportunity in 1747 with the creation of the Iron Bureau, in 1753 by a restriction of output, and again in the first year of the War through discriminatory export duties, to keep the price of her iron at an artificially high level.[5] So soon as Russian competition was fully encountered, the share of Swedish iron in the English market fell both proportionately and absolutely, not to rise again until late in the century when the Swedish iron industry at last turned away from its monopolistic and restrictive practices.[6]

[1] See H. S. K. Kent, 'The Three-Mile Limit', *loc. cit.*, pp. 550f.

[2] See below, p. 147.

[3] See below, appendix 2, Figs 6 and 7.

[4] Seven-eighths of all bar-iron exported from St Petersburg in 1766 was, according to a consular report, shipped to England. P.R.O., C.O. 388/54, 'Account of Goods exported by the English Ships anno 1766 from St. Petersburg', transmitted by Consul Swallow to the Board of Trade, March 1767.

[5] The Swedish Senate discussed again at the end of the war possible means to raise the price for export as high as could be done without driving England into buying more from Russia, or encouragring imports from the American colonies. The matter was in the end left to the mine-owners. P.R.O., S.P. 75/115, Goodricke to Halifax, 26 February 1763.

[6] The view that Sweden could have exported more to England is also taken by E. F. Heckscher, 'Un grand chapitre', *loc. cit.*, pp. 234–5. Professor Heckscher notes that after restrictive practices had been abandoned, Swedish exports to England increased concurrently with increased imports into England from Russia.

5 *Miscellaneous Imports from Scandinavia*

Iron and timber were by the mid-eighteenth century the only native produce exported by the Scandinavian kingdoms in large quantities to England. Beside these two staples other goods were of no very great importance in the legitimate trade, with the exception of Swedish pitch and tar, which were of such a high quality that even heavily subsidised imports from America could not drive them out of the English market. Sweden had in the past been practically the sole foreign supplier of these essential naval stores, which were used in caulking and in the preparation of ship's cordage. So great had English dependence on Swedish supplies become by the later seventeenth century that the export merchants, combined in the monopolistic Stockholm Tar Company, could afford to name their own price and impose their own trade conditions.[1] Most stultifying among them was the Company's refusal to ship any pitch and tar except in Swedish ships and then only at whatever time suited the Company best. There was much agitation against the Swedish monopoly, and proposals were made to import pitch and tar from the American colonies where the pine forests of North Carolina in particular showed promise of an inexhaustible source of supply.[2] The cost of shipment, however, was great, and there is moreover no reason to suppose that English merchants early in the century were prepared to desert a lucrative trade with Sweden, no matter how vexatious, and speculate in colonial ven-

[1] English grievances about the supply of Swedish pitch and tar are listed in detail by M. Postlethwayt, *Universal Dictionary of Trade and Commerce* (4th ed., London, 1774), vol. 2, s.v. 'Naval Stores'. See also for a contemporary account Robert Jackson's 'Memoir on the Swedish Tar Company', ed. J. J. Murray, in *Huntington Library Quarterly*, vol. 10, no 4 (1947). Murray's introduction to the memoir suffers from an uncritical acceptance of contemporary statistics. For a Swedish account, see Heckscher, *Sveriges Ekonomiska Historia*, I, 2, pp. 436f.
[2] Postlethwayt, *Dictionary of Commerce*, *loc. cit.*, and also vol. 1, s.v. 'British America', section 'Carolina'.

tures.[1] But conditions changed suddenly when Parliament intervened. A naval squadron which was to be fitted out against France in 1703 could not be made ready for sea as there was insufficient pitch and tar available, and the Stockholm Company refused to ship any despite the intervention of the British envoy with the Swedish court. The danger to British preparedness was obvious, and a contemporary bitterly observed how much 'it was in the power of the king of Sweden to forward the fitting out of the royal navy of England, or to keep it in harbour'.[2] What had long been urged was now at last done: an Act was passed[3] giving a substantial bounty to importers of colonial pitch and tar which encouraged American production to such an extent that within a few years the English market was glutted, prices for the colonial produce stood, at least for a time, at one-third of those formerly paid for the Swedish, and quantities were re-exported to the Mediterranean, to Spain, Portugal, Holland, and even to Hamburg and Bremen.[4]

American pitch and tar, however, could not wholly replace Swedish. Their quality was poor, and the various Acts extending the bounties for further periods became ever more stringent in laying down that payment would only be made on produce conforming to a prescribed standard of purity.[5] Despite these regulations, improvement appears to have been very slight or nonexistent, and the bounty on pitch was eventually lowered from

---

[1] Postlethwayt notes in the article on Naval Stores that the freight from the Baltic and North Sea was only about one-third of that from the American colonies.

[2] The strategic consequences of this refusal are discussed by Sir Herbert Richmond, *Statesmen and Seapower* (Oxford, 1946), p. 102. The quotation about the effects of Swedish intransigence is taken from a despatch by Dr John Robinson, British envoy to Sweden, printed in Postlethwayt's article on Naval Stores.   [3] 3 & 4 Anne c. 10.

[4] The effects on supply and re-exportation are noted by J. Gee, *The Trade and Navigation of Great Britain Considered* (2nd ed., London, 1730), pp. 144–5, and by Postlethwayt in his article on Naval Stores. The statistics of the trade are entered in P.R.O., Cust. 3/20, and Cust. 14/1 *a*–1 *b*, imports from American colonies (chiefly Carolina), and from Sweden to London, to the Outports, and to Scotland, and re-exports of goods to the countries noted above on this page. The breaking of the Swedish monopoly made such an impression in England that Russian exporters of iron and naval stores were threatened by publicists so late as the end of the century with the same fate that befell the Swedish monopolists when England developed her colonial resources. See D. Gerhard, *England und der Aufstieg Russlands*, pp. 54–5.

[5] 5 Geo. I c. 11; 8 Geo. I c. 12; and 2 Geo. II c. 35. See also Gee, *Navigation of Great Britain*, p. 145, that experts had to be sent from England to the colonies to demonstrate the proper manufacture of pitch and tar before any improvement occurred.

£4 to £1 for the last.[1] It is unlikely that after that time much colonial pitch was imported as its price came to be about on a par with Swedish.[2] The original bounty of £4 on colonial tar continued to be paid, and it may be assumed that practically all the shipments indiscriminately entered in customs accounts under the combined heading of pitch and tar consisted in fact practically wholly of tar. Some 6,000 lasts were imported from America in 1750, as against some 800 of pitch and tar from Sweden.[3] The prices for that year are not available, but in the following year colonial tar was bought by the Navy Board at £6 per last, Swedish at £9 10s. 0d., and pitch at the unity price of £13 2s. 6d. That the demand for Swedish tar persisted is shown by the prices ruling in 1754 when 350 lasts of pitch and tar were imported at the high price of £11 10s. 0d. per last for tar, while colonial tar remained at £5 13s. 6d.[4] So soon as hostilities began in 1755, imports from Sweden increased, and prices for colonial and Swedish tar rose. Imports from America initially also increased, only to fall again by 1757 to reach their lowest point in 1760 when they were actually overtaken by supplies from Sweden. While the prices paid for American tar rose steeply, those for Swedish advanced little on the immediate pre-War price and fell well below it in 1760–1 when imports reached their highest point.[5]

As was to be expected, purchases by the Navy Board for the royal dockyards were heavier during the War than in time of peace; what seems surprising at first sight is that the Board should have bought throughout the War Swedish pitch and tar, rather than colonial as was its invariable practice in normal years.[6] The reason for this change from colonial to Swedish supplies was most probably a very simple one. Contracts for stores were placed by the Board

[1] The last of pitch or of tar was of 12 barrels of *c.* 32 gallons each, or of *c.* 30 cwt dry-measure. Although the Acts specified measurement by the last for pitch, this was generally measured by merchants and the Navy Board by the ton of *c.* 2/3 last. The Act lowering the bounty on pitch was 2 Geo. II c. 35.

[2] Pitch and tar prices at the Deptford and Woolwich naval yards are tabulated by Beveridge, *Prices and Wages*, p. 675. It is to be understood that the prices given by Beveridge are only approximations to the market price, as special factors influenced contract prices for royal dockyards.

[3] See appendix 3.   [4] Beveridge, *Prices and Wages, loc. cit.*

[5] Appendix 3; and Beveridge, *Prices and Wages, loc. cit.*

[6] On the purchasing policy of the Navy Board, see Beveridge, *Prices and Wages*, pp. 618–19, 662 and 666.

before the beginning of the sailing season for delivery later in the year, and so long as war made communications with America uncertain it was more prudent to order supplies of a known high quality brought from the Sound under convoy. During the War, then, Swedish pitch and tar came to be much sought-after, if not essential, naval stores.

That certainty of supply in war appears to have been a main consideration when switching so widely from colonial to Swedish pitch and tar may also be inferred from the distribution of shipping in the trade.[1] Pitch and tar were both contraband of war, and liable to seizure by French privateers even when carried in Swedish ships.[2] During the earlier years of the War, pitch and tar were therefore almost entirely carried in English ships which had the protection of convoying warships. In 1759 there was a change in the distribution of shipping. Slightly more than half was carried in Swedish vessels in that year, and during the remaining years of the War nearly all the pitch and tar sent to England went in Swedish bottoms. The re-emergence of Swedish shipping in the trade coincided with the withdrawal of French privateers from the North Sea towards the end of the 1759 sailing season, as they were needed in helping to mount the planned French invasion of the British Isles in the following year, an invasion in which Thurot, who has already been noted as the commander of the most successful privateering fleet in the North Sea, met his death when leading a foray on Ireland.[3]

[1] The relative shares of English and foreign shipping in the trade are as usual to be found in P.R.O., Cust. 3/50–70, and Cust. 14/1*a* and 1*b*.

[2] Pitch and tar had been expressly declared a contraband of war by England in 1744, and instructions were accordingly given to warships and privateers to bring up any neutrals loaded with these naval stores. On the instructions, see Sir Ernest Satow, *The Silesian Loan and Frederick the Great* (Oxford, 1915), pp. 121–2. Sweden countered this declaration by a royal proclamation of 16 July 1756 to the effect that neither pitch nor tar were contraband, and that she reserved the right to trade freely in them. The proclamation is laid in under date 13 September 1756 in Swed. S. Arch., Diplomatica, Anglica 1, Brev till Wynantz från Kanslikollegium o. a. ämbetsverk i Sverige, and is enrolled in Utrikes Expeditions Registratur, 1756, f. 174. As will be seen below, England enforced her declaration on pitch and tar as contraband by captures at sea, and the Admiralty Courts upheld the British contention by condemnations.

[3] The action is described in some detail in the *London Gazette Extraordinary*, 3 March 1760.

The pitch- and tar-trade itself differed in no essential detail from the iron- and the timber-trade. English merchants with connections in Sweden through the iron-trade bought pitch and tar as occasion arose, and had it shipped as part of a mixed cargo.[1] There is little likelihood that they bothered to smuggle either pitch or tar as the duties on them were nominal, and customs returns of imports may for once be taken at something near their face value.[2] They agreed in any case very closely with the Swedish export figures which showed further that the trade was still of some consequence to Sweden, despite American competition, as nearly a quarter of total Swedish tar exports were taken by Great Britain during the War.[3]

Like Sweden, Norway had never ceased to supply England with some pitch and tar, but the quantities were smaller and rarely exceeded 200 lasts in the years between 1750 and 1770.[4] Scotland, which had closer connections than England with the Norwegian ports of Bergen and Trondheim from which pitch and tar were mostly shipped, received about the same amount from Norway whereas her imports from Sweden were no more than an odd last or two.[5] The East Country, Russia, and Holland were other sources of supply, but there again the quantities were small and by the mid-century quite negligible. This pattern of imports stayed unchanged until the American Revolution temporarily cut England off from

[1] There are numerous records of ships carrying pitch and tar as part of their cargo. See, for examples, Dan. S. Arch., T.K.U.A., Engl. C, 266, Bernstorff to Bothmer, 18 March 1758 and enclosures, which instances i.a. the cargoes of a number of ships from Sweden; and also, P.R.O., S.P. 75/114, Titley to Halifax, despatch of 16 November 1762 in which a list of prized ships is given. Arrangements for shipping tar from Stockholm to London are discussed in the Finlay–Blount correspondence in Swed. S. Arch., Enskilda Samlinger, Arkivfragment, Arkivbildare, Jennings correspondence.

[2] The duty on pitch was at the time of the Seven Years War 10s. 9d. per last when imported by British subjects, and 11s. 5d. when imported by foreigners; the duty on tar was only 1s. 2d. per last irrespective of the nationality of the importer. See Baldwin, *The British Customs*, pt 1, pp. 49 and 62 on duties, and *ibid.*, pt 2, p. 19, on the premiums given on colonial pitch and tar.

[3] Heckscher, *Sveriges ekonomiska historia*, II, 1, pp. 333ff., and *ibid.*, II, 2, appendix, table 8. See also J. J. Oddy, *European Commerce...detailing the Produce and Manufactures of Russia, Prussia, Sweden, Denmark and Germany* (London, 1805), p. 301, that Swedish tar was irreplaceable for high-quality work.

[4] See the relevant entries in P.R.O., Cust. 3/50–70, and Cust. 14/1 *a* and 1 *b*.

[5] Beawes, *Lex mercatoria*, p. 828, details the Norwegian ports from which pitch and tar were shipped to Scotland.

some of her colonial supplies, and she had to draw more heavily on Scandinavia. By that time, however, Canada had become the principal source of pitch and tar from the colonies and British dependence on Swedish supplies was therefore never again as acute as it had been in the seventeenth century.[1]

Of further imports from Scandinavia which entered England legitimately, little remains to be said. They were neither large in quantity or value, nor had they any particular strategic importance.[2] One group consisted of such odds and ends as wooden tubs and trays, boat-hooks, oars, handspikes, and even wooden spoons which found their way into the customs accounts at the rate of 100 or 200 every year, suggesting if nothing more that some customs officers were punctilious over details, or some merchants honest. During the War an occasional bale of sailcloth turned up, and some hundredweight of hemp and flax which were of no consequence whatever compared with the amounts that reached England from Russia, the East Country, and also Holland. Denmark and also Sweden shipped a few hundred Pounds-worth of hides which were admitted into the country despite the danger of the introduction of cattle-disease which raged in some years in Scandinavia. The British envoys sent warning whenever it broke out, but the government in London took no action to bar the import of hides in those years.[3] Beef itself, salted and packed in barrels ready for provisioning merchantships and warships, was imported occasionally from Denmark where it was a staple article of trade. One such shipment of about 600 barrels reached London in 1758, and there is evidence that some 10,000 barrels captured in the preceding year as prize goods also were Danish.[4] England had declared salt beef a contra-

---

[1] The steep rise in colonial pitch and tar shipments after the Seven Years War was entirely due to Canadian supplies reaching the British market. Pitch and tar were both in effect enumerated commodities as they did not qualify for the British bounty unless offered to the Navy Board for first refusal.

[2] The customs ledgers are the principal source of reference for imports of the commodities discussed in the remainder of this chapter.

[3] P.R.O., S.P. 75/106, Titley to Holdernesse, 25 December 1759, is an example of such a warning, yet hides continued to be listed in the customs ledgers as imports from Denmark-Norway.

[4] P.R.O., Cust. 3/57, section Prize Goods, and S.P. 75/102, Titley to Holdernesse, 28 May 1757, that Bernstorff had complained to him about substantial seizures of salt beef by English privateers.

band of war in the 1740s despite Danish protests, which were rejected on the grounds that it was of direct use to the enemy's navy. Denmark, in fact, had complained during the War of the Austrian Succession that provisions shipped by neutrals were regarded by England as contraband, and seized by her privateers. The London Court of Admiralty condemned provisions as contraband, and in at least one instance a case involving a Danish ship was taken further to the Court of Appeal which upheld the decision of the lower Court on the grounds that provisions were of direct use to the enemy's navy.[1] Titley warned the government after the big seizures of 1757 that this ruling might do more harm politically than the military advantage warranted, as the estates of the powerful royal favourite, Count Adam Gottlob Moltke, supplied the French Navy under contract with the larger share of all the salt beef shipped from Denmark.[2] This warning was effective, and Danish ships laden with beef for France were later tacitly allowed to pass unmolested.[3]

Norway had like Denmark one staple article of ship's provisions for export, in her case unsalted, sun-dried cod known as stockfish which was shipped every season to England in some quantity.[4] There was hardly a year in the middle decades of the century when at least 1,000 Hundred, each of 120 fish, were not declared at the customs, and in some years as many as 4,000 Hundred at an official value of 28s. to 32s. the Hundred, were entered in the

---

[1] This case had some other features of interest, and is discussed in Nicolas Magens, *Insurances*, vol. 2, p. 638.

[2] P.R.O., S.P. 75/102, Titley to Holdernesse, 14 June 1757; and S.P. 75/103, same to same, 28 February 1758 and 18 March 1758. See also Moltke Archives, Breve fra fransk Ambassadør J.-F. Ogier, Mémoire: Conditions auxquelles l'on pourroit livrer annuellement des viandes salées en France pour la Service de sa Majesté très Chrétienne. Remis au mois d'octob. 1755.' And also, letters from Ogier to Moltke, dated 3 July and 23 August 1757, and draft reply Moltke to Ogier, 4 July 1757.

[3] After 1757 salt beef no longer appeared as prize goods in the customs ledgers except for an odd hundredweight, although Denmark continued to ship it regularly to France in unarmed ships. It is obvious from Titley's despatches that he had privately assured Bernstorff of England's acquiescence in the trade. See P.R.O., S.P. 75/103, Titley to Holdernesse, 27 May 1758; and S.P. 75/105, same to same, 24 April and 15 May 1759.

[4] The value of dried cod as ship's provisions must have been regarded highly as it was imported despite the heavy duty of £1 2s. 4d. per Hundred whether on British or foreign account. See Henry Saxby, *The British Customs* (London, 1757), p. 152.

customs returns. Scottish imports of Norwegian stockfish were so small that they are not worth noting. During the War years, some few shipments from Sweden are also recorded, and one may safely assume that further odd quantities which reached English ports ostensibly from Russia had in fact originated in Norway or Sweden.

One last article of import from Scandinavia that need be considered, not so much for its value, but rather for the light it throws on certain trade practices, is copper. Both Sweden and Norway had in the past supplied England with much copper while her own mines in Cornwall remained neglected. At the end of the seventeenth century, copper-mining was resumed and British imports dwindled to negligible amounts.[1] British interests in Norwegian copper-works were given up,[2] and Swedish copper which had once been used even in the English coinage, now only appeared on the English market, when at all, a few tons at a time, selling at the competitive price of around £100 the ton.[3] These occasional intrusions of Swedish copper may have been engineered by English merchants as a warning to intending monopolists who were attempting to gain control of English copper production.[4] If that was so, then English importers combined long-term business policy very advantageously with quick profits when importing, as they usually did, minted copper from Sweden. Sweden had instituted in the seventeenth century a copper coinage with which she persisted after the world price of copper had risen above the face-value of her coin, which stood in a fixed relation to an irredeemable paper currency.[5] Prohibitions on the export of copper coin were, as is

[1] Hamilton, *Brass and Copper*, pp. 57, 60, 61 and 277.   [2] See above, ch. 2, p. 14.
[3] Hamilton, *Brass and Copper*, p. 279. The price given by Hamilton for unworked copper compares reasonably with the price of simple copper utensils in use at dockyards as tabulated by Beveridge, *Prices and Wages*, p. 679.
[4] Hamilton, *Brass and Copper*, pp. 279–80, and see also Beawes, *Lex mercatoria*, p .840, about arrangements for the purchase of copper in Sweden. That Swedish copper was imported into England in the eighteenth century to deter local attempts at monopoly is regarded as likely by E. F. Heckscher, 'Den svenska kopparhanteringen under 1700-talet', *Scandia, Tidskrift for Historisk Forskning*, 13, pt 1 (Stockholm, etc., September 1940), pp. 71–2.
[5] E. F. Heckscher, *De svenska penning-, vikt-, och måttsystemen* (3rd ed., Stockholm, 1942), *passim*. Heckscher also discusses in his *Sveriges ekonomiska historia*, II, 1, p. 375, the history of the copper and silver coinage and their relation to the paper currency, and confesses that the reason for the persistence with a copper coinage after the rise in value of copper is unknown.

87

seen, ineffective, and after experimenting for a short time with copper–silver bimetallism, Sweden finally went over to a silver coinage.[1] It would appear that merchants took advantage of the differences in value between copper ingots and copper coin which they did not scruple to smuggle out of the country – nor, for that matter, did the English customs authorities ask any awkward questions if they knew of Swedish regulations.

The official valuation of all these miscellaneous imports from Scandinavia – copper, stockfish, hemp and flax, pitch and tar, hides, and other minor items – was on the average in the 1750s and 1760s only around £30,000 annually. This valuation cannot have been so far off the actual landed cost which may be assumed as slightly greater. Two-thirds or more in official value of all these imports consisted of pitch and tar, and, as has earlier been shown, by far the greater part of this joint entry was tar. The official value of pitch and tar stood at £8 to £10, a value at which these naval stores were assessed late in the seventeenth century. The actual price had in the meantime sunk and then risen again to stand at around £9 for Swedish tar, and at *c.* £13 for pitch at the time of the Seven Years War. The official value of the main item in this list of minor trade goods was therefore closely related to the actual price in England, and the remaining items did not greatly affect the total sum. There was, no doubt, some smuggling, but even an inordinate allowance for it would still leave expenditure on all these various imports at a fraction of the amounts laid out for timber and iron, the great staples of legitimate trade, let alone the smuggling trade.

[1] The prohibition on the export of minted copper in 1743 is noted by Stavenow, *Sveriges Historia*, vol. 9, p. 293.

6 *The Export Trade*

The economic policies of the Scandinavian kingdoms were bearing hard on the legitimate British export trade to Denmark and Sweden in particular. Restrictions and outright prohibitions on the entry of goods had multiplied since the later sixteenth century until the scope for open trade had been narrowed considerably by the mid-eighteenth century. Yet despite the rising Scandinavian manufacturing enterprises, British merchandise still found a market though it was not always the legitimate one. This is not surprising, as the well-established British industries could turn out goods of better quality and at a lower price than the infant manufactures of Denmark and Sweden – Norway remained largely a primary producing country – and the price difference between Scandinavian and English goods was often great enough to make smuggling attractive.[1] England also had some goods to offer which native Scandinavian industries could not supply; she had minerals which Scandinavia needed, foodstuffs that were in short supply, and some colonial wares for which the Scandinavian countries had to rely on foreign sources. British supplies therefore remained in demand despite Scandinavian protectionist measures for home industries and for their own colonial trade, and the goods exported were of such variety that the customs declarations of ships leaving England, or arriving at the Sound and in Scandinavian ports, read today rather like pages from a mail-order firm's catalogue.

The cargoes of three ships may serve as an illustration of the diversity of exports to Scandinavia. The brig *Trenne Brödre* of Bergen, returning to her home port from London early in 1760,

---

[1] Comparative costs of English and Danish cloth are given by Nielsen, *Wirtschafts-geschichte*, p. 250. A survey in 1766 showed that Denmark could not compete with England in the production of cloth. English cloth was thought to be 'unbelievably inexpensive', and Nielsen also notes that it was smuggled into Denmark via Hamburg, the Duchies and Altona (p. 248).

carried a mixed cargo, consigned to some twenty people, of knives, files, saws and other hardware, printed cottons, woollens, cloths, woollen yarn whose export from England was actually prohibited, and fruit, flour, malt, and more beside: Claus Reimers, one of the consignees, had shipped to him two nightcaps and one flat-iron; Fru Sophie Thommesen received a pair of spectacles and sixteen straw hats.[1] A second ship, the English snow *Friendship* which reached Bergen late in 1756 from an unspecified English port, had aboard stone coal, lead in strips and in bulk, coarse cloths, grindstones, window-glass, bottles, pots and pans, hops, malt, and hemp. The master declared that the whole cargo was being shipped on his own account, and he or his principals in England, must have felt certain that there was a market for every single item.[2] Finally, the brig *Lark* from Hull arrived at Gothenburg in May 1750 with potatoes, malt, grain, butter, stone coal, and bricks. This cargo had been indented by a group of Swedish merchants.[3]

Among the merchandise just described were some items like hardware and haberdashery and millinery whose import into the Scandinavian countries was prohibited, yet they were in these instances openly declared at the ports of destination. This was not likely to have been a mistake on the part of the importers who were undoubtedly armed with import licences. Merchants who were persuasive enough to convince the authorities that prohibited goods could not be supplied at the time by home manufacture or from native sources were given dispensation from the prohibitions, and English merchandise could enter through such a loophole when it would normally have been excluded from legitimate trade.[4] There is no direct evidence that dispensations were issued in Sweden, but the occasional customs entries of fine cloths which

[1] Nor. S. Arch., Bergen port book (Toldbog), 1760, I, entries 1 and 42.
[2] *Ibid.*, 1756, I, entries 294 and 430.
[3] Gothenburg Provincial Archives, city accounts and port books, 1750, f. 663 *v.* & *d.*
[4] Dan. S. Arch., Rentekammeret, Københavns Civiletatskontors-Kopiprotokol 1748–50, nr 779, entry of 7 March 1750; *ibid.*, 1750–2, nr 902, entry of 3 February 1752; also, Kopiprotokol for Aalborg og Viborg Stifters Kontor 1756–8, nr 202, entry of 15 October 1757; and see also Rentekammeret, Relations- og Resolutionsprotokol, 1757, nrs 46, 137 and 266. In these enrolments of import licences for normally prohibited goods are instanced various qualities of cloth, of printed cottons, silks, linens, and haberdashery. The licences are made out for definite quantities and are granted to particular merchants.

were on the prohibited list suggest that Sweden also relaxed on occasion her restrictions on English goods.[1] A trickle at least of goods that one would not have expected to meet with except in the smuggling trade found its way therefore quite legitimately to the Scandinavian markets. Still more English goods on the prohibited lists were bonded in Danish and Norwegian ports for re-export as it was the policy of the Danish–Norwegian administration to encourage the *entrepôt* trade especially of Copenhagen and Elsinore.[2] Swedish ports do not appear to have possessed bonding facilities for prohibited goods, and the pattern of the English export trade also suggests that the *entrepôt* trade in such goods was not encouraged by Sweden.[3]

Dispensations from import-prohibitions, and bonding facilities for prohibited imports, introduce the first of several complications when attempting to assess the extent of legitimate British trade with the Scandinavian countries, as one cannot simply write off as clandestine trade those shipments of British merchandise whose importation into Scandinavia was normally not permitted. Yet this difficulty, upsetting though it is, was of little consequence when compared with another and more serious obstacle to reaching any hard-and-fast conclusions on the extent of legitimate trade. The fundamental difficulty in assessing the quantity and possibly also the range of British exports lies in the nature and in the accessibility of contemporary statistics. Port books in England and in Scandinavia from which statistics can be extracted are known either to have been destroyed or exist today only in broken series, and when available are often so badly damaged and illegible that they cannot safely be used. Entries from the port books were originally the basis of contemporary English and Scottish customs accounts

[1] Imports into Gothenburg are tabulated in Ivan Lind, *Göteborgs Handel och Sjöfart 1637–1920* (Göteborg, 1923), pp. 90–7, tables 17–20, 'Införsel från Olika Länder 1750–1765.' Entries in the Gothenburg port books show that the cloth imported in those years from England appears to have been only of the better qualities. This impression is further strengthened by the description of Anglo-Swedish trade in the article 'Sweden' in Postlethwayt's *Dictionary of Commerce*, vol. 2.

[2] Danish–Norwegian *entrepôt* trade is discussed in some detail in Schovelin, *Fra den Danske Handels Empire*, vol. 1, pp. 82ff., and in Olsen, *Danmark-Norge*, p. 19.

[3] It is apparent from Lind, *Göteborgs Handel*, pp. 22–3, that the importation of prohibited goods for re-export was not permitted at least in Gothenburg, and there is no reason to assume that other Swedish ports had better bonding facilities.

which have so far been one of the sources for assessing the scope of the import trade, but the surviving port books and the contemporary annual accounts are unfortunately of little help when it comes to the export trade, as changes in customs policy during the seventeenth and early eighteenth centuries led to irregularities in port entries for outward-bound goods. Outward duties on practically all exports had progressively been abolished since the later sixteenth century by a series of Acts which culminated in the virtual freeing of the export trade from all duties by 1722.[1] The Act of the preceding year which freed the export trade did indeed lay down that all goods exported had to be declared at the custom house, but there is no doubt whatever that this regulation was not strictly observed. Evidence from the scattered and incomplete series of Scandinavian records shows that, on the one hand, goods from England whose export was not prohibited turned up in Scandinavia without any entry of them having been made in the English ledgers.[2] And, on the other hand, there is at the least a suspicion that English merchants made over-entries at the English custom houses either to raise their credit by impressing others with the extent of their trade, or merely to mislead competitors about the state of the market.[3]

These warnings about their reliability should alone suffice to make one approach the available statistics on the export trade with the greatest caution. Further difficulties in interpreting the records are still to be noted when various export goods come to be dealt with, and the conclusion is inescapable that at least a

[1] Saxby, *British Customs*, pp. 278ff., cites the various Acts by which practically all export duties were abolished. The final in the series of these Acts was 8 Geo. I c. 15, which came into force in 1722.

[2] Large shipments from England of bricks and of salt are entered in the Gothenburg port books for 1750 (see Gothenburg Provincial Archives, city accounts and port books, 1750, *passim*) without there being any corresponding entries of exports in the English or Scottish customs ledgers. Similarly, the Bergen port books (Nor. S. Arch., Bergen Toldbøger, 1756 I, and 1763 I and II) show that linens were imported in 1756 and 1763 in some quantity from Scotland in Scottish ships, yet there are no entries of linen exports for those years in the Scottish customs ledgers. The quantities involved were too large to have been covered by British customs entries of unspecified goods at value.

[3] The likelihood of that having happened is also noted by Clark, *English commercial statistics*, p. 55.

quantitative estimate of the export trade can only be given within very wide limits. A qualitative assessment also suffers from the defects in the records, and an account of the legitimate export trade to Scandinavia must therefore more often than not be impressionistic rather than elaborate in detail.

Much of the trade was in small quantities of a large range of goods. One group consisted of dress and similar articles among which the straw hats of Mrs Thommesen and the nightcaps of Mr Reimers have already been instanced.[1] Linens, manufactured silk, and printed cottons are entered in most years as exports to Denmark–Norway at a combined official value of about £1,000 per year for linen and cottons, and around £2,000 for silks.[2] No mention of these goods being exported to Sweden is to be found in the 1750s and 1760s, but they may be partly concealed in the recurrent entry of 'Goods sevl. sorts' to the real value of some £500 which is met with year after year.[3] Another item in this group is tanned or 'wrought' leather, shipped to Denmark–Norway to the official value of £2,000 to £3,000.[4] Tanned leather was one of the few commodities on which an export duty was still payable, and it may be assumed that the customs authorities were fairly watchful when it came to declarations of such dutiable goods.[5] The export of tanned leather allows an interesting sidelight on the state of Danish–Norwegian manufacture, or, possibly, communications. Denmark was herself an exporter of hides, and imports of tanned leather either by Denmark or by Norway show up the ineffectiveness of their mercantilist practices.

Next may be taken foodstuffs which went to Sweden and to Norway – the entries in the British customs ledgers are as usual for Denmark–Norway, but Denmark as a food exporter herself had no need of them except possibly of fish. Walter Titley at Copenhagen had had hopes of fish becoming a British export item to

[1] See above, p. 90.
[2] P.R.O., Cust. 3/50–70, and Cust. 14/1 *a* and 1 *b*, exports from London and out-ports to Denmark–Norway.
[3] *Ibid.*, exports to Sweden.
[4] *Ibid.*, exports to Denmark–Norway. There are only a few entries relating to insignificant quantities exported to Sweden.
[5] Saxby, *British Customs*, p. 292. The duty was only 1*s*. per hundredweight.

Denmark, but the Norwegian fisheries should have proved sufficient for Danish requirements.[1] There are occasional entries on the Scottish customs ledgers of exports of herring to Denmark–Norway in small quantities,[2] but it is quite likely that they were taken further into the Baltic by Scottish vessels which were plying a trade from Norway to the Baltic with Norwegian fish.[3] The trade in herring from Scotland can therefore be regarded as no more than a token one, and that was also the opinion of the Danish envoy in London who reported to Copenhagen that the Scottish herring fisheries were being encouraged after the Scottish Rebellion of 1745 not so much for any profit that might come from them, but as a means 'de civiliser par là les Ecossais, qui par cette Pêche ont quelque Moyen de s'occuper utilement'.[4]

Of some importance, though, was the trade in grain, that is, in wheat, rye, barley, bigg or beer corn, flour, and malt, and to it may be added exports of hops. None, so far as can be gathered, went to Denmark. Norway appears to have taken the bulk of barley and wheat, and smaller quantities of other grain and malt, while Sweden received large shipments of malt and lesser quantities of other grain.[5] Norway was dependent on grain imports which she largely received from Denmark who had a monopoly of supply for Southern Norway, whereas the northern districts which were served mainly by the ports of Bergen and Trondheim could obtain their requirements from any source.[6] British grain exports were encouraged in normal years by a bounty, and it may therefore be assumed that the quantities recorded in the customs ledgers were at least not under-estimated.[7] In those years of the mid-century when there was no British embargo on exports,[8] the official value

[1] See above, ch. 2, p. 19.
[2] P.R.O., Cust. 14/1 *a* and 1 *b*, 1755, 1756, 1757 and 1762.
[3] Bang and Korst, *Tabeller*, vol. 2, pt 2, pp. 521–761, tables on goods traffic from Norway, *passim*.
[4] Dan. S. Arch., T.K.U.A., Engl. B, 103, nr 170, 6 March 1753.
[5] P.R.O., Cust. 3/50–70, and Cust. 14/1 *a* and 1 *b*. The different kinds of grain are separately entered in the customs ledgers.   [6] See above, ch. 1, p. 8.
[7] D. G. Barnes, *A History of the English Corn Laws 1660–1846* (London, 1930), pp. 10–11. The provisions of the Bounty Act of 1689 are fully discussed in these pages.
[8] Embargoes were placed on grain exports from late 1756 to 1759. See Barnes, *Corn Laws*, pp. 31 and 37.

which was closely related to the real value was on the average as high as £10,000 for exports to Denmark–Norway, and £12,000 to £15,000 for Sweden.[1] The greatest single item was invariably malt, and in an isolated instance Sweden received over £20,000 worth of malt alone.[2] Most of the grain shipments were in British vessels from the out-ports, and it was not unusual for grain cargoes to be directly bartered for timber or more rarely for other Scandinavian merchandise.[3] The English agent at Porsgrund in Norway of a Newcastle firm wrote early in the century to his principals that he could exchange any quantity of barley for timber with which he would freight as return cargoes all ships sent to him.[4] English and Scottish ships to Bergen in the mid-century brought in grain and returned with timber and iron cargoes.[5] Ships to Gothenburg came into port with grain and malt, and left within a few days on return to England with iron and also timber.[6] Traffic through the Sound shows that the Swedish East Coast ports imported English grain, malt shipments as usual being particularly heavy.[7] There is a suspicion though, that the quantity of malt exported may have been over-estimated in the British port books and customs ledgers. The export bounty made it worth-while to steep malt in water to let it swell to as much as ten times its normal volume, and it could well have been that any loss in the quality and the sale price was more than compensated for by fraudulent bounty claims.[8] Like

---

[1] The official values for customs purposes had been determined in the early 1690s and remained unchanged in the eighteenth century. Actual average values for grain are to be found in Beveridge, *Prices and Wages*, pp. 81–4, 535–44, and 566–9. London prices for 1762 are in [Anderson], *Origin*, vol. 3, p. 303. See also Basil Williams, *The Whig Supremacy 1714–1760* (Oxford, 1945), p. 102.

[2] P.R.O., Cust. 3/56, exports from the out-ports to Sweden in 1756.

[3] That this happened may be seen from the Gothenburg and Bergen port books, cited above, which often show English or Scottish ships arriving in port with grain and leaving for home with timber and with iron.

[4] Nor. S. Arch., Privatarkiv nr 67, James Bowman, Porsgrund, 1707–39, bundle 1, copybook, letter of 12 February 1714.

[5] Nor. S. Arch., Bergen port books (Bergen Toldbøger), 1760 I, entries 23 and 43, 26 and 44, 25 and 52, 27 and 53, 28 and 86, *et al.* All these entries relate to British ships which brought in grain and informed the port authorities that they would only unload if they could exchange it for timber. The outward entries show that they were successful in their dealings.

[6] Gothenburg Provincial Archives, Gothenburg port books (Räkenskaps Böker), 1750, entries on ff. 855v., 712v., 750d. and 751v., etc.

[7] Bang and Korst, *Tabeller, passim.*   [8] Barnes, *Corn Laws*, p. 16.

other merchandise, grain was also smuggled when it proved worth-while. That was the case in the years 1757 and 1758. Bad harvests in England and added demand for war supplies led in those years to an embargo on grain shipments out of the country.[1] The authorities suspected that smuggling was going on, and that ostensible coastwise shipments to Scotland were in fact destined for Scandinavia. The Collector at King's Lynn, for example, was warned that the records showed grain shipments to Scotland from the out-ports to be greater than 'the consumption of Scotland seems to require, and that such corn is therefore design'd to be exported clandestinely'. Immediate returns of quantities entered for Scotland, and of the names of the ships and their masters were to be sent to London.[2] The Commissioners in London had good reason to be sus-picious as the Sound Toll Registers show that English grain was indeed shipped to Sweden despite the embargo.[3] There is no record to be found of the consul at Elsinore having been instructed to report illicit shipments, nor are there any indications that offenders had been prosecuted.[4] On the contrary, when Danish–Norwegian ships were found with grain aboard on sailing for home, the intervention of the Danish envoy with Newcastle sufficed to get them released.[5]

Other foodstuffs that were regularly exported to Norway and to Sweden have already been noted: potatoes, butter, and cheese were always in demand, and the Norwegians at least had as well a taste for less homely fare – how else can one account for ship-ments from London in a single year of £1,000 worth of gingerbread?[6] English cheese was also regarded as a delicacy. An English visitor

[1] See above, p. 94, n. 8.
[2] Custom House, King's Lynn, letter book 1758, 21 February 1758.
[3] See tables relating to these years in Bang and Korst, *Tabeller*.
[4] The consul at Elsinore actually complained that he was not required to report on illicit shipments from England, and suggested that all British shipmasters should be ordered to report to him with their charterparties so that he could keep some check on illicit trade by comparing bills of lading with Sound Toll declarations. P.R.O., S.P. 75/96, Titley to Newcastle and enclosures, 26 May 1753.
[5] Dan. S. Arch., T.K.U.A., Engl. B, 109, Bothmer to Bernstorff, 6 March 1759. Bothmer advised Bernstorff that he had obtained the release of Norwegian ships caught leaving with grain cargoes, and that he had been equally successful in the past by applying directly to Newcastle.
[6] P.R.O., Cust. 3/55, exports from London to Denmark–Norway. There can be no doubt that this shipment went to Norway which imported gingerbread in large quantities from Denmark – see Steen, *Kristiansands Historie*, p. 335.

to a Norwegian estate late in the century has recorded that on his offer to perform any commission for his hosts on returning to London, both asked eagerly: 'Send us a Gloucester cheese!'[1] The total value of these miscellaneous food shipments to Norway and Sweden cannot easily be assessed. English and Scottish sources make this section of the export trade appear to have been worth only £1,000 or £2,000 in a normal year, but Scandinavian records give the impression that it was rather more extensive. Hardly a ship seems to have arrived in Swedish and Norwegian ports without, for example, some tons of potatoes, yet the entries of potato exports in the English and Scottish customs ledgers are few and far between. It is possible, of course, that Irish potatoes were transhipped for Northern Europe in English and Scottish ports without passing through the customs, and more likely still that masters of ships did not bother to declare the export of odd lots of foodstuffs. English sheep, for example, whose export was actually prohibited, were taken out of the country as ships' provisions without any hindrance from the customs authorities, and without any customs entries being made. There is no reason to expect customs entries for other foodstuffs unless the ship's master stood to gain an export bounty by declaring his cargo.

When it came to the export of minerals and mineral products, masters of ships and exporters generally had very good reasons to be as evasive as they could and no doubt knew how to be. Most goods in this category were either still charged with an export duty, or were not allowed to enter the Scandinavian countries. Coal, lead and tin paid export duties; salt, glass, and ironware were generally prohibited imports. This leaves grindstones as the only considerable mineral export article to pay neither duties in England, nor to be barred from legitimate trade.

Grindstones from the Northumberland quarries in particular, but also from Derbyshire, Cumberland, and elsewhere had so great a reputation that they were shipped to all parts of Europe.[2] Denmark–Norway received according to English records between

---

[1] Cited from E. D. Clarke's *Travels in Denmark, Sweden, Norway, etc.* (London, 1824), by A. B. Polak (contributor) in *Nordsjøkulturen – Britisk Kunsthaandverk (i Norge) 1650–1850* (n.p., 1955), p. 23.

[2] J. Campbell, *A Political Survey of Great Britain* (London, 1774), vol. 2, p. 22.

£1,000 and £3,000 worth annually at value, and the Sound Toll Registers show that the Swedish Baltic ports also imported English grindstones.[1] They do not appear to have been charged with any imposts at the Sound, and may well have been regarded as ballast, for which they would have been very suitable. It is more than likely that the quantities exported to Scandinavia were greater than English customs accounts indicate, as ballast, if they were shipped as such, was hardly an item to receive much attention. A contemporary noted that grindstones shipped from Newcastle were the best available, and that 'scarce a ship stirs from this port without them'.[2] Newcastle alone should in that case as one of the main ports in the Scandinavian trade have shipped a considerable amount, and London was at least one other port from which grindstones were exported to the Northern countries.[3]

English salt which had earlier in the century been of some importance in the legitimate trade to Scandinavia was barred from Denmark–Norway because, so it was said, its qualities as a preservative were so poor that it adversely affected Danish meat and Norwegian fish exports.[4] English writers very naturally extolled its fineness and held it to be equal to the best Spanish and Portuguese salt whose importation to Denmark–Norway was allowed.[5] Despite the prohibitions, salt was still shipped to the double kingdom at an annual official value of a few hundred to as much as three thousand Pounds.[6] It was hardly an article that could easily be smuggled, and the explanation for its continued export lies most probably in a despatch written by Titley from Copenhagen in 1753. Titley had heard rumours of a project to establish a private monopoly for the import of all salt into Norway, and protested against it on the grounds that it 'would be very detrimental to the

---

[1] Bang and Korst, *Tabeller*, vol. 2, pt 2, Tables of shipments from England to Sweden, *passim*.

[2] Postlethwayt, *Dictionary of Commerce*, vol. 2, s.v. 'Northumberland'.

[3] P.R.O., Cust. 3/50–70, exports from London to the Scandinavian countries.

[4] Moltke Archives, Breve fra fransk Ambassadør J.-F. Ogier, Mémoire: 'Conditions auxquelles l'on pourroit livrer annuellement des viandes salées en France' etc. October 1755.

[5] Campbell, *Political Survey*, vol. 2, pp. 25ff.

[6] P.R.O., Cust. 3/50–70. There are no customs entries apart from insignificant amounts from London and Scotland, and all the salt shipped to Scandinavia seems to have come from the Liverpool region.

British Navigation as Our Ships carry great quantities of foreign salt to Norway'.[1] Some of it may possibly have been foreign, but there can be little doubt that most if not all was Spanish and Portuguese only in description to the Danish–Norwegian customs authorities. The salt-works near Liverpool were regarded as producing especially fine white salt, and there is evidence of Danish–Norwegian ships loading it for return journeys.[2] Again, it is unlikely that they would have advertised this by entering salt for export, and the quantities shipped were undoubtedly far greater than the records would suggest.

Glass exports to Denmark–Norway were under a similar handicap to salt. The importation of glass to Denmark–Norway had been prohibited in 1760 to protect a native industry which had in part been introduced by British glass-workers.[3] Yet glassware to the value of £2,000 to £3,000 was still entered in the English customs ledgers as being destined for Denmark–Norway, and one may safely assume that at least some of it was to be smuggled.[4] Small shipments of ironware may as well have been intended for the smuggling trade, though import licences for it were on occasion obtainable in Denmark and Norway, and possibly in Sweden.[5] These shipments were computed in the customs ledgers at actual value which rarely exceeded £1,000. Of somewhat the same order was the export trade in tin, but the export duty, though less than 5% of the official value, probably led to under-entries at the custom house.[6] It is strange that in some isolated years the entries for tin exports shot up from £1,000 to £5,000, £6,000 or £7,000,[7] and one wonders whether customs supervision was especially strict, and informers especially active in such years, as the result of periodic pressure by the Pewterers' Company which had a vested interest in hindering the export of its main raw material.

The remaining exports in this category were lead and coal. The official value of lead exports to Scandinavia was normally in the

[1] P.R.O., S.P. 75/96, Titley to Newcastle, 12 May 1753. [2] See above, ch. 3, p. 46.
[3] See below, appendix 5. [4] P.R.O., Cust. 3/50–70.
[5] Imports of ironware into Denmark–Norway and Sweden are listed in the Gothenburg and Bergen port books which have been cited. The declared value of shipments from England is as usual to be found in the customs ledgers.
[6] Saxby, *British Customs*, p. 299.
[7] Instances of such high export figures are in P.R.O., Cust. 3/57, 61, *et al.*

vicinity of £7,000 or £8,000, and higher in some of the War years. The actual value was about twice the official,[1] and under-entries may again be expected with an export duty of £1 per foder, so that the real value cannot have been less than £20,000 in most years.[2] The customs entries for coal exports were in the pre-War and War years at about the same level as for lead, but rose steeply after the Seven Years War to £20,000 or more per year. The official and the actual values were closely related, with the latter slightly higher.[3] This branch of the export trade differed from others in that the duties were exceptionally high, standing until 1757 for the Newcastle chaldron at 6s. when shipped in British ships, and at 17s. in foreign. A sharp increase brought the duties from 1757 until the late 1760s, when they rose again, to 7s. and 21s. respectively, that is, to about 50% at value for British shipping, and to well over 100% for foreign.[4] It is no wonder then that the trade was carried on almost entirely in British vessels.[5] The high duties make one suspect once again that exports were much greater than British records make them appear, and Danish and Norwegian estimates do indeed bear out that suspicion.[6] There is one curious feature in the Danish and Norwegian records that have been examined. Coal is almost invariably stated as having been carried in Scottish ships, and the Sound Toll Registers also give the impression that the carrying trade in coal was a Scottish near-

---

[1] The official value of lead for export was £10–£11 per foder, and a comparison with the price tables in Beveridge, *Prices and Wages*, pp. 202, 298, and 679 gives the approximation to actual value.

[2] Saxby, *British Customs*, 293. One foder of lead equalled one ton.

[3] For actual values, see Beveridge, *Prices and Wages*, pp. 90, 146, 195 *et al.*

[4] Saxby, *British Customs*, pp. 283–4, and 646. Note that T. S. Ashton and J. Sykes, *The Coal Industry of the Eighteenth Century* (Manchester, 1929), p. 247, are mistaken in their statements on the export duties on coal. The authors failed to note the Act of 9 Anne c. 6 which consolidated earlier export duties on coal, and the duty then imposed is to be added to that of 12 Anne c. 9 and of succeeding Acts. The Newcastle chaldron measured 53 cwt.

[5] P.R.O., Cust. 3/50–70 and Cust. 14/1 *a* and 1 *b*, entries of British and foreign shipping to the Scandinavian countries.

[6] [E. Pontoppidan], *Oeconomiske Balance eller Uforgribelige Overslag paa Danmarks naturlige og borgerlige Formue* [*etc.*], (Copenhagen, 1759), pp. 144–5; also, Steen, *Kristiansands Historie*, p. 336; and despatches on coal shipments in Dan. S. Arch., T.K.U.A., Engl. B, 113, Bothmer to Bernstorff, 21 December 1764; also P.R.O., S.P. 75/112, Titley to Bute, 25 April 1761; and *ibid.*, S.P. 75/115, Goodricke to Halifax, 26 February 1763.

The Export Trade

monopoly. Yet coal shipments from Scotland itself were, according to the Scottish customs ledgers, quite negligible, practically all coal being shipped from the English out-ports. There may of course have been some unfathomable and quite proper reason for this Scottish predilection for carrying coal, though a less charitable view can be taken: the coastwise duty on coal from England to Scotland had long ago been abolished,[1] and it is probable that Scottish colliers were in the habit of declaring their cargo from English ports for shipment to their Scottish home ports, and then veering farther out to sea and sailing to Scandinavia when well clear of the English coast. Most of the shipments went to Denmark–Norway where coal was used extensively in salt- and glass-works, for lime-burning, in smithies, and for heating.[2]

The next large section of the export trade comprises colonial wares. Tobacco, coffee, brown and some refined sugar, rice, dyes and spices entered into it. The smaller items can be disposed of quickly. The dyes and spices shipped mainly from London to both Denmark–Norway and Sweden were indigo, cochineal, ginger, pepper and pimento. There is no record to be found that any of these had been imported from England before the War. The first mention of substantial indigo shipments to Denmark–Norway occurred in 1759, and to Sweden in 1760. The quantities entered in the customs ledgers rose quickly, the official value being at the beginning of the Seven Years War £400 for Denmark–Norway, to reach more than £1,000 by the end of the War, and £1,000 for Sweden to reach over £5,000 by 1765. It is known that France had earlier supplied the Scandinavian countries with indigo and other dyes and spices, and the interruption of French trade and the loss of French colonies led therefore to England taking over this branch of trade. Later records indicate that England continued to supply Scandinavia in increasing amounts with these colonial wares.[3]

[1] Saxby, British Customs, p. 284. There is no record to be found of the amount of the coastwise bond on coal, and bond may actually not have been taken. If it was still demanded, then it would quite likely have been lower than the export duty and it was therefore worthwhile to pay and forfeit the bond.
[2] Pontoppidan, Oeconomiske Balance, loc. cit.
[3] The English customs ledgers show in the later years of the War entries of shipments from London to the Scandinavian countries of 'French' coffee, sugar, indigo, and of other drugs and spices. These were probably both prize goods and produce from

Exports of brown and of refined sugar to Denmark–Norway and to Sweden had been quite negligible before the War, as the Danish sugar colonies in the West Indies could supply much of Scandinavia, and Sweden obtained the balance of her requirements from France. During the later part of the War occurs the first mention of sugar shipments at an average annual official value of some £5,000. The importation of foreign sugar into Denmark–Norway, though not of course into Sweden which then had no colonies, was prohibited without any possibility of special import licences being available, and English records may be misleading about shipments which might have been intended for another country. Other possibilities are as usual smuggling, or that sugar was bonded for re-export at Elsinore and Copenhagen.[1]

Denmark–Norway also began to take during the last years of the War shipments of rice which amounted on the average to more than £2,000 at official valuation. The impression is again that it had earlier been obtained from France, and, as in the instance of dyes and spices, England kept her place in this trade which became later on very much more substantial.[2]

The pattern repeats itself with coffee exports. There are no records of any shipments before the War, and the first entry in the English customs ledgers occurs in 1758 and is not very large.[3] From that year on shipments are continuously recorded at ever-increasing value. The official value stood at about one-half the actual

captured French colonies. Special mention of the export of French colonial goods ceased after the war, and colonial goods exported from Britain to Scandinavia were the produce of British colonies.

[1] The Danish West Indian trade for the period of the Seven Years War is described in detail by Jens Vibaek, 'Dansk Vestindien 1755–1848' (offprint of a major section from Brønstead (ed.), *Vore Gamle Tropekolonier* (Copenhagen, 1953), vol. 2, *passim*). For the trade in sugar, see also P. P. Sveistrup and R. Willerslev, *Sukkerhandels Historie, passim*. Sweden did not acquire a tropical colony until 1784.

[2] The quantities of rice shipped from England to Scandinavia from 1752–62 are tabulated in P.R.O., C.O. 390/9, f. B. 29. For later shipments, see the customs ledgers. The trade was not very large, and rice shipments to Scandinavia until the later 1760s accounted for only 1% or 2% of the total re-exports of colonial rice.

[3] Denmark–Norway had obtained coffee from France, as did Sweden in the years when the importation of coffee was allowed. The annual value of coffee imports from France into Denmark–Norway was assessed at £20,000, and it therefore appears that England drove France completely out of the market. See P.R.O., S.P. 75/104, Goodricke to Holdernesse, private, 23 December 1758.

value,[1] and an adjustment to this actual value brings one to the quite respectable sum of £20,000 per annum by the end of the War. London was the main centre of supply for Denmark–Norway, while the out-ports shipped the greater quantity to Sweden. The explanation would appear to be that London, taking the lion's share of timber, loaded more ships for the return journey to Denmark–Norway, and the out-ports, having the larger share of the iron-trade, supplied more cargoes for Sweden.

Tobacco exports, the last in this category, present rather a pretty problem in trade evaluation. Tobacco is well known to have been one of the smuggling staples,[2] and customs records of exports are therefore particularly suspect. Quite apart from the usual tricks associated with smuggling, there was the added problem of shippers being deliberately misleading about their destination and the size of their cargo as they were well aware of foreign consuls and informers trying to get a lead on tobacco shipments which might contribute to the smuggling trade. The shippers had good reason to be worried if they had clandestine dealings in mind: consuls were becoming more numerous in England, and could appoint as many vice-consuls as they pleased in any port within their consular territory. They could and did build up a network of news gatherers as well as informers. This was not the end of it so far as intending smugglers were concerned. Envoys themselves with their legation staffs kept an eye on legitimate or illicit trade to their country, and relied on friendly merchants to keep them informed on trade

---

[1] The real value has as usual been estimated from the tables in Beveridge, *Prices and Wages*, p. 421. The interesting discussion of English eighteenth-century trade statistics by W. Schlote, *Entwicklung und Strukturwandlungen des englischen Aussenhandels von 1700 bis zur Gegenwart* (Jena, 1938), pp. 17ff., in which coffee is singled out as an illustration, is unfortunately based on incorrect assumptions. Schlote had failed to find the English series of customs ledgers, i.e. Cust. 3/1–80, and his discussion is therefore needlessly conjectural. He also mistook the rateable for the official value, and made confusion worse confounded. Finally, Schlote is mistaken in his estimates of contemporary prices, and his arguments are therefore based very largely on wrong premises.

[2] Smuggling and customs frauds in the tobacco-trade were so serious that they attracted the attention of Parliament, which appointed in 1733 a committee of inquiry whose report and evidence are in *R.H.C.*, 1st series, vol. 1, pp. 601ff. Later parliamentary committees also investigated the tobacco as well as other smuggling trades. For their reports, see *J.H.C.*, vol. xxv (1745–6), pp. 101ff., and *R.H.C.*, 1st series, vol. 11, pp. 228ff.

conditions and on intended smuggling. Although reports by Danish–Norwegian and Swedish consuls in England during the eighteenth century are few and far between, they still show how useful consuls could be in curbing smuggling to their country. There is, for example, a very full and revealing report in 1771 from London by the Danish consul von Passow on his network of informers. He had even recruited customs officers in London and the out-ports.[1]

Straightout smuggling or intended smuggling is, however, only one factor which makes it so difficult to arrive at any reasonable estimate of tobacco exports, particularly of exports to Scandinavia. The import duty on tobacco into England was heavy, and at the mid-century added about 200% to the landed cost.[2] This duty was drawn back on re-export. It was therefore very profitable to enter tobacco for export, obtain the remission of duty, and then smuggle it back into England. Just this procedure was known at the time to have been established practice.[3] The Isle of Man, one of the great supply-centres of smugglers' goods until its administration passed from private ownership to the Crown in 1765, was a well-known staple for enumerated colonial goods that had first been shipped to it from England to be smuggled back into England. No drawback on tobacco was allowed for the Isle of Man, and dishonest dealers were therefore noted for clearing shipments from Bristol and Liverpool for Norway as the normal course of a Norway-bound ship would take it close enough to the island to make unloading by lighters practicable. The clearance papers for Norway provided the alibi for being in the vicinity of the Isle of Man if an English revenue cutter should be about.[4]

[1] Dan. S. Arch., Kommercekollegium, Konsulatsreporter fra London o. a., 1753–1806, Rapport, v. Passow, 30 August 1771, and other reports in this bundle.

[2] For duties and drawbacks, see Saxby, *British Customs*, pp. 244–6. Prices are noted in the various parliamentary reports cited above, p. 103, note 2, and by J. M. Price, 'The Rise of Glasgow in the Chesapeake Tobacco Trade 1707–1775', *William and Mary Quarterly*, 3rd ser., 11, no 2 (April 1954).

[3] See *R.H.C.*, 1st series, vol. 1, report into frauds and abuses in the customs, 1733, *passim*.

[4] B.M., Add. MS 38,462 (vol. 273 of Liverpool MSS), ff. 20–30, 'An Impartial Enquiry of the State of the Isle of Man', n.d. (*c*. 1750). An appended note shows that the report was written by one Captain Mercer, commander of a revenue vessel.

On the one hand, then, there is the probability of under-entries in the English and Scottish customs ledgers for shipments to Scandinavia, not so much due to concealment of quantity as that would have meant loss of drawback, but to misleading declarations about destination to throw consuls and informers off the scent when intending to smuggle to any one country. And, on the other hand, there is the likelihood of shipments having been entered for export to Scandinavia without their having got much farther than the Isle of Man, or some hidden beach in England. No solution to the problem of assessing the extent of the tobacco-trade can under such circumstances be easily thought of, and one might be tempted to fall back on the rough-and-ready one of assuming that one factor cancelled out the other, and that the customs ledgers could then serve as some guide. The impression given by the ledgers in conjunction with other records is that this would be unwise when attempting to assess quantities, though the ledgers most probably indicate the trends of the trade faithfully enough.

The trend was for the trade to become more extensive with the years, and for Scotland to participate in it to an increasing extent. In 1755, the first year for which Scottish figures are available, the ledgers show entries of exports from England to Denmark–Norway and Sweden of £12,000 worth of tobacco at the official valuation, and of £1,800 from Scotland. The figures rose year by year with hardly a break to £22,000 for England in 1764, and to £19,000 for Scotland. They were in the following year £26,000 for England, and £27,000 for Scotland. England later regained the lead, and the 1770 figures of £45,000 and £20,000 respectively are more representative.[1] The Seven Years War therefore allowed Britain to gain the lion's share of Scandinavian tobacco imports.

The value of tobacco exports to Scandinavia may well have been rather greater than the customs ledgers would indicate. Scandinavian sources give the impression that legitimate trade was heavy, and smuggling heavier still.[2] One definite estimate of actual exports to Denmark has been found, and it reinforces the impression gained

---

[1] P.R.O., Cust. 3/50–70, and Cust. 14/1 *a* and 1 *b*.
[2] See, for example, Heckscher, *Sveriges ekonomiska historia*, II, 2, pp. 643–4 and 657, and Olsen, *Danmark–Norge*, p. 49.

from scattered sources. Cosby, who was Titley's assistant in Copenhagen for a time,[1] reported in March 1765 that the most exhaustive enquiries into the extent of British trade with Denmark had shown that tobacco imports were worth about £50,000 Sterling.[2] This account must have referred to the preceding, and possibly to earlier years, as well. Yet the actual value of tobacco exports to both Denmark and to Norway as computed from the English and Scottish customs ledgers for 1764 was no higher than about £18,000, the highest figure then reached.[3] The remainder of Cosby's report dealing with other merchandise can be checked against independent sources, and is reliable. His comments on the tobacco-trade must therefore inspire some confidence, and his estimate of its extent accords better with the impression gained from all the available, though in part fragmentary, sources, than from the customs ledgers on their own.

Some of the most puzzling aspects of Anglo-Scandinavian trade have been left till last. They are met with in the cloth-trade. Denmark, as has already been noted,[4] had imposed earlier in the century prohibitions on the importation of all types of woollen goods; in Norway, their entry from any country but Denmark was discouraged by heavy duties; Sweden had either outright prohibitions on the importation of some types of cloth, or prohibitive duties on others. The effect of the prohibitions in Denmark and Sweden could be mitigated by import licences, but these were issued very sparingly indeed. In short, open trade in cloth with Denmark and with Sweden would appear to have been virtually stopped, and with Norway at the least crippled. Entries in the English and Scottish customs ledgers show in confirmation that exports of cloth to Sweden were no greater than could be accounted for by import licences, a fact which incidentally confirms the impression given earlier that exporters did not generally declare goods for a country to which they were to be smuggled.

[1] See above, p. 13, note 1.
[2] P.R.O., C.O. 388/95, Cosby to Pownal (Secretary, Board of Trade and Plantations), 16 March 1765.
[3] P.R.O., Cust. 3/64, exports from London and out-ports, and Cust. 14/1 *b*.
[4] See above, ch. 1, p. 6.

It was well-known at the time that cloth was smuggled in large quantities into Sweden as well as into Denmark and Norway.[1] Cloth for smuggling into Denmark would not, on analogy with Sweden, have been declared in England as exports, and the quite substantial entries of shipments to the double kingdom should therefore refer largely to Norway alone where cloth could be imported on payment of duty. Some was shipped to Denmark to be imported on licence, and more was probably bonded at Elsinore or Copenhagen either to be transhipped to the Eastern Baltic or, most likely, to be smuggled into Sweden. The impression given by available records is, however, that Denmark took only a small quantity in legitimate trade, and that the bulk went to Norway. The amount of total shipments entered annually from 1750 to 1759 in the English customs ledgers – entries from Scotland were negligible – was on the average £30,000 at official values. The real values of the various types of cloth shipped to Denmark–Norway were, so far as they can be checked, close to the official values, and the figures in the customs ledgers can be accepted as an approximation to the extent of legitimate trade.[2]

For a country like Norway, £30,000 was a reasonable sum to have spent on open imports of English cloth which, a contemporary noted, was greatly preferred to Danish.[3]

About half of the recorded exports were low-quality stuffs which East Anglian clothiers manufactured extremely cheaply. These would have been intended for the poorer people. Of the rest, a

[1] Olsen, *Danmark–Norge*, pp. 145–6; O. A. Johnsen, *Norwegische Handelsgeschichte* (Jena, 1939), p. 337; Lind, *Göteborgs Handel*, p. 22 and note 1; and B.M., Egerton MS 2696 (Gunning Papers), ff. 258–65, Gunning to Conway, 4 May 1767; and P.R.O., S.P. 75/118, Cosby to Sandwich, 23 February 1765.

[2] The official values have again been compared with Beveridge, *Prices and Wages*, pp. 90, 146, 195, 293 and 458. The description of the cloths which entered Beveridge's tables (see his index under 'cloth') has been compared with the specifications of various types and qualities as noted by H. Heaton, *The Yorkshire Woollen and Worsted Industries* (Oxford, 1920), pp. 145, 179, 198 and 266–9. This comparison showed that cloths in Beveridge were in fact generally the same as some of the cloth types in the customs ledgers. There are, however, other types of cloth listed in the customs ledgers for which no real values could be obtained, and it has been assumed that the relation of their official to their real value would be similar to that of the cloths for which real values were found.

[3] Dan. S. Arch., Generalmagasinet, nr 633.36, Indberetning fra Faktor Herman Hoe, dat. 10 June 1760.

good third consisted of minikin bays and 'short cloths', two of the best and most expensive English cloths for which there was hardly a substitute to be had from Denmark.[1] They were just the type of cloth one would expect the wealthier people to have bought at any price.[2] Most of the shipments were in Danish–Norwegian ships, which is easily explained as only the cargoes brought in by native vessels were allowed to be put in bond.[3] Thomas Fearnley, who has been met with earlier as an English timber- and general merchant living in Norway, explained to one of his correspondents at Hull that bonding facilities took some of the risk out of the trade because cloths which did not sell could be returned to England without any duty having been paid.[4]

Recorded exports to Denmark–Norway rose steeply in 1760 from the previous £30,000 to £45,000, then to £50,000 in 1761, and to nearly £80,000 in 1762. This increase in the export figures is not easily explicable. Smuggling might have been made more difficult by the greater number of warships about, and demand had to be met by open trade; demand itself may have increased with the prosperity which the War brought to the Norwegian timber and shipping industries; the war scare in Denmark of 1761 and 1762 when a Russian attack seemed imminent could have led to stockpiling and to heavy buying for the army; finally, Danish merchants might have engaged more heavily in the *entrepôt* trade and shipped cloth on their own account to the Eastern Baltic.

The high level of recorded exports was not maintained for long beyond the end of the War. There was already some falling off in 1763 and 1764, and in 1765 the export figure had sunk to as low as £21,000. The wave of post-War bankruptcies which had hit Danish merchanthouses severely might explain such a low figure if Danish merchants had indeed been active earlier in re-exporting English cloth to the Baltic. It is probable that they did, as subsequent increases in the recorded exports to Denmark–Norway were

[1] P.R.O., S.P., 75/118, Cosby to Sandwich, 23 February 1765.
[2] S. Tveite, 'The Norwegian Textile Market in the 18th Century', *Scandinavian Economic History Review*, 17, 2 (1969), has an interesting discussion on the demand for high-quality textiles on p. 171.
[3] Schovelin, *Fra den danske Handels Empire*, pp. 82ff.
[4] Nor. S. Arch., Fearnley Papers, f. 58, letter of 24 March 1754.

The Export Trade

accompanied by a corresponding fall in English export figures to Russia and the East Country.[1]

Smuggling of cloth has so far only been mentioned in passing, and it invites closer attention. That it took place is undeniable, but how great it was in relation to legitimate trade can of course never be known. There is evidence that it was extensive. The Danish–Norwegian authorities were forced in 1755 to publish a proclamation condemning the practice of selling at public auctions prohibited imports like cloth, silks, and printed cottons.[2] A general search of retail shops was made in the following year in Copenhagen which brought to light so much contraband goods that the heavy penalties for having it in possession could not be enforced without putting practically every trader behind lock and bars. Fines had instead to be substituted for imprisonment and confiscation of all property.[3] Three years later, the Danish bishop Pontoppidan, a reliable writer on economic conditions, had to confess that the smuggling trade in cloth made it impossible to assess the balance of trade in Denmark.[4] English envoys reported that illicit imports of cloth were heavy both in Denmark and in Norway.[5] Thomas Fearnley, in letters from Christiania and Frederickshald, gave advice to his correspondents in England about methods of smuggling. His arrangements were not always successful, and he had to complain to a Hull firm about its inefficiency. The firm had failed to warn him that every piece in a shipment of cloth would 'measure something More than Specifyed in the Inv.e', and he had for lack of proper arrangements not taken the usual precautions, with the annoying result that the customs officers had found '4 a

---

[1] Schovelin, *Fra den danske Handels Empire*, pp. 87ff., notes that transit bonding in Copenhagen fell off considerably after the war, and it may be assumed that smaller cloth imports for re-export had something to do with it. See also the tables of exports to Russia and the East Country in P.R.O., Cust. 3 and Cust. 14/1 b, for the relevant years.

[2] Dan. S. Arch., Kongelige Forordninger og Aabne Breve, 1755, Placat dat. 20 October 1755.

[3] Bro-Jørgensen, *Industriens Historie*, p. 110.

[4] Pontoppidan, *Oeconomiske Balance*, p. 140.

[5] P.R.O., S.P. 75/96, Titley to Newcastle, 26 May 1753. This despatch refers to reports sent to him by consuls Fenwick and Wallace. Also, S.P. 75/118, Cosby to Sandwich, 23 February 1765; and *ibid.*, consular report from Wallace of Bergen to Sandwich, 26 February 1765.

5 Yds on each p.e diff.ce which made me look Ridicolos'. For smaller woollen goods like stockings there was 'Little Vent...out of Shops', he advised another correspondent, as 'the Generality is furnished privately by Oppt.y of Ships...in the Summer Season'.[1]

In the summer season and out of it, smuggling and customs frauds never ceased. The export duties in England on coal and on other minerals, the bounty on corn, the drawback on tobacco inevitably led to irregularities which were reflected in faulty customs entries. Import duties and prohibitions in the Scandinavian countries added their own effects to the confusion in trade statistics. To set under such circumstances any definite limit to the extent of the export trade to Denmark–Norway and Sweden is plainly impossible, though one is perfectly safe in assuming that it was larger than the English and Scottish customs accounts make it appear to have been. The customs ledgers may be relied on, however, in so far as they show that the range of export merchandise was wide, and there is no reason to doubt that cloth and woollens generally, tobacco, coal, and corn including flour and malt, were the staples of the trade. The money value of all exports may also be taken as having been no less than the adjusted values based on the customs accounts, that is, about a £100,000 annually in the first years of the Seven Years War, and somewhat more as it progressed, yet to apportion shares within those sums to each particular country is more than can safely be done. Sweden is made to appear by available contemporary statistics to have been of less importance in the trade than Denmark–Norway because there are no customs entries crediting her with cloth imports. It would be strange indeed if the lack of open imports was not remedied as in the case of Denmark–Norway by more intensive smuggling since there was not much to choose between the Swedish and Danish textile industries in size and efficiency.

On the whole, then, one is left with the impression that British exports more than held their own in value despite the increasingly restrictive policies of the Scandinavian countries. The growth of

[1] Nor. S. Arch., Fearnley Papers, ff. 31–2, letter of 17 September 1753; and f. 157, letter of 24 July 1766.

native manufacture may possibly have affected such traditional export goods as cloth, but a diminution compared with earlier times in the cloth- or salt-trade was at the least offset by the extension of younger trades such as those in coal and in tobacco and other colonial wares. Individual British merchants who wrote pamphlets about the 'falling off' in exports to Scandinavia were quite likely justified in their complaints – their particular merchandise may have been hit hard – and British envoys protesting against trade restrictions did no more than was expected of them. The successful merchants had no reason to advertise their good management and astuteness by rushing into print and thereby manufacturing historical records, but their presence on the scene can be both deduced by inference and proved by direct evidence. The inference remains, and available records support it, that the majority of British merchants trading with Scandinavia were successful in their various enterprises and in expanding exports to Scandinavia. The Seven Years War moreover allowed them to acquire a share of the former French export trade, and these gains they retained after the War.

The despairing admission by the eighteenth-century Danish historian and divine, Erik Pontoppidan, that all his labours to strike a true balance of trade for his country had been in vain because of the extent of smuggling, can be echoed with added poignancy by present-day historians. Contemporary English and Scottish statistics for every branch of Anglo-Scandinavian trade noted in the customs ledgers have been shown to be suspect or definitely misleading, and responsible officials in the office of the inspector-general of customs and excise as well as publicists and members of Parliament cannot have helped knowing that the annual returns of imports and exports were an unreliable guide towards assessing the balance of Britain's trade. What made the position in England particularly aggravating was the indulgence in tea-drinking which the English more than any other European people fell into during the eighteenth century. This would have been a harmless enough habit if tea had been just another article of trade freely imported by whoever chose, but since the import of tea was a monopoly of the East India Company and was moreover subject to high duties, interlopers and smugglers saw the opportunity of reaping a rich harvest. So soon as the Ostend Company which served in the earlier years of the century as a cloak for English interlopers had been forced to cease operations in the China trade, Sweden became a haven for interloping British traders who were instrumental in founding a Swedish East India Company, while in Denmark the virtually defunct East Asiatic Company took on a new lease of life and entered on its most prosperous period by concentrating on the trade in tea.[1] Neither Sweden nor Denmark

---

[1] For the Danish company, see K. Glamann, 'Studier i Asiatisk Kompagnis Økonomiske Historie 1732–1772', in *Historisk Tidsskrift*, 11th series, vol. 2 (Copenhagen, 1949); and *ibid.*, 'The Danish Asiatic Company, 1732–1772', *Scandinavian Economic History Review*, 8, 2 (1960); also, Olsen, *Danmark–Norge*, p. 21 and *passim*. An English view

were tea-drinking countries, and a substantial part of the large
tea shipments to Copenhagen and to Gothenburg were ultimately
destined for the English market.¹ These shipments very obviously
did not figure in the British customs ledgers, and the balances of
trade arrived at every year were thus still further thrown out.

The popularity of tea in England dates from the early eighteenth
century, and it became such a favourite drink among all classes
in the country that 'even the beggars and their brats, if they can
steal any thing to purchase coarse sugar, drink it once or twice
a day'. But for smuggling, tea-drinking would hardly have become
such a widespread habit as the price of legally imported tea was
high, and it was therefore 'especially the damnified teas imported
[illicitly] from Gottenburgh' at a lower price which were said
to have contributed most to the spread of the tea-drinking habit.²
The high price of East India Company tea was due mainly if not
entirely to heavy import and excise duties which tended to rise
inexorably every few years till they reached a practically prohibitive
level by the time of the Seven Years War.³ They stood then at
about 100% *ad valorem* for a lower-priced tea such as Bohea
which was the most commonly used quality in England, and at
somewhat less for the more expensive teas such as Hyson and
Singloe.⁴ In contrast, Denmark only laid a duty of 1% on tea

of the background to the company's formation is given in *British Diplomatic
Instructions, Denmark*, pp. xv and 82–4. For the Swedish company, see Heckscher,
Sveriges ekonomiska historia, II, 2, pp. 693–5. English views on the company
are noted in *British Diplomatic Instructions, Sweden*, vol. 2, pp. viii, ix, xii and *passim*.
The article on Sweden in Postlethwayt's *Dictionary of Commerce*, vol. 2, gives a
useful summary of contemporary English opinion on the company.
¹ This fact is succinctly stated by H. B. Morse, *The Chronicles of the East India
Company trading to China 1635–1834* (Oxford, 1926), vol. I, p. 295: 'But in the
four countries engaged in this trade [i.e. Denmark, Sweden, Holland and France]
it is notorious that tea has never been – is not now and was not then – a popular
beverage; and the greater part of the continental importation was smuggled into
England, the high duty levied there being an incentive to the "free trader".'
² Postlethwayt, *Dictionary of Commerce*, vol. 2, s.v. 'Smuggling'. See also W. Kennedy,
English Taxation 1640–1799 (London, 1913), p. 161, n. 2, citing a pamphlet by
Arthur Young that tea and with it sugar had become a necessity.
³ There were complaints that the East India Company did not import tea in sufficient
quantities, and that the scarcity at the London auctions drove up the price beyond
that at the continental auctions. See *J.H.C.*, vol. xxv, pp. 106–7.
⁴ The computation of the tea duties was fairly complicated. The duties consisted of
customs and excise charges levied *ad valorem* and on quantity. Rebates were given

which was to be re-exported, and of $2\frac{1}{2}\%$ on the small quantity that remained in the country.[1] The other substantial Continental importing countries, that is, Sweden, France and Holland, were equally content to levy low duties and to profit indirectly from a re-export trade. The resulting position as it affected England was summed up in a report of a parliamentary committee of inquiry into illicit trade: 'Tea is a very principal article of Excise and Customs, and claims the first attention...being highly valuable in proportion to its bulk and weight; easily purchased, at a low rate, and to any amount, in the foreign ports of Europe; and so highly taxed in this kingdom, as to be a great object of temptation to those who are disposed to defraud the revenue of their country.'[2] And, as several parliamentary reports and many other documents show only too clearly, there were few traders not disposed to take advantage of the cheap tea to be obtained from the Continent.

Among the suppliers of tea for smuggling into England, Denmark and Sweden came to be pre-eminent at the time of the Seven Years War. When the Scandinavian companies entered the field in the 1730s, the smuggling trade in tea was already well organised thanks to the pioneering work of the Ostend, the Dutch, and the French companies. The evidence collected in 1733 by a parliamentary committee on smuggling shows how far the trade had progressed in a very short time, and how well the Danish and Swedish companies found the ground prepared for their advent.[3] Tea- and brandy-smuggling, the committee noted, generally went together, brandy being used to fill up any space left on board the smuggling vessel by a short cargo of tea.[4] At a later date, as will be shown

for prompt payment so that the total duties chargeable could vary for the same amount of the same quality tea. Tables for computing the duties are in Saxby, *British Customs*, pp. 347–9, and 353. For the amounts payable per pound of tea of various qualities, see *R.H.C.*, 1st series, vol. 11, first report of the committee on illicit practices used in defrauding the revenue, 1783, pp. 220 and 261; and *ibid.*, third report, p. 287.   [1] Glamann, 'Studier', *loc. cit.*, p. 396.

[2] *R.H.C.*, 1st series, vol. 11, first report on illicit practices, 1783, p. 230.

[3] *R.H.C.*, 1st series, vol. 1, frauds and abuses in the customs, pp. 601ff. The organisation of the smuggling trade may be gathered from the evidence in appendix 26, pp. 645. See also A. L. Cross (ed.), *Eighteenth Century Documents relating to the Royal Forests, the Sheriffs and Smuggling: Selected from the Shelburne MSS in the William L. Clements Library* (New York, 1928), pp. 308: 'Report of the Commiss.r.s of Excise; on Smuggling.'   [4] *R.H.C.*, 1st series, vol. 1, frauds and abuses, p. 610*a*.

below, smugglers from Scandinavia conformed so explicitly to accepted practice that brandy was shipped from France to Denmark and Sweden to be smuggled from there to England. To return, however, to the evidence before the parliamentary committee. In the ten years preceding the enquiry, a quarter of a million pounds of tea and more than half a million gallons of brandy had been seized by customs officers alone, and more besides by excise officers.[1] Some 2,000 people had been prosecuted for smuggling, and over 200 vessels had been confiscated. A convicted smuggler told the committee that he alone had handled annually 15,000 to 20,000 pounds of tea to supply merely the City, Westminster, and Southwark. His stocks which came from Holland were escorted from the beaches by armed gangs, and watchmen at the City gates corroborated his evidence to the extent of telling of their fights with bands of armed men who invaded London by night with large quantities of tea.[2] Surveyors and collectors of customs handed in written evidence of the methods used by smugglers. The collector of Colchester, for example, gave an account of his seizure of a load of tea which had been hidden inland, only to be robbed of it again by an armed gang assisted by country folk equipped with flails and pitchforks.[3] The collector of Yarmouth reported that ships from Holland and France with cargoes of tea, brandy and tobacco had bills of lading made out for Bergen in Norway, and gained immunity from seizure by that subterfuge when they were boarded by customs officers close to the English coast.[4] Other smuggling vessels beat off attempts to seize them, customs officers had been killed in such affrays, and, when smugglers actually were caught, confederates released them forcibly from prison.[5] The evidence gave in all a picture of near-anarchy on the coasts and along the smugglers' routes inland even when allowance is made for understandable overstatements by officials anxious to excuse their lack of success in putting down the smuggling trade. That smugglers were prepared to take risks is explicable as the profits in their trade were great, and demand for tea seemingly inexhaustable.

[1] *Ibid.*, p. 610*b*.
[2] *Ibid.*, pp. 610*b* and 646–7.
[3] *Ibid.*, p. 647.
[4] *Ibid.*, p. 647.
[5] *Ibid.*, pp. 610*a* and *b*, and 645ff.

One English wholesale supplier of tea for smuggling from Dunkirk assessed the total amount of money paid on the Continent by English smugglers for tea alone at £800,000 annually, a sum that would at a rough estimate have bought three and a half million pounds of tea. This sum of £800,000 annually was mentioned to the Commons committee on smuggling of 1745–6, and had, according to the evidence to the committee, been assessed so early as 1736 by one Hanning who was recognised at the time as one of the principal suppliers of tea at Dunkirk. The sum would have been far larger ten years later when the committee sat. Hanning was further stated to have collected information on the smuggling trade from all his associates, who were said to have organised the smuggling trade along proper business lines. The information was originally intended for Sir Robert Walpole in return for a free pardon for a murder committed by Hanning, and was now given to the committee by one Samuel Wilson, grocer, a self-confessed former smuggler who had taken the benefit of an Act of Indemnity of 1736. The evidence by Hanning–Wilson was corroborated by one Abraham Walter, dealer in tea, who sprang it on the committee that Hanning was his brother. Walter had been his associate, but like Wilson had taken the benefit of the Act of Indemnity of 1736. Now he only dealt in legally imported tea, or so he said, and was therefore free to tell all about the shady doings in his past and of dealers in general who had not seen the light and were still smugglers' accomplices. Further evidence given the committee showed that at the 1745 London sales, the cheapest Bohea tea cost the dealer 4s. 8d. after payment of duties, and was retailed at anything over 6s. The same quality tea sold at the same time for 2s. in Holland, and for less in Gothenburg. Smugglers retailed it in England at 4s.[1] All that Parliament could think of doing when faced with such evidence was to pass more and more Acts increasing the penalties on smuggling and tightening up the law on hovering, and, as a last hope, to pass Acts of Indemnity offering a pardon to smugglers who gave themselves up within a specified time.[2]

[1] *J.H.C.*, vol. xxv, report of committee into causes of smuggling, 1745–6, p. 104.
[2] A number of Acts touching on the tea-trade are listed in Morse, *East Indian Company*, vol. 2, pp. 114–17. For the penal Acts, see W. Addington, *An Abridgement of Penal Statutes...to 1786* (3rd. ed., London, 1786), sections 'Customs', 'Smugglers', and 'Tea'.

The succession of Acts of Parliament against smuggling and hovering and the like were no deterrent to the fraternity of Continental East India merchants, illicit traders, and English distributors of smuggled tea with their bands of hired ruffians. The 1733 committee had hardly laid its report before Parliament when the first of the Danish East Asiatic Company's ships took on her cargo of tea at Canton, the only port in China apart from Macao at which Europeans traded at the time. The ship, of so far unprecedented size in the China trade, was on charter to the Danish company, and loaded more tea than the combined cargo of the two ships which had been sent out by the English company that season.[1] The first of the Swedish ships did not appear at Canton until two years later, in 1736, and one of them was recognised as a former Ostender which had also masqueraded as a Prussian, and was in fact owned by English interlopers.[2] From then on, there was hardly a year in which Danish and Swedish ships did not load at Canton, often taking on more tea than the English ships which loaded a higher proportion of silks.[3] Further, the Scandinavian ships were reported to have loaded mainly the cheap Bohea tea which was most in demand for smuggling.[4] A typical distribution of tea shipments from Canton to Europe may be instanced. In 1750, the combined English fleet of 7 ships loaded some 21,000 peculs of tea; the 8 French and Dutch ships between them 24,000 peculs; and the 4 Danish and Swedish ships 25,000 peculs.[5] From the English shipments, a deduction must be made for re-export to the colonies

[1] Morse, *East India Company*, vol. 1, p. 229. Note also that Macao was a Portuguese trading settlement from which only a little tea was shipped. All other European nations were by that time required to trade from Canton.

[2] *Ibid.*, p. 247; Morse notes only a single ship but cf. Lind, *Göteborgs Handel*, pp. 191–2, table 61, that a second Swedish ship was at Canton as well. This ship, the *Rex Sveciae*, is noted by Postlethwayt, *Dictionary of Commerce*, vol. 2, s.v. 'Sweden', to have been specially built for the China trade.

[3] Lind, *Göteborgs Handel*, pp. 191–2, table 61, gives the names and approximate cargoes of all Swedish ships which traded to Canton. For Danish ships, see Morse, *East India Company*, vol. 2, *passim*.

[4] J.H.C., vol. xxv, evidence of R. Sclater, dealer in tea, p. 103. The earlier-cited witness Samuel Wilson stated that the advent of the Swedish and Danish companies had drastically lowered the price which smugglers had to pay for tea on the Continent (p. 104). See also Glamann, 'Studier', *loc. cit.*, p. 395, that Bohea tea was the mainstay of the Danish company's trade.

[5] Morse, *East India Company*, vol. 2, p. 292. The pecul of tea weighed 136 pounds.

so that only part of the total amount was available for home consumption. What remained was by every account insufficient to meet the demand for tea in England where people had become 'so habituated to it, that they can't leave it off'.[1] The deficiency was made good by smuggled imports, and increasingly so by such imports from Scandinavia.

The evidence for smuggling of tea from Scandinavia is extensive and incontrovertible. Some of it may be gathered from a second parliamentary committee of inquiry which investigated the smuggling trade in 1745-6. Among the witnesses were several who as self-confessed smugglers had earlier taken the benefit of the Act of Indemnity recommended by the previous committee, but were still curiously well-informed about the latest doings of their former comrades. That may not have been much of a surprise to the committee when it heard these witnesses describe themselves as dealers in tea, as druggists, and as grocers. The tenor of their evidence, and of that of the customs authorities, was the same: England was ringed by a chain of ports from which tea was smuggled into the country. The main centres of the illicit trade were Ostend and Flushing; the Channel Islands which were still, like the Isle of Man, outside English customs jurisdiction; the Isle of Man itself; Gothenburg; Copenhagen; the Norwegian ports; and the Danish Faeroe Islands north of the Orkneys. The witnesses further agreed that the tea most in demand for the illicit market was Bohea which was bought on the Continent at 2*s*. to 2*s*. 4*d*. per pound, and sold in England for 4*s*. 6*d*. to 5*s*. per pound, and that Bohea was the quality mainly shipped from Canton by the Danish and Swedish companies which, the committee was told, had become the most important of the four Continental companies supplying England with smuggled tea.[2]

Independent evidence corroborates in detail what the committee was told by customs officers, by reformed or perhaps not quite so quiescent smugglers, and by other merchants. Titley and Goodricke reported in despatches from Copenhagen that tea was shipped from Denmark and Sweden to England and the Isle of

---

[1] *J.H.C.*, vol. xxv, p. 106, evidence of R. Sclater.
[2] *J.H.C.*, vol. xxv, pp. 104ff.

Man;[1] a British naval officer spying out the Swedish defences mentioned smuggling from Gothenburg;[2] the British consul in Bergen, Alexander Wallace, reported on smuggling from Norway – he had intimate and painful knowledge of it as one of his own ships had been seized in England;[3] a Danish merchant house with English connections obtained the right to bond tea in the Faeroes for re-export;[4] customs seizures of tea from Scandinavia are noted in custom house and other correspondence;[5] and, to give a final piece

[1] P.R.O., S.P. 75/96, Titley to Newcastle, 12 August 1752; *ibid.*, same to same, 26 June 1753; S.P. 75/112, Titley to Weston (secretary of the Northern Secretary of State), 2 June 1761, with enclosure listing in detail the cargo of a Danish East Indiaman. From endorsement may be seen that Weston had passed the list on to the East India Company which was thus kept informed of likely smugglers' supplies; S.P. 75/112 Titley to Holdernesse, 18 August 1761; S.P. 75/115, Goodricke to Halifax, 26 February 1763: Goodricke notes in this despatch that English dealers alone, not counting others buying on English account, had over the last five years bought at an average 800,000 pounds of tea annually at the Gothenburg auctions at an average price of 2s. 6d. per pound, and that commissions had already been placed by British buyers for a like amount at the sales later that year.

[2] P.R.O., Ad. 1/4352, report by Lieutenant H. Angel, secret, August 1754. See also P.R.O. 30/8, bundle 80, 'The Earnest Address of Edward Stockley, late of Liverpool, merchant, for...the Benefit of the fair Trader' (pamphlet, dated 1759), in which the author admits that he himself had special knowledge of smuggling to the Isle of Man. According to him, the greater part of the tea and chinaware taken to Man came directly from Gothenburg in Swedish ships.

[3] P.R.O., S.P. 75/118, Wallace to Sandwich, Bergen, 26 February 1765. Note also that Fearnley, who has cropped up in the timber- and iron-trades, smuggled tea from Norway – see Nor. S. Arch., Fearnley Papers, ff. 75, 83, 86–7, *et al.* Further, see P.R.O., Ad. 1/3834, Wallace to Cleveland (secretary, Admiralty), 21 September 1757, in which Wallace describes shipments of East India goods from Copenhagen to Norway, from where they were smuggled to England.

[4] Dan. S. Arch., Coll. Mallingiana, Toldkammeret, 1, Resolution of 29 April 1766 ang. Nils Ryberg; and *ibid.*, Resolution of 26 April 1768. Note that the Faeroes were believed to have been used also as a staging-place for tobacco and other goods shipped from England and Scotland with benefit of drawbacks, and smuggled back into England. Special legislation was therefore passed by 5 Geo. III c. 43, abolishing drawbacks for shipments to the Faeroes.

[5] Custom House, King's Lynn, letter book, Commissioners of Customs to collector, 14 August 1764, concerning disposal of tea seized from a Norwegian ship; *ibid.*, same to same, 9 September 1764, same subject; and *ibid.*, W. Wood (secretary, Custom House, London) to collector, 31 August 1756, in which Wood writes at length about the slackness of preventive measures, and warns the collector that great quantities of tea had been bought recently at Gothenburg to be run into England. Further, see Dan. S. Arch., T.K.U.A., Engl. C, 266, Bothmer to Bernstorff, 16 September 1760, that a Norwegian ship with a cargo of tea had been confiscated when on her way to Man, and that he would intercede for her with Newcastle who had been helpful on similar occasions. Also, *ibid.*, Engl. A. II, 31 b, consul v. Passow to Bernstorff, London, 20 November 1764, that direct tea smuggling to England from Norway and Copen-

of direct evidence, Swedish customs records show the declared value of East India goods entered annually for export to England and Scotland.

The Swedish customs figures need some interpretation before their significance becomes clear. They are for exports from Gothenburg, which was the place of shipment for East India goods imported by the Swedish company, and refer therefore in effect to total East India re-exports from Sweden.[1] Unfortunately, the records do not distinguish between the various East India goods exported, but other and later records show that tea was then the major commodity shipped by the Swedish company, and this had been the position in the preceding years.[2] There are no entries for the Isle of Man, which may be assumed to have been comprehended in the general classification of England and need therefore not be regarded as an omission. The amounts with which England itself is credited appear quite large enough,[3] yet they do not accord with the supposition that the Swedish company was mainly in the trade as an illicit auxiliary to the English East India Company. Large shipments from Gothenburg to Holland, Germany and, in the years preceding and succeeding the War, also to France are annually recorded. The Dutch invariably took the major portion of Swedish East India goods. Shipments on German account were at that time about on a par with recorded English purchases, and France normally bought on her account somewhat larger quantities. This accords well with what is known about the organisation of the smuggling trade. The smugglers were largely supplied by wholesalers in the Channel ports among whom there were, incidentally, a number of English merchants. Tea to be smuggled from the Channel ports would

hagen was very extensive, and that within the last few months four ships and their cargoes had been confiscated in the London region. Three of the ships were loaded on account of the prominent London timber-merchant Claus Heide. Further, Swed. S. Arch., Diplomatica, Anglica I, Brev från Kanslikollegium till Wynantz, 8 February 1753, concerning release of a Swedish ship confiscated with a cargo of tea. Further, B.M., Add. MS 38,463, ff. 195–7, 201 and 217–18; and *ibid.*, Add. MS 38,462, ff. 67–78. All these contain eyewitness accounts of shipments of tea from Sweden and Denmark to the Isle of Man and the Channel Islands.

[1] The tables of exports are in Lind, *Göteborgs Handel*, p. 184.

[2] *Ibid.*, p. 23.

[3] The amounts for 1755, 1760 and 1765 were respectively 210,000; 526,000; and 616,000 daler s:m. (*silvermynt*).

have been bought on French, Dutch, and probably German account, while tea to be smuggled directly into England or via the Channel Islands and the Isle of Man was credited to English account. That this was so beyond reasonable doubt may be inferred from shipments credited to the various countries after the Isle of Man came under British customs jurisdiction late in 1765: the figures of shipments for England, including the Isle of Man, dropped radically, while those for Holland and France rose steeply. It further appears that at least by a later date the direct trade to England was financed by London merchants. This may be inferred from a report headed 'Goods exported from Gothenburg, 1785'[1] in which nearly all East India goods shipments from Gothenburg are credited to London.

There is, then, no difficulty in reconciling shipments from Sweden to Holland, France and Germany with the assumption that they were in fact destined for England, particularly when it is remembered that Holland and France were themselves tea-importers through their own national companies, and in neither country was tea a popular beverage. Scandinavian exports to these countries may therefore safely be regarded as having swelled the stocks of Dutch and French tea to be smuggled to England. What happened to the bulk of the tea shipped from Sweden to Germany – some was re-exported to Russia – remains more conjectural, though the quantities involved make one suspect that much of it was also destined for the English market as the Germans were not a tea-drinking people. It is probable that the Austrian Netherlands were included in the term 'Germany', and no difficulty remains if that was so as the Flemish ports are known to have been supply centres for the smuggling trade.

The contention that tea imported by the Swedish company was almost wholly intended to reach ultimately the English, and to a lesser extent the American, market, is paradoxically lent additional weight by the complete lack of evidence concerning buyers at the Gothenburg East India auctions. The company's records of its trading activities and its sales were invariably destroyed each year, and it is believed that this was done not only to ensure secrecy

[1] B.M., Add. MS 38,346, f. 95, v. and d.

about the company's affairs, but to protect buyers of tea and other East India goods to be smuggled into England. Apart from tea, silk may have been a minor article in the smuggling trade.[1]

The Danish company organised its sales differently from the Gothenburg auctions which were thronged with foreign buyers. Only Danish merchants were permitted to bid at the Copenhagen sales, and their names are known, though there are few known records of the actual disposal of the tea bought by them.[2] That some at least found its way to England via Norway and the Faeroes has already been noted, and there can be no doubt that more shipments went to England by the other route via Holland and the Austrian Netherlands. Shares in the company were held in the Dutch and Flemish ports from where smuggling to England was carried on, and it may well have been that they were held by wholesale suppliers for the illicit market who profited both from the Danish company's trading ventures and from their own more private ventures across the Channel.[3]

Further evidence of the Danish Company's role as an illicit auxiliary of the English East India Company can be gathered from the fact that it was well supplied with English bills drawn by Danish tea buyers on some of the foremost London merchants who had connections with Amsterdam, though no legitimate ones with the Baltic, and on Amsterdam houses that had connections with London.[4] How closely both the Danish and Swedish companies

[1] P.R.O., Ad. 1/3866, J. Burrow, Collector at Whitehaven, to Admiralty, 18 March 1763.

[2] Glamann, 'Studier', *loc. cit.*, pp. 393ff., gives a number of names of the principal buyers at the Copenhagen auctions. See also H. Furber, *John Company at Work* (Harvard, 1951), p. 111, on British merchants settled in Copenhagen who participated in the China trade. And also, Moltke Archives, bundle Asiatisk Kompagni, Auktionsforretninger 1769–70 (*sic*). In this bundle is a marked catalogue of a Copenhagen auction held in 1761 at which the principal buyers were the merchant houses Fabritius; Isselin; Borre & Fenger; Ryberg; Wewer; Tutin; Black; and Chippendale. Each of these houses traded with England and Western Europe.

[3] Glamann, 'Studier', *loc. cit.*, pp. 353ff. It is also of some interest that the company appointed as its representative in England a Mr Clifford, a member of the great Amsterdam merchant and banking family, who specially settled in London to take on the company's commission. See P.R.O., S.P. 75/118, Titley to Grafton, 23 July 1765.

[4] Dan. S. Arch., Asiatisk Kompagni, Inden og Udenlandske Breve 1753–9, entries of bills of exchange, ff. 435–6, 445–6, 524–5, 631–6, 662–77, *et al.*

were tied to the English market is further seen by fluctuations in the rate of exchange which were brought about directly by the turn-over at the Gothenburg and Copenhagen sales.

This dependence of the Danish and Swedish money markets on sales of tea for smuggling to England was well appreciated at the time. The Danish Wholesale Merchants' Society in a memorial of 1759 gave a detailed account of customary practices in negotiating bills of exchange, and noted in particular that the course of exchange was sharply affected after the Copenhagen East Asiatic Company sales when English bills glutted the market.[1] The same sensitivity of the money market was observed in Sweden. Richard Blount, noted earlier in connection with the iron-trade, wrote in 1745 to his Stockholm correspondent, Jennings, that he had just had advice of the two Swedish East Indiamen which had loaded during the past season in Canton. One had missed its voyage home, but the other was due at Gothenburg: 'Altho' your Exchange is fallen on the Report of one of your Chinamen being returned, I am of opinion it will advance again when they know She is the only Ship they are to expect this Year.'[2] And again, in later years when the two Scandinavian companies were even better established, Titley in a despatch from Copenhagen of 1761 advised the Northern Secretary that the sale of the cargoes of two Danish East Indiamen was expected to affect the course of exchange favourably.[3] The following year he reported that Denmark was near bankruptcy, and only the coming East India sales, principally of tea, would save the exchange from falling yet lower.[4]

The Seven Years War affected the illicit trade in tea in two ways. The French East India Company was forced out of the China trade and the amount of tea for smuggling into England would therefore have been diminished if the Scandinavian companies and presumably also the Dutch company had not stepped into the breach

[1] Danish Business Archives, Aarhus (Erhvervsarkivet), Kiøbenhauns Grossereres Protokol 1759–74, ff. 84–91, 'Erklaring paa det indgivne Memorial af 27 Februarii 1759 og Forslaget.'
[2] Swed. S. Arch., Enskilda Samlinger, Arkivfragment, Arkivbildare, Jennings Correspondence, Blount to Jennings, London, 14 May 1745.
[3] P.R.O., S.P. 75/112, Titley to Holdernesse, 18 August 1761.
[4] P.R.O., S.P. 75/114, Titley to Bute, 18 May 1762.

by increasing their shipments from Canton.[1] This they did with a will. Tea was therefore available from Scandinavia in larger quantities for the English market, and smuggling need not have fallen off for lack of supplies. Smuggling, however, may have become more difficult as more warships were active in the waters around England. A London merchant complained to a Swedish correspondent about this unfortunate effect of war on the smuggling trade,[2] but one wonders whether some of the small privateers did not come to the rescue and combine patriotism and their lawful pursuits with free trading in tea or in whatever else brought sufficient profit. Customs officers, at least, were convinced that this was the case, and regarded the small privateer as no more than a 'licensed smuggler'.[3] On balance, the deterrent effect of warships on smuggling was quite likely offset by other warships helping out with running smugglers' goods to England. The exact amount of tea smuggled into England through the good offices of the Danish and Swedish companies will of course never be known, but minimum estimates can be given. In 1755, for example, East India goods bought at the Gothenburg sales on British account alone were valued at about £40,000; in 1760, after allowance is made so far as possible for the depreciation of the Swedish currency, their value was about £60,000; and by 1765 it had risen to about £80,000.[4]

[1] Lind, *Göteborgs Handel*, pp. 180–1, table 61; and Morse, *East India Company*, vol. 5, pp. 72, 87, 100–1, 108, and *passim*.

[2] Swed. S. Arch., Enskilda Samlinger, Arkivfragment, Jennings correspondence; Blount to Jennings, London, 29 May 1744: Referring to the coming Gothenburg auctions, Blount advises that he had arranged for Jennings to draw on Clifford & Sons at Amsterdam, and continues that 'This high Exchange is an evident Proof of the decay of your Trade...Sales of Tea I believe will be low as our Ships cannot carry on the Smuggling Trade from Gothenburg as they used to do in time of Peace.' See also, *R.H.C.*, 1st series, vol. 11, report on distilleries in Scotland, 1798, p. 748, that smuggling was hampered by the large number of armed vessels along the coast.

[3] P.R.O., Ad. 1/3866, memorial of Commissioners of Customs to Lords Commissioners of Treasury, London, 9 September 1758. Note also that other papers in this bundle of letters from the Custom House, London, give numerous instances of smuggling of tea by small privateers.

[4] The amounts in Swedish currency are in Lind, *Göteborgs Handel*, p. 184, table 63 a. Rates of exchange are occasionally noted in diplomatic correspondence, as in P.R.O., S.P. 75/104, Goodricke to Holdernesse, 25 July 1758; and *ibid.*, same to same, 23 December 1758; and *ibid.*, same to Halifax, 16 August 1763: and see also, Postlethwayt, *Dictionary of Commerce*, vol. 2, article on Sweden. For Danish and Norwegian exchange rates on England see also Royal Library, Copenhagen, Wasserschleben Arkiv, Ny kgl. Samling, MS no. 700, copies of journals, 1758–.

There are no figures available for the Copenhagen sales, but one has the impression that they cannot have been less, as the Danish company operated generally on a larger scale than the Swedish. These figures must be augmented by sums paid for tea which had been bought in Scandinavia on Dutch or other account so that the total sum paid by Britain for tea originally shipped by the Danish and Swedish companies was probably not less and possibly greater than that laid out for all other imports from Scandinavia.[1]

When smuggling of tea into England was at least temporarily made unprofitable later in the century by a drastic lowering of the import and excise duties, both the Danish and Swedish companies fell on evil days, as, incidentally, did the Dutch and French companies. The Danish East Asiatic Company practically deserted the China trade for the time and eked out some existence by its trade with Bengal. The Swedish East India Company had less to fall back on and was eventually wound up.[2]

Tea-smuggling, it has earlier been mentioned, went hand in hand with smuggling of spirits. The heavy excise duty in England made brandy in particular a very acceptable clandestine import,[3]

[1] Stavenow, *Sveriges historia*, vol. 9, p. 290, writes that the Swedish company's re-exports were on an average during the years 1756–9 valued at four million daler s:m. The exchange stood at that time at between 5 to 7 dalers s:m to the Pound. Note also that for the period of the American War of Independence, Heckscher believed the value of re-exports by the company to have been no less than the combined values of exports of all Swedish home produce and manufactures.

[2] The occasion for the temporary setback to tea-smuggling was Pitt's Commutation Act of 1784 (24 Geo. III c. 38) which followed on the recommendation of a parliamentary committee of enquiry into smuggling (*R.H.C.*, 1st series, vol. 11, pp. 263ff.) that only a drastic reduction in duties could stop smuggling. Pitt's reasons for lowering the tea duties may be gathered from his 'Proposed Review of the Smuggling Laws...,' in Cross (ed.), *Documents*, pp. 237ff. The views of the English East India Company are given in 'Three Reports of the Select Committee appointed by the Court of Directors...on the Export Trade...laid before...the Privy Council' (n.d., 1793. Pamphlet in Cambridge U.L., class-mark Ddd. 25. 170). The East India Company held the Swedish company to have been 'by far the best regulated and most prosperous in Europe' and its progress in the past so rapid that 'if the Commutation Act had not intervened, that Company must have swallowed up most of the China trade' (p. 84). Note incidentally that Furber, *John Company*, p. 110, is mistaken in stating that the Swedish company traded only to China. It sent some ships to India, but unlike the Danish company did not establish any factories there, nor keep up a regular connection. The interruption of the profitable smuggling trade therefore left it with fewer resources for carrying on trade than the Danish company.

[3] Saxby, *British Customs*, pp. 233–4, gives both the duties and the regulations on import.

and the Scandinavian countries were not slow to take advantage of the opportunity to add yet another commodity to their range of smugglers' goods. An English merchant settled in Norway advised a correspondent in Newcastle already early in the century that he had been granted bonding privileges for French brandy so that English ships could load it for their home ports. Customs officers, he added, would not look for brandy in ships from Norway, and his new venture ought to develop so well that his correspondent might advertise it among his acquaintances with every confidence in its success.[1] This pioneer of a new trade route for brandy from France to England helped to lay the foundations of what was to become a thriving business, which finally attracted the attention of the Northern Secretary of State who ordered the consul at Bergen to enquire into the extent of brandy smuggling via Norway. Needless to say, the consul himself was involved in the smuggling trade and reassured London that after exhaustive enquiries very little could be found out about it, and that it must be small.[2] The Bergen port books, however, give the impression that the trade was fairly extensive. The port books of Gothenburg show further that Swedish merchants also engaged in it, and there seemed to have been hardly an English ship that did not load French brandy beside its main cargo of bar-iron and of tea.[3]

Smugglers did not only run goods into England, but were also active in smuggling prohibited exports out of the country. Live sheep were in the category of prohibited exports to make the establishment in foreign countries of a cloth industry dependent on fine English wool more difficult.[4] Swedish sheep husbandry, however, was given great encouragement by the importation of a flock of thirty English sheep early in the century, and this flock

[1] Nor. S. Arch., Privatarkiv no 67, James Bowman, 1707–39; bundle 1, copy book, Bowman to R. Harris, Porsgrund, 26 November 1713.

[2] P.R.O., S.P. 75/118, Wallace to Sandwich, Bergen, 26 February 1765.

[3] For an example, see Gothenburg Provincial Archives, port books, 1750, f. 665 v., that one J. C. Selbe was shipping practically a full cargo to Scotland in a Scottish ship. See also Lind, *Göteborgs Handel*, pp. 176–7, table 60*a*, for shipments of French brandy and wine to England. Titley had earlier warned London that French 'wines' were being smuggled from Norway to Scotland – see P.R.O., S.P. 75/95, Titley to Newcastle, 12 August 1752. There is further evidence of brandy-smuggling from Norway in the Fearnley Papers.

[4] A list of all prohibited exports is given in *R.H.C.*, 1st series, vol. 11, pp. 292ff.

was augmented from time to time by further shipments.[1] Wool
itself was another prohibited export, yet it continued to leave the
country and was regularly imported into Sweden where, an English
publicist avowed, the cloth industry was based on wool smuggled
from Scotland which had in turn been carried north from England.[2]
Neither the smuggling of sheep nor of wool to Scandinavia can
have been of great dimensions, and its effect on the balance of
trade would have been insignificant when compared with the illicit
trade in tea or in cloth. It had, though, a significant effect on the
establishment of a Swedish textile industry.

How impossible it is to strike any balance of trade beyond saying
that the Scandinavian countries exported very much more to England
than they received in return will have been appreciated after the
appraisal of smuggling and of customs frauds which between them
invalidated contemporary trade statistics. The Seven Years War
had nothing to do with this position beyond increasing the share
of the Swedish East India and the Danish East Asiatic Companies
in the international smuggling trade in tea, which tipped the
balance of trade still further against England. The Seven Years War
had, however, one very decided effect on a concomitant of trade,
that is, on shipping. Danish–Norwegian, and to a lesser extent
Swedish, ships supplanted British carriers in the timber- and iron-
trade, due entirely, as has earlier been shown, to the War, and
freights which had been earned by British owners were now paid
to Scandinavia.[3] Outside the North Sea and the Baltic, Scandinavian
ships were equally in demand as neutral carriers of British goods.
Prussia had no fleet worth talking about and could therefore not
interfere seriously with Swedish shipping, and the few enterprising
British privateers who sailed under Prussian colours were more of
a nuisance than a menace. There are only one or two known cases
of Anglo-Prussian privateers attacking Swedish ships carrying

[1] G. H. Stråle, *Alingsås Manufakturverk* (Stockholm, 1884), p. 40, and Gothenburg
Provincial Archives, port books, 1725, ff. 816*d* and 817*v*.
[2] Postlethwayt, *Dictionary of Commerce*, vol. 2, s.v. 'Sweden'; see also, Stråle, *Alingsås
Manufakturverk*, p. 260, on the use of English wool in Swedish industry; Lind,
Göteborgs Handel, pp. 90–7, tables 17–20, for imports of English wool into Gothen-
burg; and *R.H.C.*, vol. 11, 1st series, 'Report on...Exportation of Live Sheep and
Lambs, Wool, etc.', 1788, pp. 308 and 316, wool-smuggling to Sweden.
[3] See above, chapters 3 and 4, *passim*.

cargoes to Britain, and some *contretemps* with homeward-bound ships occurred on a few more occasions.[1] Danish–Norwegian ships carrying British goods were invariably safe from the attentions of these privateers, and made the most of their privileged status. Denmark had farsightedly secured her shipping in the years preceding the War against capture by the feared Barbary pirates through a series of treaties with the Barbary states, and her ships were therefore in an excellent position to carry British goods in the Mediterranean from which British ships were driven by French privateers soon after the outbreak of war.[2] The number of Danish–Norwegian ships was very great, and the Danish envoy could assert after the Seven Years War without being contradicted that British trade with the countries in the Mediterranean region would have been wiped out but for the assistance given it by some 400 ships of the Danish–Norwegian merchant fleets.[3] The income derived from this carrying trade, which was mostly on English account, amounted by a contemporary estimate to 14 million Rixdaler for the years 1755–70.[4] The Rixdaler at that time was worth about 4s. to 4s. 6d. which gives one the respectable sum of some £3 million earned by Denmark and Norway by carrying freight for British merchants. This intrusion of the Danish–Norwegian merchant fleet into British trade did not go unnoticed in England, and an English merchant in 1761 especially sent a memorial to the Lords Commissioners of trade in which he wrote that he had recently been in the Mediterranean where he had found British trade at the mercy of Danish–Norwegian fleets, which had entirely replaced British merchantmen.[5]

It was not only Danish and Norwegian ships which were active during the Seven Years War as carriers of British goods, and of imports into Britain. Swedish ships also took part in the carrying trade, though their part was a smaller one, as the Swedish merchant fleet was not as large as the Danish–Norwegian, and a proportion of it continued to be confined to trade in the Baltic. Nevertheless, so early as October 1755 Swedish ships were offered for charter

[1] See next chapter.   [2] Schovelin, *Fra den danske Handels Empire*, vol. 1, p. 20.
[3] *Ibid.*, p. 22.   [4] *ibid.*
[5] P.R.O., C.O. 388/49, f. Hh. 26, 'Memorial of James Clark'.

in London,[1] that is, before British ships were seriously threatened by French warships or privateers. What attracted them so early was the rise in freight rates, and once they had established themselves in the carrying trade, Swedish ships were used constantly throughout the War by British exporters and importers. The position of the neutral carriers was well described after the War by Cosby, Titley's assistant in Copenhagen, when he wrote that Denmark–Norway – and he could as well have included Sweden – had 'gained considerably by carrying for other Nations in time of War which they look on as their harvest, and therefore view with pleasure anything that tends to a rupture'.[2]

There was little to offset the increased Scandinavian earnings from shipping services during the War apart from marine insurances which were taken out in London by Scandinavian owners. The Danish East Asiatic Company often insured in London in preference to Amsterdam which was the main insurance mart for Scandinavia, and individual shippers appear to have done the same now that their vessels were carrying more British cargo.[3] The income from this source seems to have been small as the attraction of Amsterdam remained strong until the post-War series of Dutch bankruptcies lowered the financial prestige of Holland and made the stability of the London market appear all the stronger in contrast. In the meantime, freight charges paid by British merchants to Scandinavian owners had to be added virtually undiminished to Scandinavian earnings from open and illicit trade, and, once again, the balance inclined in favour of the Scandinavian countries. Trade with Denmark–Norway and Sweden was indeed by mercantilist conceptions a losing trade.

[1] Swed. S. Arch., Diplomatica, Anglica I, Wynantz till Kanslikollegium, despatch of 3 October 1755.   [2] P.R.O., S.P. 75/118, Cosby to Sandwich, 22 February 1765.
[3] J. O. Bro-Jørgensen, *Forsikringsvaesenets Historie i Danmark indtill det 19. Aarhundrede* (Copenhagen, 1935), pp. 201–5. See also Moltke Archives, bundle Asiatisk Kompagni, Korrespondance og Aktstykker: insurances negotiated in London between 1744 and 1757 on account of Count Moltke for his shares in cargoes in the East Asiatic Company's China trade. Some Swedish ships and cargoes were, like Danish–Norwegian, insured in London since at least the 1730s, but Swedish shipping was throughout the eighteenth century of less importance than Danish–Norwegian and the sums spent in London on insurance must have been small – see T. Söderberg, *Försäkringsväsenets historia i Sverige intill Karl Johanstiden* (Stockholm, 1935), pp. 181ff.

8 The First Armed Neutrality: Anglo-Scandinavian Disputes over Neutral Rights

British merchants and manufacturers could not have helped feeling satisfied with the course of Anglo-Scandinavian trade during the Seven Years War. Sweden and Denmark, although in treaty relations with France, continued to send to England their forest and mining produce which were all-important to many industries and not least to ship-building on which the outcome of the War might well depend. For the 'free trader' there were gratifyingly large supplies of tea from the Scandinavian companies to make good the loss of shipments from France and from Flanders. And for the export merchant there was moreover the timely help from the Scandinavian merchant fleets in carrying British and foreign cargoes through enemy-threatened seas into which the dwindling number of British merchantmen could only venture at great risk. So far, so good. The War, however, was not being fought merely to maintain the *status quo* of British trade. Once it had broken out, it was intended to become the means for curbing the economic power of a rival, a resolve bluntly stated by a publicist when writing in 1757 'That the great object of a maritime nation should be, to take advantage of any rupture with another trading state, to destroy and distress their shipping and commerce, and to cut off all resources for naval armaments'.[1] That great object could obviously only be attained if the neutrals were not allowed to give the enemy the aid which England herself expected from them, that is, naval stores and shipping services. Just those two essentials for carrying on a war and for remaining solvent during it could be obtained from

[1] M. Postlethwayt, *Great Britain's Commercial Interest Explained and Improved* (London, 1757), vol. 2, p. 347.

Sweden and Denmark–Norway, and both the Scandinavian powers were therefore bound to come into conflict with England if they should attempt to trade with France and to carry her goods. This they meant to do. Denmark, as will be seen later, had expressly used the argument with France that she would be of greater use to her as a neutral carrying French goods than as a co-belligerent. Sweden hoped to have it both ways: to carry on trading with France as a neutral not at war with England, and to fight for her own ends against Prussia as a pensionary of France. England, in turn, recognised that these were the aims of Denmark and Sweden and was determined to thwart them.

The time for stopping the Scandinavian neutrals from helping France did not come until war had been formally declared, as contraband regulations, blockades and other sanctions could not be made effective before then. During the months of 1755 and 1756 while English and French fought in America and manoeuvred for position in India, British naval commanders had therefore to face a period of galling inactivity in which Danish–Norwegian and Swedish shipping enjoyed a close season utilised at least by Sweden to ship arms to France.[1] Some impetuous officers could not stand by and watch the neutrals get away with helping the enemy, and lashed out against them in defiance of established legal practice. There was an incident in late August of 1755 in the Sound itself when a Swedish ship bound for France was boarded by a British naval party searching ostensibly for deserters, though in fact for a cargo of cannon known to be on the way to France.[2] Sweden protested, and Denmark joined in the protest as her territorial waters had been violated. England apologised, a young lieutenant was dismissed the service, though he was later re-instated at the request of the king of Denmark, and the incident was closed. It served as a warning, though, that England would not allow the

[1] Shipments of Swedish cannon to France continued during the war, and the Admiralty received from time to time detailed intelligence reports about them. See for immediate pre-War and later shipments P.R.O., Ad. 1/4121, 'Intelligence for Lord Anson', no date, no signature (sent from office of Secretary of State), bound in under months September to October 1756. Also, B.M., Add. MS 15956 (Anson Papers), ff. 61–2.

[2] The importance of this incident in the development of International Law is discussed by Kent, 'The Three-Mile Limit', p. 547.

neutrals to cross her when war came, and the Scandinavian powers understood the incident as such.[1]

England could not have done much else than apologise, but she had in any case every reason at that time to be conciliatory and to step warily. The quest for alliances had begun, and there was a rather misplaced hope that Denmark could be won over to the English side. How unlikely that was should have been apparent to Cabinet, which was warned of Danish and Swedish intentions by Titley at Copenhagen and by the well-informed intelligence agents whom England employed at Stockholm where, it will be remembered, no English envoy was stationed at the time. The despatches of Titley and the reports of agents from Stockholm – some of the reports were sent directly to London, but the majority went to Titley who either sent them on to London, or more often included the gist of them in his despatches – were remarkably accurate, and Cabinet was fully informed through them of the Danish–Swedish–French negotiations which resulted in the Armed Neutrality Convention of 1756.

There were actually two distinct groups of agents in Sweden. The first was simply patriotic British merchants and ships' masters who were living in Stockholm and Gothenburg or were there temporarily. They usually sent reports on shipping, trade, arms shipments and also fortifications and warships to the Admiralty, the Secretaries of State, or occasionally to the Board of Trade or the customs authorities, and sometimes directly to a minister: Pitt was sent quite a few such reports. The other group was made up of professionals, that is, agents who were paid for their services, and foreign diplomats who wanted to make themselves agreeable to the British government for various reasons, or had been instructed by their own governments to 'co-operate' with British colleagues or their agents. Representative of the former, that is of agents paid

[1] Swed. S. Arch., Diplomatica, Anglica 1, Kanslikollegium to Wynantz, 1 September and 9 December 1755, and Kanslipresidenten to Wynantz, 9 September 1755. Also, Dan. S. Arch., T.K.U.A., Engl. C, 264, Bernstorff to Rantzau, 23 August, 13 September, 11 October and 11 November 1755; and *ibid.*, Engl. B, 106, Rantzau to Bernstorff, 31 October 1755 and 20 February 1756. Also, P.R.O., S.P. 75/99, Titley to Holdernesse, 23 and 30 August, and 4 November 1755; and Potenger (secretary of Holdernesse) to Titley, Hanover, 29 August 1755; and Holdernesse to Titley, 4 November 1755.

for their services, was a young Swedish nobleman at the Court in Stockholm, Baron Karl Gedda, who signed his reports as 'Wilkinson'. He was a member of a Swedish diplomatic family, and had been educated at Oxford. He received a salary out of Newcastle's secret service fund, and hoped that he would be employed eventually either as a Swedish diplomat in Britain, or a British diplomat abroad. Gedda was anything but discreet, and was soon well known in Stockholm as a British agent. Various Swedish ministers and politicians used him to transmit messages to London on the Swedish political situation, on the conduct of the War, on intended legislation that might affect England, or simply told him whatever they wanted London to believe.

Of the foreign diplomats who made themselves useful to London the most active earlier during the War was the Dutch envoy in Stockholm, de Marteville. He was the regular go-between of the queen of Sweden, the redoubtable sister of Frederick II of Prussia, and England. Titley did not entirely trust him, and believed that he had pro-French sympathies. Whether that was so or not, de Marteville's reports were both accurate and useful. Titley gave no evidence for his occasional denunciations of de Marteville, and it seems to have been a case of personal dislike. He let Holdernesse know, for example, that de Marteville was merely keeping in with England because he wanted to be transferred to London as the Stockholm climate did not agree with him, and hoped that the British government would press the States-General to appoint him to the London embassy if it fell vacant. De Marteville may have been right about the Stockholm climate: he died in Stockholm, and Titley arranged passage home for the widow, generously lending her money for all her expenses. There were other foreign diplomats in Stockholm who transmitted information to England and they will be mentioned later; de Marteville's death, therefore, did not lead to an interruption of reports from that quarter.[1]

From all this it can be gathered that French diplomatic moves in Sweden were no secret to the British government. France had

[1] Representative examples of intelligence reports and the like from Sweden chosen from among a great number are in P.R.O., S.P. 75/99, Titley to Holdernesse with enclosed intelligence reports, 28 October 1755; *ibid.*, 75/100, same to same, 6 January and 6 and 20 March 1756.

been trying since the summer of 1755 to make Denmark and Sweden commit themselves to joining her in the expected war in Europe, and, failing that, she encouraged concerted Danish–Swedish naval preparations against the threat of British interference with neutral shipping.[1] Suffice it to say in this context that France was successful in making the Scandinavian powers agree to join in an Armed Neutrality Convention, and that Denmark and Sweden were fitting out impressive-looking, though as the event showed far from impressively handled, naval squadrons which were to link up as a Neutrality Fleet that was to cruise in the North Sea for the protection of Scandinavian shipping.[2] England could not know how innocuous the Neutrality Fleet would turn out to be and suspected that it might reinforce the French navy, or at least convoy Scandinavian merchantmen to and from France. The alarm over the intentions of Denmark and Sweden became in fact so great that on a rumour of the Danish fleet being sighted in the summer of 1756 making for the Channel, Cabinet hurriedly recalled a squadron from the Atlantic.[3] The rumour was soon shown to have been

[1] The best short accounts of the negotiations which resulted in the Neutrality Convention of 1756 are in G. Carlquist, *Carl Fredrik Scheffer och Sveriges politiska förbindelser med Danmark åren 1752–1765* (Lund, 1920), chs 4–6; and in Th. Boye, *De vaebnede Neutralitetsforbund* (Kristiania etc., 1912), ch. 4. A good deal of the source material has been printed in the *Recueils des Instructions données aux Ambassadeurs de France*, vols 2, 8 and 13; in P. Vedel (ed.), *Correspondance Ministerielle du Comte J. H. E. Bernstorff* (Copenhagen, 1871); and in Freiherrn A. F. v. d. Asseburg, *Denkwürdigkeiten* (Berlin, 1842) who was Danish envoy to Stockholm at the time of the negotiations. The views on the negotiations of a leading Swedish politician of the time are in A. J. von Höpken's *Skrifter*, ed. J. Silverstolpe (Stockholm, 1890–).

[2] The public text of the Convention is in P.R.O., S.P. 75/101, bound in under date of 12 July 1756.

[3] The rumour originated with the master of a Swedish ship who reported on running into Portsmouth that he had sighted nine Danish warships flying the French flag coming down the Channel. The Admiralty took it in bad part when it later found that the supposed Danish warships were merely a fleet of Dutch merchantmen, and kept the Swedish ship in port for nearly a year. See Dan. S. Arch. T.K.U.A., Engl. B, 106, Rantzau to Bernstorff 3 August and 22 September 1756, and *ibid.*, Engl. C, 264, Bernstorff to Rantzau, n.d., that he could assure Holdernesse that there was no truth in the rumour. Also, Swed. S. Arch., Anglica I, Wynantz to Kanslikollegium, 6 and 13 August, 10 September, 2 and 5 November 1756, and 11 March 1757. The squadron which was recalled was Keppel's. English concern over the Scandinavian naval armament led her so early as February 1756 to ask Russia to intervene at Copenhagen and Stockholm. Russia obliged, and obtained a declaration from Bernstorff that the Neutrality Fleet would on no account be joined with the French

quite unfounded, but Holdernesse, the Northern Secretary, was in the meantime very circumspect when Rantzau, the Danish envoy, and Wynantz, the Swedish chargé d'affaires, called to inform him of the signing of the Neutrality Convention, of which Holdernesse was already well aware, and to assure him that it was directed not only against England but against any power that might interfere with Scandinavian commerce.[1]

Holdernesse might have suspected after listening to the separate representations of the Danish and Swedish diplomats that their two governments did not see eye to eye about the purpose of the Convention. Rantzau and Wynantz had both asked in their interviews for an English declaration on contraband, but only Rantzau on that occasion brought up the old vexed issue of the right of neutrals to carry the goods of the enemy, in other words, the long-disputed principle that Free Ships made Free Goods. And when Holdernesse had studied the text of the Convention which had been handed to him, he should have noticed that this issue had not been explicitly raised in it.[2] As it turned out, Holdernesse missed this point. Denmark and Sweden, as it happened, did not at all agree on what to claim from England, and on the lengths to which they would go to protect their trade with France against British interference. Sweden was the more determined, or rather, one section of the governing party in Sweden was the more prepared, to risk war with England, and it was this Swedish faction, then in the ascendant, which had been pressing during the negotiations with Denmark for a joint Scandinavian declaration that Free Ships made Free Goods. Denmark, whose foreign policy was firmly under the direction of the shrewd and pacific Bernstorff, would have

navy. See P.R.O., S.P. 91/62, Hanbury Williams to Holdernesse, St Petersburg, 6, 9 and 16 March, and 11 May 1756; and Holdernesse to Hanbury Williams, 2 and 6 February, and 13 April 1756.

[1] Sweden as much as Denmark was doing her best to convince England that the Convention was not directed against her, and Wynantz was given special orders to assure Holdernesse of Sweden's peaceable intentions. See Swed. S. Arch., Anglica I, Kanslipresidenten to Wynantz, 27 April and 9 July 1756.

[2] How great Sweden's annoyance was that Denmark had not agreed to writing the principle of Free Ships, Free Goods into the Convention may be seen from an instruction to Wynantz never to leave Rantzau out of sight in case he raised the issue on behalf of Denmark. Sweden would then also do so. See Swed. S. Arch., Anglica I, Kanslikollegium to Wynantz, 5 May 1756.

nothing to do with such a declaration. Bernstorff had pointed out to the Swedes that England was not likely to concede now what she had consistently refused to recognise in the past, that is, that the neutral flag covered the goods of the enemy, that Free Ships made Free Goods. If the Scandinavian powers insisted on the principle, Bernstorff believed that England was bound sooner or later to contest it by arms, and Bernstorff had no intention of seeing Denmark go to war so long as peace could be made to pay handsomely in increased trade. He therefore firmly refused to sign a convention that would in effect contain a *casus belli*, and suggested to the Swedes that it should instead be worded in such a way that complete freedom to carry enemy goods could be claimed when the opportunity offered, but that England should not be required to subscribe to the principle or given a pretext to reject it outright. In the meantime, every case of trade obstruction should be examined on its merits; but the convention which Bernstorff eventually signed neither specified what would be regarded as an obstruction to trade nor what was to be the nature of the reprisals which, Denmark and Sweden informed England, would be taken if she interfered with their shipping.

There was, though, one article in the convention which might have appeared particularly threatening, and that was the seventh. It stipulated that merchantmen were to be convoyed, but it was obvious that Denmark and Sweden could not commission a Neutrality Fleet and have as well sufficient warships for convoy duty. Titley and the agents from Stockholm had reported fully and accurately on the numbers and armaments of the warships in their respective countries, and it cannot have taken the Admiralty long to have seen through the threat. It turned out soon enough that generally only frigates were available for the very occasional convoys, and frigates were no deterrent except to a small privateer. The Dutch early in the War found out that convoys were no protection to their shipping when a large fleet of Dutch merchantmen including its convoying warships was brought up. Later in the War, the same thing happened again to the Dutch, and a Danish convoy suffered a like fate. The Danish case which will be described more fully later in this chapter showed that the Fighting Instructions of the Danish Navy – and there is no reason to doubt that those of the Swedish or for that matter Dutch Navy were in any way different – laid it down that merchantmen need not be protected by their convoying warships against a stronger force.[1]

No matter how determined the text of the Neutrality Convention might have made Denmark and Sweden appear to be to stand no nonsense from England, there was really nothing much in it to alarm her. On the contrary, one of the provisions of the Convention spared England from having to protect her shipping in the Baltic, which was closed to the warships of the warring powers and in which none of the unspecified reprisals mentioned in the Convention were to be taken. Denmark and Sweden proclaimed as well by separate decrees neutral zones along their North Sea coasts in which hostilities were not to be permitted.[2]

Of all this, Holdernesse seems to have realised nothing. He recognised, though, the one obvious fact, that Denmark and Sweden had commissioned a fleet that might prove dangerous, and he may have feared as well that the Scandinavian powers would throw in their lot completely with France unless England showed them some consideration. The Neutrality Convention had been specific on only one point which called for an immediate and definite concession from England, and that was on contraband. Contraband, Denmark and Sweden claimed, should be only those goods listed in the Treaty of Utrecht of 1713, and in support of their claim issued additional and separate instructions to their shipping.[3] If the Scandinavians got their way, pitch and tar which had in the last

[1] On Danish convoys, see Dan. S. Arch., T.K.U.A., Engl. B, 107, Bothmer to Bernstorff, private, 21 October 1757, and *ibid.*, same to same, 12 September 1758; as also *ibid.*, Admiralitets og General-komissariets Collegium, Kongelige Resolutioner, 'relation' of 26 April and 'resolution' of 5 May 1760. For Swedish convoys, see Swed. S. Arch., Ämneserier, Handel och Sjöfart, ser. III, Konvoj-väsendet, 'Transunt af det till Kungl. Maj:sts från Admiralitets Collegio...Bref [dated] 8 August 1760 ang. Convoyen.' The Fighting Instructions of the Danish Navy are in Dan. S. Arch., Søetaten, Kongl. Ekspeditioner, 1759–60, Instruks no 180; the relevant article is the fourteenth.
[2] On the problems this gave rise to, see Kent, 'The Three-Mile Limit', pp. 545–51.
[3] See Dan. S. Arch., Kongl. Forordninger 1756, 'Reglement und Verordnung betreffend was die commercirende Unterthanen...in Ansehung der Schiffahrt zu beobachten haben. 6 Aug. 1756'; and Swed. S. Arch., Kungl. Maj:ts Förordningar, 1756, 'Kungiörelse hwarefter de Handlanda och Sjöfaranda...hafwa sig at rätta. 16 Jul. 1756.'

war been declared contraband by England,[1] could in this be freely carried. Although Holdernesse did not commit himself publicly, Swedish ships bound for France with pitch and tar – no case of a Danish–Norwegian ship carrying it has come to notice – were allowed to go free. Wynantz accepted this as the first step towards a complete overthrow of English pretensions, and wrote jubilantly to Stockholm that victory was in sight.[2]

Wynantz was mistaken. The policy of leniency towards the Swedish ships was soon abandoned, and Swedish complaints were disregarded. Titley at Copenhagen had found out how precarious the much advertised Danish–Swedish accord really was, and in his despatches gave Holdernesse to understand that a stronger line might well be taken.[3] An attempted *coup d'état* in Sweden at about the same time showed up the weakness of one partner to the Neutrality Convention,[4] and Cabinet must have come to the conclusion that all was not well in the Danish–Swedish camp and that the possibility of action from that quarter could safely be disregarded for the time being. Not only was pitch and tar now condemned as contraband, but England went further and neutral ships carrying timber to France were forced to run into English ports where the Admiralty bought up the cargo and reimbursed the shipper for the freight.[5] This was an entirely new departure in naval warfare, taken to starve the enemy's navy and merchant fleet of building-material, and it may also have been meant to impress the neutrals with England's resolve to carry on the fight against trade with France despite the Minorca disaster.

Denmark and Sweden or, for that matter, Holland, did not know what to make of this latest English move against neutral trade. The

[1] P.R.O., S.P. 95/133, 'Abstract of Papers about the Seizure of Swedish Ships', 20 October 1745.

[2] Swed. S. Arch., Anglica I, Wynantz to Kanslikollegium, 30 July 1756 and appended papers; and *ibid.*, same to same, 7, 10 and 24 September 1756.

[3] P.R.O., S.P. 75/101, Titley to Holdernesse, 24 July 1756; and also *ibid.*, intelligence report (from Gedda) dated Stockholm 10 September 1756, bound in under date.

[4] Swed. S. Arch., Anglica I, Kanslikollegium to Wynantz, 6 July 1756. Wynantz was informed by courier of the attempted *coup*, and instructed to play it down as much as possible when the news reached London; see also P.R.O., S.P. 95/102, report (from Gedda), Stockholm 13 April 1756, and S.P. 75/101, reports (from Gedda) of 25 June and 6 July 1756.

[5] P.R.O., Ad. 1/4121, Holdernesse to Lords of Admiralty, 8 July 1756.

timber cargoes forced into British ports were being paid for: England might take offence if there were protests and declare timber contraband, in which case it could be confiscated. But, if the neutrals did not protest, there was no knowing where it might end. Denmark and Sweden decided in the end to do nothing and hope for the best.[1] Timber consigned to France continued to be brought up till the end of the War and was paid for by the Admiralty, although Admiralty correspondence constantly referred to the poor quality of the shipments, which were of little or no use for naval construction, and one cannot help wondering whether Norwegian and other timber-shippers addressed unsaleable trash to France with strict instruction to masters of their ships to fall in with an English privateer.[2]

The uncertainty over timber shipments to France may have been no more than a nuisance, but Norway soon came to have a legitimate grievance about the English definition of contraband. Dried and salt fish, just like salt beef, was used as ships' provisions and could therefore be regarded as *provisions de bouche* which undoubtedly counted as contraband. English privateers looked further than that and argued that fresh fish was after all the basis of the contraband trade in salt fish and dried fish which could best be stamped out by seizing every Norwegian fishing vessel in sight – the Swedes were not conspicuous as fishermen in the North Sea and no Swedish fishing boats seem to have come their way – and condemning the cargo. The Prize Court allowed itself to be persuaded to this view, never a difficult feat, and the Norwegian fishing industry was in the end completely terrorised. Complaints to Holdernesse were of no use, and appeals to the Appeal Court were thought to be too costly.[3] There was only one consolation:

[1] The spectacle of a large fleet of Dutch timber-ships from the Baltic with its escorting 44-Gun being brought into an English port might have had something to do with that decision. See Dan. S. Arch., T.K.U.A., 106, Rantzau to Bernstorff, 24 August and 7 September 1756.

[2] See below, p. 195.

[3] Dan. S. Arch., T.K.U.A., Engl. B, 108, Bothmer to Bernstorff, 18 July 1758; and *ibid.*, Engl. C, 274, undated (after 1758) list of fishing vessels taken by privateers. Some of the ships were taking salt fish to France, and their cargoes were valued at between £1,000 and £1,500 each. For condemnations of salt beef, see *ibid.*, Engl. C, 266, Bernstorff to Bothmer, 22 July 1758.

War and Trade in Northern Seas

in no case about merchandise in dispute as contraband, that is, meat, fish, and pitch and tar, was the ship itself condemned. England plainly did not intend to go to extremes over such matters as another minor article or two of contraband, but she showed no such restraint when it came to an issue considered vital, and such an issue was the prohibition on neutral ships to carry enemy goods.

Rantzau, as has earlier been seen, had raised that issue right at the beginning of the War in Europe. Wynantz, who had kept off the topic, soon also brought it up on express instructions from Stockholm.[1] That both the Scandinavian powers should insist on the recognition of the principle that Free Ships made Free Goods gave Cabinet a splendid opportunity to play off the one country against the other. Both Holdernesse, at long last briefed by the Law Officers and probably by his astuter colleagues in Cabinet, and later Pitt himself, made the most of the different legal positions in which Denmark and Sweden found themselves over their demands that Scandinavian ships should be permitted to carry for the enemy without interference from England. Briefly, their position was this: Denmark had by treaty the undoubted right to most-favoured-nation treatment, and claimed therefore the benefit of the current Anglo-Dutch treaty of 1674 in which Holland had been given the right to carry enemy goods. For good measure, the Danes threw in as an argument a very shaky interpretation of part of their own treaty with England but did not insist on continuing that part of the discussion. While the Danes had a good legal case, the Swedes had none. The only current Anglo-Swedish Treaty of Commerce, that of 1661, was quite clear on the point that enemy goods could not be carried, and it had no valid most-favoured-nation clause which Sweden could invoke.[2]

England met the Danish demand to be admitted to the same privileges as the Dutch with a plethora of artless evasions: good manners, one must assume, did not make England give the simple

[1] Swed. S. Arch., Anglica I, Kanslikollegium to Wynantz, 5 November 1756.
[2] Cf. R. Pares, *Colonial Blockade and Neutral Rights 1739–1763* (Oxford, 1938), p. 302, n. 3, that Sweden could have claimed most-favoured-nation treatment by her treaties of 1700 and 1720. These treaties were in fact limited and their commercial clauses no longer current.

answer that the Dutch themselves despite their treaty were not being given the right to carry enemy goods. Holdernesse, Newcastle, Fox, and Pitt – by the time it came to Bute the argument had run dry – told the Danes instead that their interpretation of their own treaty was incorrect; that their interpretation of their own treaty was correct but not their interpretation of the Dutch treaty; that their interpretation of both treaties would be correct if there were such a valid Dutch treaty, but there wasn't; that Denmark herself had not allowed neutrals to carry enemy goods when she was at war with Sweden; that they were right on every point, but could not claim any benefit from their treaty as they had failed to honour it themselves by not supplying England with troops; and if Denmark insisted that England was breaking faith, she could only reply *tu quoque*.[1]

The Swedes were handled far less playfully. Wynantz was bluntly told Sweden had no case whatever, which happened to be correct, and that no argument would do Sweden any good.[2] Wynantz in an interview with Holdernesse pointed out that Spain, although she had no treaty rights to that effect, had recently been given quite gratuitously the right to carry enemy goods, and that the Swedish government insisted on being given the same rights as any other neutral power. Holdernesse does not appear to have been briefed on that point and, according to Wynantz, let it slip out that England did not expect the Spanish carrying trade to be of any benefit to France as Spain could not supply her with naval stores nor had she much to offer her in general shipping services. Rantzau he told the next day that Spain was in special treaty relations with England who always honoured her obligations.[3]

[1] Dan. S. Arch., T.K.U.A., Engl. B, 106, Rantzau to Bernstorff, 28 December 1756; and *ibid.*, 107, same to same, 21 February and 5 July 1757; and *ibid.*, Bothmer to Bernstorff, 13 December 1757; and also for conversations with Newcastle and Holdernesse prior to declaration of war, see *ibid.*, 106, Rantzau to Bernstorff, 16 and 23 April 1756. These are a selection of the better examples from the most pertinent documents.

[2] Swed. S. Arch., Anglica 1, Wynantz to Kanslikollegium, 7 September and 28 December 1756, and 26 July 1757. Again, the examples can be multiplied.

[3] Swed. S. Arch., Anglica 1, Wynantz to Kanslikollegium, 28 December 1756; and Dan. S. Arch., T.K.U.A., Engl. B, 106, Rantzau to Bernstorff, 28 December 1756. The instructions to privateers and warships are in the *Gazette* of 6 and 10 July, and the additional instructions about Spanish ships in the *Gazette* of 5 October 1756.

The difference in approach to the Danish and Swedish claims for Free Ships, Free Goods was of course not due to Denmark having a good case and Sweden none, but to political considerations. Cabinet never quite lost hope despite every rebuff that Denmark might be persuaded to forsake her French alliance and come over to the English side, and year after year Titley was given yet another set of instructions to conlude a subsidy treaty for Danish troops.[1] It was a forlorn hope, but Cabinet clung to it. And even if there was no longed-for treaty with Denmark, it could only do good to hold out to Denmark the vaguest possible promise that sometime in the far, far future England might recognise Denmark's claim to Free Ships, Free Goods; and to withold any promise from Sweden. The two of them, Cabinet had been told by Titley and was to be told later also by Goodricke, were not happy in each other's company, and seemingly different treatment by England might make them even less happy to continue on the same side of the fence. Whenever the opportunity offered, Rantzau and his successor Bothmer were therefore given to understand that England failed to see why Denmark associated herself with Sweden over such an issue as neutral rights since the Danish and Swedish treaty positions were so very different. The implication, always there though never spoken out aloud, was that Denmark had something to hope for, and would be best advised not to prejudice her chances by making common cause with a country that had no claim to be considered.[2] It is hard to decide whether Rantzau saw through the English stratagem and therefore ignored it, or continued to champion Sweden in his conversations with Cabinet ministers because he was too obtuse to catch their meaning. On the whole, one inclines to the second alternative. Bernstorff, not happy from the first about Denmark being harnessed to Sweden, disapproved of Rantzau's Swedish proclivities. He must have seen that Rantzau could not prejudice the Danish case which was hopelessly lost, yet he clutched at the straw London pushed his way. Rantzau was instructed to cease speaking on behalf of Sweden, and was given a very broad

[1] See next chapter.
[2] A good example of this argument occurred in a conversation between Pitt and Bothmer, reported in a despatch to Bernstorff on 13 December 1757, in Dan. S. Arch., T.K.U.A., Engl. B, 107.

hint to keep aloof from Wynantz.[1] Only once was he ordered to act in concert with Wynantz in presenting in 1757 a joint memorial on Free Ships, Free Goods, and on the outrages of English privateers. Bernstorff cannot have promised himself anything from that move, but he made it to appease France which was pressing him to take a firm stand with England. France had already agreed in principle to concede to the neutrals the privilege of Free Ships, Free Goods if England would do the same, a course that could cost France nothing and from which she could only gain immeasurably. If Bernstorff should be able to cajole England into granting his demands, France would overlook Danish pusillanimity in having neither joined her in the War, nor taken a stand independently or with Sweden against British attacks on neutral commerce.[2] Since France was meant to be paying subsidies to Denmark in return for effective aid – France was rather forgetful about transmitting the money – Bernstorff could do no less than fall in with the French proposal to associate with Sweden in presenting a strong demand to England for redress of their grievances. England temporised, as an outright refusal of a joint Danish–Swedish demand would have spoilt her game of playing off Sweden against Denmark, and the repeated requests for a written answer were met with evasions.[3]

Neither Denmark nor Sweden could have expected that England would concede that Free Ships made Free Goods, but they might reasonably have hoped to meet with some consideration in their complaint about privateers bringing up every Danish–Norwegian and Swedish ship they could lay hold of, and about open piracies. Holdernesse and Pitt did indeed promise that proved piracies would be dealt with adequately, and some privateers-cum-pirates

[1] Dan. S. Arch., T.K.U.A., Engl. C, 264, Bernstorff to Rantzau, 12 February 1757.
[2] Dan. S. Arch., T.K.U.A., Engl. C, 264, Bernstorff to Rantzau, 26 July 1757; and also Swed. S. Arch., Anglica 1, Kanslipresidenten to Wynantz, 15 July 1757. It may be noted that France had in her treaty with Denmark conceded the right to Free Ships, Free Goods, but on the outbreak of war refused to implement that part of her treaty unless Denmark obtained an undertaking from England on that issue.
[3] Dan. S. Arch., T.K.U.A., Engl. B, 107, Rantzau to Bernstorff, 16 August 1757, and Bothmer to Bernstorff, 20 December 1757. Also, Swed. S. Arch., Anglica 1, Wynantz to Kanslipresidenten, 27 September 1757. See also P.R.O., 30/8 (Chatham Papers), bundle 40, Holdernesse to Pitt, 13 August 1757.

were caught and hanged.[1] The few known prosecutions, however, touched only the fringe of the problem. Privateers had to commit actual robberies to qualify for the gallows, and therefore soon found a less risky method of relieving the Scandinavian neutral of his money without overstepping the letter of the law. It will be remembered that the Anglo-Scandinavian treaties provided for ships' passports which were to be issued in time of war by the neutral partner to the treaties on a sworn declaration by the ship's master that no contraband or enemy goods were carried. The passport was to save the ship from molestation, but since the Scandinavian powers both disputed the nature of contraband and claimed the right to carry enemy goods, passports could obviously not be accepted by Britain as safe conducts. Every Scandinavian ship on the way to or from French or enemy-occupied ports was therefore liable to be brought up, and once in an English port might have to wait for a year or longer before its case reached the Prize Court. The expense in wages and harbour dues during the enforced wait was large, and the added loss in the earning capacity of the ship and the temporary withdrawal of the capital value of the cargo could easily lead to the owners' bankruptcies. This meant that the main complaint of Danish–Norwegian and Swedish merchants or their agents was not so much over the seizure of ships to which they soon became resigned as an inevitable consequence of war, but over the unnecessarily long delays before a Prize Court decided the case of a ship that might be brought before it. Time after time, Wynantz and Bothmer or Rantzau tried to persuade owners to allow the case of a seized ship to go before the Prize Court so that a definite ruling on some disputed article of contraband might be obtained, but they nearly always refused to submit their case for a decision by the Court and preferred to make private arrangements or settlements with the captor to save time. This is

[1] Swed. S. Arch., Anglica I, Kanslikollegium to Wynantz, 6 August 1756; and also Dan. S. Arch., T.K.U.A., Engl. C, 264, Bernstorff to Rantzau, 4 January 1757; and *ibid.*, Engl. B, 107, Bothmer to Bernstorff, 25 November and 16 December 1757; and *ibid.*, 108, same to same, 18 August 1758, advising that Admiralty had offered rewards for information on piracy incidents; and also *ibid.*, same to same, of 12 December 1758, that Pitt himself had advertised in the *Gazette* for information on an act of piracy in which a Danish ship was robbed in the Channel. Four privateers-cum-pirates were later caught and hanged: see *ibid.*, 109, same to same, 13 March 1759.

not at all surprising when one considers the costs to which owners were put when they actually waited for the Court to hear the case. The cases of two Danish ships, *Den Ringende Jakob* and *Eenrom*, were quite typical. Both were acquitted, but the owners lost over the first £875 11*s*. in costs of suit, demurrage, and expenses, and over the second £427.[1] To make the position worse, there was no possibility of reimbursements to Scandinavian owners for such losses even on acquittal, since seizure on suspicion alone was held justified so long as Denmark and Sweden claimed rights of carriage not recognised by England. On the contrary, Scandinavian owners were loaded with the full costs of an unsuccessful claimant, and privateers or warships were therefore under no restraint whatever from bringing up the most innocent Scandinavian merchantman suspected of sailing to or from an enemy port.[2]

Under such conditions, blackmail flourished. The captain of a Scandinavian ship might offer to pay a ransom to avoid being brought into port, and would be the more agreeable to do so when he had a cargo aboard that could be disputed in earnest. If ransom was either not offered or not accepted and the ship taken into port, there was still a chance to escape the long delays and the uncertainties of Prize Court actions by compounding with the captor for the value of the cargo or ship in dispute.[3] The opportunities for blackmail given by ransoming and compounding are obvious, and the Scandinavian complaints about the practices of British privateers – ships of the Royal Navy seem to have been both less high-handed and more honest – are only too understandable.

One remedy for such abuses, and the Scandinavians pressed for it time after time, would have been the speeding-up of Prize Court procedure, but for the present England gave every appearance of

---

[1] P.R.O., S.P. 75/107, Goodricke to Holdernesse, private, and enclosed papers, 13 February 1759.

[2] Bernstorff himself took up the case of owners having to pay the full costs of a suit in which they were acquitted, but got nowhere. See P.R.O., S.P. 75/101, Titley to Holdernesse, 8 January 1757, and *ibid*., 103, same to same, 23 December 1758. Also, see Ad. 1/3882, for legal opinion on the seizure of Danish–Norwegian and Swedish ships, dated 1 December 1757.

[3] There was a risk when compounding or paying ransom of being brought up by another privateer and having to go through the same procedure again, and a few Scandinavian ships suffered that way, but it was a rare occurrence. There was after all everything to be said against milking the cow dry.

being determined to remain unaccommodating. England must have believed that the neutrals were knuckling under, and that the danger had passed of their combining to any effect against the English trade war. The Danish–Swedish Neutrality Convention was a dead-letter by the second year of the War in Europe, and the combined Neutrality Fleet took the sea for only a few weeks; Holland was playing her own hand, and by all accounts was not likely to fall for French blandishments designed to make her join with other neutral powers who, Holland saw, could not agree among themselves; Russia was heavily engaged on land against Prussia though, like Sweden, at peace with England, and would not willingly engage at sea as well; and Spain, the only remaining neutral with a fleet that might cause anxiety had been bought off by concessions.[1] In fine, so soon as England had taken their measure, she ceased worrying seriously about any ill-effects her actions against the trade of the neutral powers might have. And, so far as complaints were concerned, England herself had a few of her own with which to take some of the wind out of the neutrals' sails.

English complaints to Denmark and Sweden were, one has the impression, meant to be more of a diversion than a means of accomplishing anything useful by gaining concessions from the Scandinavian powers. Whenever Bernstorff took Titley to task over English behaviour towards neutral trade, the answer came sooner or later that Denmark by her own action in admitting French privateers to Norwegian ports, and in allowing them to sell their prizes there, had invited reprisals and should therefore not be surprised that England could not accede to requests from a country which was behaving in an un-neutral fashion. What Titley on instructions from London proposed was, that Denmark should close the ports to all privateers and thus conform to the English definition of strict neutrality.[2] There was something to

[1] For the diplomacy of the time, see the next chapter.
[2] France had arranged so early as 1755 to base privateers on Norwegian and Swedish North Sea ports, and after some intrigues was given permission to sell prizes in Scandinavia without prior condemnation in French ports. See Moltke Archives, bundle 'Breve fra...Ogier', Ogier to Moltke, 26 June [1756], and undated draft reply; and undated memoir by Ogier for Moltke [late May–early June 1756]; also P.R.O., S.P. 75/99, Titley to Holdernesse, 23 August 1755; *ibid.*, 102, same to same, 2 April 1757; and *ibid.*, 109, copy of Danish order tightening up the regulations on

this argument as English privateers had no need to use foreign North Sea ports as bases or for the sale of prizes, while the French could only operate with any profit in the North Sea so long as they were given facilities in Norway or, for that matter, in Sweden who also had opened her North Sea ports to them.[1] Bernstorff's replies were as automatic as Titley's complaints, that the thing had been done before, and was therefore a traditional right of neutral powers. Sweden would no doubt have given the same reply if she had been tackled on the subject, which no one bothered to do. As to the sale of prizes without condemnation in Court, Bernstorff similarly cited precedents and Titley was eventually ordered to desist from bringing up that topic as English privateers were doing in the Mediterranean what the French were doing in the North Sea.[2] There it would have stopped if English warships and privateers had not allowed themselves to be tempted by the undefended state of the Norwegian coast to penetrate into Norwegian harbours and to violate Norwegian territorial waters in search of French privateers and of British ships they had captured. This in turn furnished Denmark with material for complaints which were sometimes acknowledged by the dismissal of naval officers responsible for too flamboyant exploits, and at other times rejected on the plea that the provocation had been too great.[3]

the reception of privateers and the sale of prizes in Norway, bound in under date 8 February 1760. The order for the reception of privateers etc. in Norway is in O. A. Johnsen, *Norges Historie* (Kristiania, 1914), 5, p. 15.

[1] The Swedish regulations are in P.R.O., Ad. 1/3833, laid in under year 1756. See also Swed. S. Arch., Anglica I, Kanslipresidenten to Wynantz, 17 March 1756, that England could have the same facilities as the French if she applied for them. This was never done, presumably because there was no need for facilities in Sweden, and a request would have weakened the English case.

[2] Calendar of Home Office Papers, 1760–5, p. 72, entry 333.

[3] One case that led to particularly acrimonious exchanges was that of Captain Webb in *H.M.S. Antelope. Antelope* in company with two privateers captured a French privateer in a Norwegian harbour, and a shore-party pursued escaping French sailors. See Dan. S. Arch., T.K.U.A., Engl. C, 266, Bernstorff to Bothmer, 26 January, 5 and 26 August, and 19 December 1760; 7 September 1761; and 20 April 1762; also P.R.O., S.P. 75/106, Titley to Holdernesse, 15 September 1759; and *ibid.*, 109, same to same, 19 January 1760, and also in same volume bound in under date 20 August 1760, memorial by Bothmer, and also Holdernesse to Titley, 22 August 1760, and Titley to Holdernesse, 6 September 1760. There are more cases than the few here noted. See for further examples Ad. 1/4124–5, *passim*, and S.P. 110/85 *passim*, and Kent, 'The Three-Mile Limit', *passim*.

No disciplinary action was taken on any of these occasions against privateers who, one suspects, were a law unto themselves as they had the backing of important financial interests which the government did not want to displease. Pitt managed, it is true, to get a Privateering Act through the House in 1759 that gave him some control over the smaller privateers which had infested the Channel. Titley was instructed to make the most of the new regulations about privateering, and to impress on Denmark England's willingness to stamp out any abuses.[1] If that was really so, it is strange that the Act only curbed the smaller and generally owner-operated privateers. These were not likely to have commanded the sympathy of the privateering syndicates which financed the larger vessels. The small free-lancing privateers were moreover reported by customs officers to be operated by mere smugglers and robbers, and had aroused the anger of insurance underwriters. The Danish envoy kept Copenhagen constantly informed on what was to Denmark literally a vital issue. London merchants, as well as insurance brokers, Bothmer reported to Bernstorff, had held meetings at which they resolved to put pressure on the government to curb privateering excesses. In turn, the privateering syndicates had protested against any attempt to interfere with their enterprises in which they had invested over £2 million. In the past year, 1758, so the report continued, the privateering syndicates had only captured £100,000 worth of French shipping. If they could not have their way with the neutrals from whom over £2 million worth of goods alone were taken in the past year, the syndicates threatened to withdraw from the privateering business, and Britain's war effort, let alone her earnings, would suffer greatly.[2] It is clear when one considers the contents of the Act to restrain privateering in conjunction with these reports that Pitt was not prepared to try conclusions with the powerful privateering syndicates. His actions

---

[1] The Privateering Act was 32 Geo. II c. 25. It had some effect in stamping out piracy, and the English consul at Elsinore reported that he had heard of hardly any cases of robberies since the Act was passed. See P.R.O., S.P. 75/106, Fenwick to Titley, Elsinore, 1 September 1759, and S.P. 75/105, Titley to Holdernesse, 26 March and 7 April 1759.

[2] Dan. S. Arch., T.K.U.A., Engl. B, 108 and 109, Bothmer to Bernstorff, 8 December 1758 and 6 April 1759.

against the small independent privateers simply served to pacify opinion at home, and could be represented abroad as proof of his concern over legitimate grievances of the neutrals although it was in fact nothing of the sort.

It is obvious from the course of this and of other disputes that neither treaties nor custom were allowed to stand in the way of England's determination to drive French trade off the seas in whatever guise it might show itself. England could be persuaded to make a concession to one or the other neutral in return for something of greater value, but she steadily kept in sight her goal of destroying French trade and would, as later in the case of Spain, or of Denmark and Sweden in the early days of the War, withdraw whatever concession she had thought it politic to make so soon as she possibly could. On occasion and when the mood took it, Cabinet might consider the neutrals even after the necessity to humour them had passed, as, for example, by paying until the end of the War for all the timber which was brought up although Denmark–Norway, Holland, and Russia would have had to bow to any British dictate on contraband in the last years of the War. By an occasional timely concession but generally by a show of force and by sheer good luck, Cabinet was able to the last to avoid an open conflict with the Scandinavian powers.

One issue which might have led to an open conflict between England and Denmark arose over what later became known as the Rule of the War of 1756, and its subsequent corollary the Doctrine of Continuous Voyage. Neither Rule nor Doctrine need be discussed as they have attracted a number of expositors and commentators,[1] and only a reminder of what it was all about is needed. France, like other colonial powers, reserved to herself the right of trade between mother-country and colonies. She knew

---

[1] See in particular O. H. Mootham, 'The Doctrine of Continuous Voyage, 1756–1815', *British Year Book of International Law, 1927*, pp. 62ff., and Pares, *Colonial Blockade, passim*. Pares has to be used with caution as he had not seen the Danish archives and relied on intercepted despatches in the Record Office. The most important instructions and despatches were sent in cypher, and these are not at the Record Office. The Danes knew that England was intercepting their correspondence and therefore on occasion sent deliberately misleading information etc. *en clair*, following it with cyphered corrections. Pares unfortunately fell into the self-same trap which Bernstorff and Bothmer had prepared for the English Cabinet.

War and Trade in Northern Seas

that England would attack her colonial trade and might interrupt it, and therefore opened it on the outbreak of war to friendly powers which could supply her colonies and take off their produce. Trading with the enemy – contraband always excepted – had in the past not stirred England into any other action than temporary and usually rather ineffective blockades,[1] and the neutrals had every expectation of getting away with it again in this war. The Rule of the War of 1756 was the English answer to French and neutral hopes of trade with the French colonies: trade closed to any nation in time of peace could not be opened to it in time of war, and the neutrals would enter the French colonial trade, and, incidentally, the French coasting trade of which they were also to be free, at their peril.[2] This decision left a loophole to neutrals like Denmark and Holland whose West Indian colonies could serve as *entrepôts* for French West Indian produce, which might then be shipped with impunity as neutral property. This loophole was after 1758

[1] The British blockade of French ports in 1756, and occasional limited blockades later in the war, did not lead to disputes with the Scandinavian powers although some of their ships were taken or turned back. Blockades, so long as they were of definite ports and effectively mounted, were not regarded as being anything out of the way. See for Scandinavian acceptance of British blockades Swed. S. Arch., Anglica 1, Wynantz to Kanslikollegium, 20 August 1756, and *ibid.*, Wynantz to Kanslipresidenten, 13 August 1756; and also Dan. S. Arch., T.K.U.A., Engl. B, 109, Bothmer to Bernstorff, 13 July 1759. Conversely, when Sweden declared a blockade of the Prussian port of Stettin and took a British ship, England did not protest about it. The sequel to the Swedish blockade is interesting in showing the mistrust between Denmark, Sweden, and Russia: A Danish ship was also taken, and both the British and the Danish ships were released by the Swedes on the remonstrance of Russia and Denmark who held that the Baltic should remain entirely neutral. See P.R.O., S.P. 75/103, Titley to Holdernesse, 22 August and 26 September 1758; and also Swed. S. Arch., Anglica 1, Kanslikollegium to Wynantz, 16 February 1758.

[2] Pares is mistaken in assuming that the French coasting trade was not prohibited to neutrals by the Rule and his strictures on that point of Kulsrud are misplaced: see Pares, *Colonial Blockade*, pp. 224–5, appendix to ch. 3 and C. J. Kulsrud, *Maritime Neutrality to 1780* (Boston, 1936), ch. 2. See for proof that England regarded the French coasting trade as closed to the neutrals Swed. S. Arch., Anglica 1, Wynantz to Kanslikollegium, 17 July 1756: Wynantz writes that Dutch ships in the French coasting trade had been brought up, and released after being warned that they would in future not be permitted to take any part in a trade closed to them by France in time of peace. See also Dan. S. Arch., Engl. A. 111, 42, consul Falck to Bernstorff and appended papers, Falmouth, 9 December 1756, reporting the seizure and condemnation of a Danish ship for having taken part in the French coasting trade; and also P.R.O., S.P. 75/101, notarial depositions of 26 June and 22 July 1756 about Danish ships brought up in the coasting trade.

at least partially closed by what came to be known as the Doctrine of Continuous Voyage, that is, that goods which had commenced their voyage in an enemy ship could not be claimed as neutral property even though bought and subsequently shipped by neutrals.

Denmark–Norway with her large merchant fleet and her experience in colonial trade had been earmarked by France as a neutral power which could be relied on to keep communications with the French West Indian Islands open and, most important for France, convert their produce into money. France was too optimistic when she expected so much from Denmark, as very few Danish–Norwegian ships showed any desire to venture so far afield while there were easy pickings to be had from the carrying trade nearer home and in the Mediterranean. Denmark therefore had no occasion to make a special issue of the English prohibition of direct trade with the French colonies, and the occasional seizure of some small Danish-owned vessel caught trading between the French and Danish West Indian Islands was allowed to pass without any special complaint from Bernstorff and the Danish envoy in London.[1]

The crisis over colonial trade which did arise in 1758 after two years of silence over that issue came therefore as a complete surprise to Denmark, and the unexpected shock it gave to the Danish ministry and to Danish merchants might in part explain the virulence which was such a feature of the whole controversy. This is what happened: Denmark had for many years imported some French West Indian coffee, spices and dyes for her own consumption, and occasionally some sugar for re-export.[2] Denmark would have had to go without these imports after the English prohibitions of 1756 ruined the direct trade from the French West Indies to Europe unless she joined in the game which the Dutch were playing on a large scale and with immense success, and

---

[1] Pares, *Colonial Blockade*, p. 200, notes the condemnation of two such Danish ships, the *St Croix* Packet and the *Gode Christian*. See also Dan. S. Arch., T.K.U.A., Engl. A. III, Felckenhauer (Governor of St Thomas) to Bernstorff, 19 August 1760, that seven ships from St Thomas had been taken by British warships and privateers for trading between the Danish and French islands. They were condemned in colonial Vice-Admiralty Courts.

[2] Danish imports of French colonial produce have been noted above, ch. 6. Their supersession by imports of British colonial goods shows how effective the prohibitions on the French colonial trade were.

that was, to tranship French colonial goods in the Dutch West Indies for shipment to Europe in Dutch ships on Dutch account. The Dutch were up to some other commercial tricks as well, but these are of no interest in this connection as the Danes do not seem to have followed their mentors that far. The Dutch, in fact, engrossed the trade in French West Indian produce after 1756, and the Danes merely shipped small quantities of French colonial goods via the Danish West Indies to Copenhagen in their regular fleet of West Indiamen. The Danish circumvention of the Rule of the War of 1756 was harmless enough, the Dutch was not. It was the misfortune of the Danes to become caught up with the Dutch when English privateers in 1758 seized ship after ship returning to Europe from the neutral West Indian colonies. In the end, thirteen or fourteen Danish West Indiamen out of a total eighteen or twenty in the entire trade, were tied up in English ports.[1]

Bernstorff, when hearing of one seizure after the other, was shaken out of his customary calm and stormed at poor Titley, who in turn sent off special couriers to Holdernesse entreating him to do something, or at least to give some instructions on how to explain this latest interference with neutral trade. Bernstorff had very good cause to be alarmed. A sizeable part of Denmark's trading capital was tied up in the West India trade and in the sugar refineries which depended on it; the Copenhagen merchants had never before been so furious and were beginning to agitate for war against England, on the principle, presumably, that a terrible end is preferable to terror without end; talk at the Court itself was becoming threatening and Titley could not see where it might end. From Grand Marshal Moltke downwards, every courtier was personally interested in the West India trade, in which he had invested his money.[2]

Holdernesse gave every appearance of having been caught by surprise. The action of the privateers in bringing up ships trading between neutral ports was in effect without precedent. The Doctrine

---

[1] See list of Danish West Indiamen seized, in P.R.O., S.P. 75/105, memoir by Bothmer dated 7 February 1759, and a further complementary list in Dan. S. Arch., T.K.U.A., Engl. A. II, 30, under date 19 June 1759.

[2] P.R.O., S.P. 75/103, Titley to Holdernesse, 23, 26 and 30 December 1758.

of Continuous Voyage was as yet unknown in law, and the privateering interests seemed to be letting themselves in for heavy damages unless it could be proved in the Prize Court that the Danish or, for that matter, Dutch ships were carrying goods belonging to the enemy.[1] It was unlike the privateering syndicates to take such a risk, and one can safely assume that they had been promised beforehand some startling new departure in law which would cover them, and which of course turned out to be the Doctrine of Continuous Voyage. Holdernesse's reaction to the first news of the capture of the Danish West Indiamen shows – unless one credits Holdernesse with a Machiavellian subtlety of which there were no other signs either earlier or later – that he was alarmed, and disapproved of these new privateering ventures. He actually ransomed three Dutch ships, and offered to ransom the only Danish ship which had then been brought up.[2] This mood did not last for long. Holdernesse had either been out of step with the privateering interests in Cabinet, or opinion in Cabinet hardened against circumventions of the prohibition on trade with the French colonies. It was equally possible and even probable that Cabinet simply did not bother about the Danish ships. No more was heard of the offer to ransom that or other Danish West Indiamen, and the crisis was allowed to run its course.

Bitterness against England mounted in Copenhagen as news reached the city that more and more of the ships from the West Indies were being brought into English ports. Some ships had been taken far out in the Atlantic, and advice of the captures became known at intervals throughout the autumn and winter of 1758 till late in January of 1759. In the heat of the argument that developed, Denmark aired all her grievances of the earlier years of the War: contraband definitions, right of visit, privateering outrages, rights of carriage, and especially Prize Court procedure. The crisis which had begun over the West Indiamen widened into a conflict over neutral rights in general. Bernstorff's instructions to Bothmer became grave in tone, and Bothmer called in turn on

[1] The rule that Scandinavian ships trading to or from French ports had to pay all the costs in a suit if brought before the Prize Court would of course not have held in these unprecedented cases.

[2] Dan. S. Arch., T.K.U.A., Engl. B, 108, Bothmer to Bernstorff, 19 September 1758.

Holdernesse and Newcastle and Pitt – he had not called on any other minister but the Northern Secretary since Holdernesse some time ago protested about it – and he even went to see Münchhausen, the Hanoverian Minister in London who was believed to have special influence with the king. He received the same answer from everyone he called on, that England was acting within her rights in all matters complained of by Denmark. To rouse the temper of the Danes still further, if that was possible, England was trying to buy off the Dutch, who had carried on a campaign of their own for the release of their West India ships. The Dutch were given some concessions in their carrying trade for the enemy, but Denmark, Pitt told Bothmer, could expect nothing at all.[1]

While Bothmer went the rounds in London, Titley tried to compose matters in Copenhagen. He got nowhere. Bernstorff hinted, and Moltke more than hinted, at war. The Danish fleet, Titley reported to London, was being commissioned in the middle of winter, a thing unheard of, and the army had been put on a war footing.[2] London did not retreat one step, on the contrary, a memorial handed in by Bothmer on the Danish grievances and the Danish case for her West Indiamen[3] was answered uncompromisingly by a counter-memorial which 'had received the Sanction of those of His Majesty's Servants who are usually consulted upon the Conduct of the King's most secret Affairs...and received His Royal Approbation'.[4] The quite unusual reference to the royal approbation was the unkindest cut: Bothmer had given Münchhausen in strictest confidence a letter for the king from Frederick V who had 'faith in dealing King to King' and asked George II to intervene with his ministers before it was too late and war was decided on.[5] This now seemed to be Cabinet's answer for going behind its back directly to the king.

[1] Dan. S. Arch., T.K.U.A., Engl. B, 108, Bothmer to Bernstorff, 3 and 20 October, 5 and 12 December 1758, and *ibid.*, 109, 9 and 12 January 1759; and also Engl. C, 266, Bernstorff to Bothmer, 2 and 23 December 1758, and 16 January 1759.

[2] P.R.O., S.P. 75/103, Titley to Holdernesse, 23, 26, and 30 December 1758, and *ibid.*, 105, 6 January 1759.

[3] P.R.O., Chatham Papers, 38/8, b. 88, memoir, dated 29 January 1759.

[4] P.R.O., S.P. 75/105, memoir for transmission by Titley, 6 February 1759.

[5] Dan. S. Arch., T.K.U.A., Engl. C, 266, Bernstorff to Bothmer, 23 December 1758.

England had made it plain that she would on no account discuss issues of neutral rights or administration of justice which had been raised by Denmark in the course of the controversy. Denmark's only hope of gaining anything at this stage without going to war was to bring the discussion back to her initially straightforward demand for the release of the West Indiamen. This she did, and Bernstorff sent a proposal to London suggesting, with the usual reservations about neutral rights in the future, an immediate settlement of the issue which had sparked off the crisis. He asked that the West Indiamen should be released on full security being given for any part of their cargo in dispute, an unexceptional proposal which was legally feasible and to which Cabinet agreed in principle while insisting that certain technical conditions should be observed. Bernstorff later also asked that any agreement reached should be published as an official declaration of British policy and that cases should be tried by the Prize Court within a few weeks, but Cabinet quietly ignored that request. Bernstorff was satisfied with the British acceptance of the essential part of his proposal, and merely instructed Bothmer to remind Holdernesse when convenient that a public declaration by England would be desirable.[1]

The crisis seemed to be over, and the way clear for the release of the West Indiamen on the terms agreed between Denmark and England. It soon turned out, though, that Bernstorff had not consulted the Copenhagen merchants about the detailed terms of the settlement which would prove, so they said, quite unworkable, and all the bother had been for nothing. They would much rather be left to arrange matters themselves, and would certainly not consent to being forced into having their cases decided by the Prize Court.[2] Bernstorff had to take this in silence, as he was not to know that the Copenhagen merchants were intractable because the situation over the West Indiamen had radically changed within a week or two of his proposals for their release being accepted by England. As it happened, the Prize Court had decided on the

---

[1] Dan. S. Arch., T.K.U.A., Engl. C, 266, Bernstorff to Bothmer, 23 January and 24 March 1759; and Engl. B, 109, Bothmer to Bernstorff, 9 February 1759.
[2] Dan. S. Arch., T.K.U.A., Engl. B, 109, Bothmer to Bernstorff, 4 May 1759; and Engl. C, 266, Bernstorff to Bothmer, 19 May 1759, two differing sets of instructions, one *en clair* and the other in cypher.

first of the West Indiamen, which got off very lightly, and the privateers were disappointed of the large profit they had hoped to make out of the Danish ships. They were therefore willing to come to a reasonable agreement with the Danish owners who knew that the bargaining over the exact sums to be paid might take a little while, but certainly no longer than it would take to conform to all the regulations written into the proposed and agreed-upon Anglo-Danish settlement. Also, it would be less costly to settle directly with the privateers, and the upshot of it all was that the machinery set up by the official agreement was completely by-passed.[1]

This should have been the end of it if Bernstorff had not come to be in desperate need of making political capital out of an English concession to Denmark. France was again pressing Denmark to take a firm stand over the continual English encroachments on neutral rights, and France was Denmark's paymaster. The hold which France had over Denmark through the Danish–French subsidy treaty has already been mentioned, and Bernstorff could not ignore the promptings of the French envoy in Copenhagen although France was behind in her subsidy payments: the position of a debtor can be a very strong one, and Denmark at that time had to convince France that she was a dependable ally meriting both financial and, particularly, diplomatic assistance. The dispute with England over the release of the West Indiamen cannot have failed to have impressed France with Denmark's determination to draw the line with England somewhere, and then, to Bernstorff's disappointment, the Copenhagen merchants ignored the Anglo-Danish agreement which he might have represented as an English concession. England to all appearances had not given an inch, since the Danish West Indiamen were being set free through direct agreements with the privateers without Prize Court intervention, and Bernstorff had outwardly nothing to show for all his efforts this last winter, which France would now regard as having been designed to pull the wool over her eyes. This might not have worried Bernstorff overmuch if Denmark's relations with Sweden and Russia had not become more than usually strained in the late

[1] Dan. S. Arch., T.K.U.A., Engl. B, 109, Bothmer to Bernstorff, 18 and 25 May, 5 and 16 June 1759.

spring and early summer of 1759, that is, straight after the Anglo-Danish crisis.[1] To convince France of Danish good faith, Bothmer was instructed to press in London for a favourable declaration on the West India trade and Prize Court procedure. Holdernesse, to whom Bothmer applied, was evasive, and Bothmer therefore once again went the round of Cabinet ministers to canvass the Danish case.[2] It is hard to see why Holdernesse should have been so un-cooperative as there was no harm in making some formal statement about the earlier agreement on the release of the West Indiamen, and as to Prize Court procedure, that problem had solved itself in the meantime. The delay in having a case heard by the Prize Court had been the most constant source of complaint by all the neutrals and by the English insurers until early in 1759 when there was a change for the better. Holdernesse must have been made to see in the end that England had nothing to lose by assuring Denmark of her good intentions, and Bernstorff at long last got his declaration which he used to best effect in his negotiations with Sweden and Russia.[3] As a *quid pro quo*, Bernstorff quietly informed the British government that Danish West Indiamen would in future refuse to trade with the French West Indies.[4]

[1] Dan. S. Arch., T.K.U.A., Engl. C, 266, Bernstorff to Bothmer, 24 March 1759; see also next chapter.

[2] Dan. S. Arch., T.K.U.A., Engl. B, 109, Bothmer to Bernstorff, 10 and 20 April, and 18 May 1759.

[3] Dan. S. Arch., T.K.U.A., Engl. B, 109, Bothmer to Bernstorff, and appended memoir, 8 June 1759. Cf. this account of the 1758-9 crisis, and of its eventual settlement, with Pares, *Colonial Blockade*, pp. 284-5. Pares failed to note that the deadlock was solved by private settlements between the owners of the Danish West Indiamen or their English agents on the one hand, and the privateers on the other. There is nothing to show in the evidence cited by Pares that the crisis flared up again because of difficulties over finding money for Court security: the crisis was in fact over so soon as the first Prize Court decision on a Danish West Indiaman had been given, and what came after that was merely a stage show put on by Bernstorff for the benefit of France. Of thirteen ships named in a later list in Dan. S. Arch., T.K.U.A., Engl. A. 11, 30, dated 19 June 1759, eight had obtained release by private arrangements, only one had been before the Prize Court, and of the remaining four nothing certain was known as they were still making their own arrangements. Bothmer incidentally also mentioned that the Dutch West Indiamen followed the Danish example and solved their problems by private agreements with their captors. If that was so, doubt may be thrown on the account given by Pares of the later stages of the Anglo-Dutch crisis over the Dutch West Indiamen.

[4] P.R.O., S.P. 75/105, Titley to Holdernesse, 17 April 1759; and also Dan. S. Arch., T.K.U.A., Engl. B, 109, Bothmer to Bernstorff, 27 March 1759, and *ibid.*, Engl. C, 266, Bernstorff to Bothmer, 21 April 1759.

The long-drawn-out dispute over neutral rights which had flared up into a crisis in Anglo-Danish relations on the seizure of the West Indiamen had finally come to an end in the summer of 1759. English successes in 'the Year of Victory' made it pointless for any single neutral nation to go on demanding what England had not been willing to grant when her power at sea was still seriously disputed by France, and though complaints about this or that continued naturally till the end of the War, they were made more for form's sake than with any expectation of redress. Sweden, for example, had a grievance about English ships taking letters of marque from Prussia and bringing up Swedish merchantmen in the North Sea and Atlantic, and she protested from time to time about English privateers committing robberies. Goodricke in Copenhagen, to whom complaints were passed on by the Swedish envoy to Denmark as Sweden no longer had a representative in London, simply made polite remarks in reply and there the matter ended.[1] Denmark had more to complain about as her carrying trade was larger, and more of her ships were therefore exposed to the attentions of the privateers. The exchanges between Bothmer and the successive Northern Secretaries remained, however, very friendly after the crisis of 1758–9 had blown over, and only once more touched on the fundamental principles of neutral trade in war: Denmark then actually considered giving up her claim that Free Ships made Free Goods, and might have done so if the end of the War had not made further discussions unnecessary.

It will be remembered that Danish–Norwegian ships were very active in the Mediterranean carrying trade, and English merchants came to believe with very good reason that not only England, but France also benefited from their services, and that the ships were concealing French cargoes under coloured papers.[2] An English

---

[1] Swed. S. Arch., Anglica II, Strödda Handlingar, bundle 'Kaperier', documents in cases of ships *St Peter*, *St Johan*, *Tre Söstra*, *et al.*; also P.R.O., S.P. 75/107, Goodricke to Holdernesse, 25 September 1759, and S.P. 75/108, same to same, 1 April 1760; also, B.M., Add. MS 6817 (Mitchell Papers), Goodricke to Holdernesse, 25 September 1759; and also, Uppsala U.L., 'Neutralitet till Sjøs' MSS, Ekeblad to Ungern, 17 September 1759.

[2] B.M., Add. MS 14035 (Board of Trade papers), ff. 124 and 130, letters of 4 and 13 November 1761 inviting witnesses to an enquiry into Danish trade in the Mediterranean; also, P.R.O., S.P. 100/1, R. Wood (Mediterranean merchant) to Bothmer,

warship eventually stopped in 1761 a small fleet escorted by a Danish warship, the *Groenland*, which happened to find herself in the Mediterranean and was completing her commission by convoy duty against pirates. After some interchanges, the *Groenland* allowed the merchantmen to be taken into Gibraltar where at least one was found to be carrying French-owned cargo. The outcry in Copenhagen against the unfortunate captain of the *Groenland* and against England made Titley fear another crisis, but it came to nothing: on the contrary, Bernstorff was alarmed that the lucrative Mediterranean trade might now be seriously hampered by ships being brought up as indiscriminately as in the Atlantic, and therefore made ready to appease England. A Danish–German jurist, Martin Hübner of Copenhagen University, had recently been sent by him to London to advise on Danish cases that might come before the Prize Court. Bernstorff instructed Bothmer to put Hübner to work on drawing up the draft for a secret convention with England by which Denmark would renounce the principle of Free Ships, Free Goods in exchange for lenient treatment of Danish merchantmen. Particularly, they were to be brought quickly before the Prize Court if they should be taken into English ports for examination. Bernstorff would give the strictest instructions that Danish ships must not carry French goods under coloured papers, and would disown any ship that did. He agreed that England could treat such ships as if they were the enemy's.

Hübner was unfortunately not the kind of man Bernstorff should have asked to draw up such an *ad hoc* convention. After 'long and serious thought', Hübner produced two months later a document of fifteen articles, reserving every conceivable right to the neutral power. Bernstorff's proposals had been either completely misunderstood or, more probably, deliberately disregarded. The War was, however, practically at an end by the time Hübner had worked out what was to be in effect the legal basis of the Armed Neutrality Convention of 1780, and no more was said of a secret convention

copy, dated Whitehall 24 November 1761; S.P. 75/105, Titley to Holdernesse, 17 April 1759; and Swed. S. Arch., Anglica I, Kanslikollegium to Wynantz, 29 April 1757 and appended papers. This last shows that a few Swedish ships were also in the trade.

that would have put the seal on Danish subservience to English control over neutral trade.[1]

England, then, had been successful throughout the War in preventing Denmark and Sweden from giving France the assistance she expected from the Scandinavian merchant fleets. England had imposed her will on the two Scandinavian powers at the cost of much friction which she could afford to disregard, and of a crisis in Anglo-Danish relations that had held the risk of war with Denmark. That Cabinet ever allowed the initially simple dispute over the release of the Danish West Indiamen to develop into a crisis was due, and there is no other likely explanation, to arrogance and lack of attention. Cabinet could not know that Bernstorff would at the time go to great lengths to avoid a breach with England that might weaken his position in the Baltic where Denmark was about to be threatened with another crisis; nor, in the unlikely event of Cabinet suspecting his coming difficulties,[2] could it have known that they would not be solved. Denmark on her own may not have been considered important and strong enough to deserve consideration, but Cabinet ought to have considered the risk of a new combination of the neutrals which Denmark might be driven into joining. Bernstorff was indeed preparing to approach Holland and had made arrangements for an offer to the States-General if his proposals to England were not accepted. It was plain good luck that Cabinet

[1] P.R.O., S.P. 75/112, Titley to Holdernesse, 3 January 1761, and same to Bute, 24 November 1761, and *ibid.*, S.P. 75/114, same to same, 9 and 26 January, 2 February, and 25 May 1762; *ibid.*, S.P. 75/112, Bute to Titley, 15 December 1761, and S.P. 75/114, same to same, 23 February 1762. In this volume is also a memoir by Bothmer on the affair, bound in under date 8 April 1762. See also Dan. S. Arch., Admiralitets og General-kommissariets Collegium, Kgl. Resolutioner, order of 18 December 1760, and Relationer and Resolutioner of 12 and 25 December 1760, and of 11 and 13 November 1761; also, *ibid.*, Protocol over de fra Sø-etatens Kriegs-Cancelli Exp. Kgl. Resolutioner, 1759–60, instructions of 18 December 1760 for Captain Fisker of the *Groenland*; and vol. 1760–1, accounts of 11 November 1761; also, Søetatens Generalkriegsretsager 1762, Protocol og Documenter i Sagen...H. L. Fisker; also, *ibid.*, T.K.U.A., Alm. Afdeling, 430, 'Mémoire Préliminaire', signed by Hübner, and dated Copenhagen 6 December 1760, and Hübner to Bernstorff, London, 29 July 1762; and finally, *ibid.*, Engl. C, 274, Bernstorff to Bothmer, 20 February 1762, and Hübner to Bernstorff, London, 27 April 1762. Note that Pares, *Colonial Blockade*, p. 280, mentions that Titley was mistaken in believing that Denmark was prepared to give up her claims for Free Ships, Free Goods.
[2] Despatches from Copenhagen and St Petersburg of the time make no mention of likely Danish differences with Russia which were about to become acute.

finally got around to dealing with the problem of the Danish West Indiamen before Bernstorff's patience and diplomatic resource were exhausted. The most disturbing aspect of this crisis was Cabinet's disregard of the important Norwegian timber supplies. If it had come to a breach, the navy and merchant fleet would have been deprived of them, and trade to the Baltic would as well have become disrupted. Cabinet gauged the strength of the neutrals fairly well during the War, but in this instance England escaped from a potentially dangerous situation more by luck than by good management.

9 *Trade and Diplomacy*

England had attained an important objective when she succeeded in preventing Denmark and Sweden within a short time after the outbreak of the Seven Years War from assisting France to their full capacity with shipping and with naval stores. England had however had another objective since the early months of 1755, and that she failed to gain. She had tried to detach Denmark from her French allegiance, and to obtain Danish troops for duty in Ireland, for the defence of Hanover, or, later, as auxiliaries for the hard-pressed Prussians. Nothing that England could offer would make Denmark give up her neutrality, but no rebuff was taken as final until there was no longer any possible need for Danish military aid when, by an ironic reversal of roles, Denmark came to find herself in a position of asking for English assistance and it was England's turn to say no.

Sweden, though she was known to be firmly attached to France and was moreover hardly on speaking terms with England, was not left entirely out of account. England had to know what mischief Sweden might be planning against her or Prussia, and there was always the faint possibility that a change in government might occur and could be turned to England's advantage, but no treaty offer was ever contemplated.

In contrast to her realistic appraisal of the position in Sweden, England was indulging in wishful thinking over Denmark. Cabinet took little account of the realities of Baltic politics when it instructed Titley year after year to approach Bernstorff yet once again with a new treaty offer in the hope that the increasingly generous subsidies offered would at last make Denmark come over to the Anglo-Prussian side. Titley in turn wrote year after year to London that his every move was being frustrated by French intrigues at the Court and by the evil influence of the Grand Marshal Moltke, but Titley had been in Copenhagen for too long and was too shrewd a man not to realise that the French did not have to intrigue or that Moltke – even if he had any influence on foreign policy – could not affect the issue. Danish interests did not coincide with England's so long as Bernstorff had to consider both the dynastic claims of an absolute king, and Denmark's economic interests.

Denmark's economic interests were rather narrowly defined: she thought mainly of herself and rarely of that far-off wilderness Norway, which was looked on as a source of tax money and of soldiers for the dominant kingdom, and as a market for its goods.[1] The little that Denmark herself had to sell was not required by England, but France could be made to buy Danish salt meat while France supplied in return the salt and the colonial wares and the luxury goods which Denmark needed.

Danish manufactures would also, it was hoped, become so plentiful and well-made that they would require a market larger than Norway, and there again France as the less jealous of foreign trade than Britain was the more desirable ally. Finally, Denmark could offer shipping services if she remained neutral in a European war, and England needed them less urgently than France. Every commercial interest that Denmark had could be served by France, and Denmark had realised this so early as 1742 when concluding a treaty with France and refusing an offer made by England later in the same decade.[2]

Denmark's dynastic ambitions, Bernstorff knew from recent experience, might also be furthered by friendship with France which had shown her sympathy only such a short while ago as 1750 when she had assisted Denmark in negotiations with King Adolphus Frederick of Sweden over his Gottorpian claims, which were satisfactorily settled, and again in 1754 when France had induced Frederick II of Prussia to give up a small piece of land over which he and Denmark had squabbled for five years.[3] France

---

[1] A good description of Danish–Norwegian relations of the time may be found in Olsen, *Danmark–Norge, passim.*

[2] The instructions sent to Titley throughout the period in review are printed in Chance, *Diplomatic Instructions, Denmark*, pp. 145ff.

[3] Titley reported very fully on the Danish–Prussian dispute over the few acres of the baillage of Knyphausen. See P.R.O., S.P. 75/94, Titley to Newcastle, 29 December 1750, 27 April, 11 May, and 21 September 1751; and Newcastle to Titley, 27 August 1751; also S.P. 75/97, Titley to Holdernesse, 28 September and 22 October 1754;

had therefore succeeded twice in her championship of Danish dynastic claims, and she might do so a third time in a much more important matter, that of the claims of Peter of Holstein-Kiel, heir to the throne of Russia. The old quarrel between the kings of Denmark and the dukes of Gottorp over the Duchies was expected to reach a climax with the accession to the Russian throne of the Grand Duke Peter, head of the Gottorp House, and Bernstorff suspected quite correctly that England had been unwilling to help Denmark avert the coming crisis in her recent negotiations at St Petersburg. Titley himself was quite aware that George II as Elector of Hanover did not wish Denmark to reach a settlement of the dispute: as long as Denmark needed the English–Hanoverian guarantee of the Gottorp lands given in 1720, so long would Denmark in turn have to honour her own guarantee of Hanoverian interests in Bremen-Verden.[1] France, the other guarantor of the Gottorp lands had no particular interests that might clash with Denmark's, on the contrary, she would want to see her ally released from the distractions of the Gottorp dispute. The Reversal of Alliances and the subsequent resumption of direct diplomatic relations between Russia and France confirmed Denmark in her attitude, but had not led to her adopting it. It merely made the French connection more valuable as France could now canvass for Denmark at St Petersburg itself when the occasion should arise, and in the meantime France assured Denmark very tangibly of her good intentions by offering subsidies for a Danish army to be stationed in the disputed duchy of Holstein.

This latest French offer followed closely the fall of Bestuchev in 1758: Denmark and France both feared that Peter's partisans were in the ascendant and might divert troops from the war against Prussia to occupy the Duchies.[2] And, finally, there was Sweden

and S.P. 75/98, same to same, 8 April 1755. Titley regarded the way in which this dispute was settled as an example of France making herself useful to Denmark on every likely occasion, and reported that the settlement had made a great impression in Copenhagen as Prussia was known to be hostile to Denmark, and a settlement of the dispute had not been expected.

[1] P.R.O., S.P. 75/112, Titley to Bute, 2 May 1762.

[2] The convention for a special subsidy from France to Denmark was concluded on 4 May 1758, and Denmark shortly after moved troops to the frontiers. The text of the convention is printed in: *Danske Tractater 1751–1800* (Copenhagen, 1882), pp. 155 ff.

to be thought of, and France had great influence there. It was not so long ago that Denmark and Sweden had nearly gone to war with each other, and Danish distrust of her closest neighbour in the Baltic was still strong. Sweden's fortification of Landscrona in the early 1750s had not helped to make Denmark feel any more secure,[1] and every guarantee she could obtain against her old rival in the Baltic was more than welcome. Everything then, spoke against Denmark giving up her alliance with France in favour of one with England.

The position of Sweden was not quite so clear as that of Denmark. The foreign policy of the country was shaped not by one man but by a party in which two factions strove against each other, were watchful of the designs of an opposition, and suspicious of the intrigues of the Court. A decision for war or peace might result as much from the circumstance of factional or party strife as from the promptings of France or of Russia which had a strong interest in the country. So long as Russia was in alliance with England, Sweden was unlikely to join with France in a war against England though she might be prepared for adventures that stopped short of it.[2] England in turn trusted that Russia would keep Sweden in check, and the Convention of St Petersburg was meant not only to guard Hanover against attacks from France and Prussia but also to prevent Sweden lending warships to France.[3]

Though France could in 1755 expect neither Denmark nor Sweden to join her in a war against England, she intended to obtain a *quid pro quo* for her subsidies to the Scandinavian powers by making certain that they would be able to give her their assistance with shipping and naval stores. France turned therefore to the idea of an Armed Neutrality which was not unknown in Scandinavia where it had been attempted already twice in the preceding century.[4] The negotiations initiated and furthered by her did not go smoothly as Denmark initially could neither overcome her suspicions of

[1] P.R.O., S.P. 75/96, Titley to Newcastle, 6 January 1753.
[2] The best short account citing numerous documents is in G. Carlquist, *Sveriges politiska förbindelser*, passim, and see also Th. Säve, *Sveriges Deltaganda i Sjuåriga Kriget, Åren 1757–1762* (Stockholm, 1915), pp. 24ff.
[3] B.M., Add. MS 32859, f. 86, Hardwicke to Newcastle, 15 September 1755.
[4] The Armed Neutralities of 1691 and 1693 are described in Boye, *Neutralitetsforbund*, pp. 55ff.

Sweden, nor agree to any action that might prevent England from making concessions on neutral trade, or might even lead to retaliations. Bernstorff became finally convinced that England intended to be at least as firm on the pretensions of the neutrals in the coming War as she had been in the last, but that a mere show of strength was unlikely to provoke her.[1] Russia approved of the projected Armed Neutrality so long as it did not result in an interruption of her own trade with England, and was particularly in favour of the complete neutralisation of the Baltic which would secure part of the Anglo-Russian trade route. She even went so far as to inform England early in 1756 that no English fleet was permitted to enter the Baltic if a European war broke out, a demand which England rejected.[2]

The Reversal of Alliances altered the situation for both Sweden and Denmark. Once Russia had shown that she intended to fight on the same side as France, against Prussia though not England, Sweden was under no further outside constraint to enter the War against Prussia. Moreover her internal political complications made a diversion through war desirable. France offered to pay for a Swedish army, and France as well as Russia and Austria promised Sweden that she would receive Prussian territories. Her decision

[1] Carlquist, *Sveriges politiska förbindelser*, pp. 128ff., gives again the best short account and cites much documentary evidence. See also for conversations of Titley with Bernstorff about the Danish–Swedish negotiations, and for Titley's exposition of the British view, P.R.O., S.P. 75/99, Titley to Holdernesse, 9 September and 28 October 1755; also S.P. 75/100, same to same 6 and 20 March, and 10 April 1756, and Holdernesse to Titley, 2 April 1756. See also Swed. S. Arch., Anglica I, Kansli-presidenten to Wynantz, 9 July 1756; and *ibid.*, Kanslikollegium to Wynantz, 5 November 1756; also *ibid.*, Wynantz to Kanslikollegium, 12 October 1756, and Wynantz to Kanslipresidenten, 20 February 1756; and also Dan. S. Arch., T.K.U.A., Engl. B, 106, Rantzau to Bernstorff, 16 and 23 April, 18 May, 21 and 24 August 1756; and Engl. C, 266, Bernstorff to Rantzau, 8 May 1756. The Danish and Swedish diplomats gave their views on English reactions to the Convention in their reports, and were instructed on how to represent it at London. See also P.R.O., S.P. 91/62, Holdernesse to Hanbury Williams, 6 February 1756, on English instructions to induce Russia to help prevent any breach of the peace by the Scandinavian powers; and B.M., Add. MS 32864, ff. 176–9, which consist of intercepted despatches between Rouillé and the French envoys in Scandinavia.

[2] P.R.O., S.P. 91/62, 'Déclaration Sécretissime (of Convention of St Petersburg), dated 1 February 1756, signed by Bestoucheff and Woronzoff, with the rejection of this interpretation of the Convention by Holdernesse to H. Williams, 30 March 1756.

Trade and Diplomacy

was a foregone conclusion, and Sweden was ready to enter the War at any time after the spring of 1757.

Sweden's decision to enter the War completely altered the complexion of the Armed Neutrality Convention. Denmark was as determined as ever to remain neutral, and her association with Sweden in the Neutrality Fleet could therefore hardly continue after Sweden entered the War. The Neutrality Fleet had only put to sea in 1756 for a few weeks at the end of the sailing season, and its North Sea cruise in 1757 lasted little longer, the Swedish squadron having been temporarily recalled when on its way to join the Danish as an English fleet was rumoured to be sailing for the Baltic. This was the last joint cruise, and the Neutrality League had effectively come to an end. Sweden was at war with Prussia before the year was out, and Denmark remained neutral.[1]

While England was prepared to write off Sweden as a potential Protestant ally, she never became accustomed to the fact that Denmark was a client of France, bound to her by subsidies and self-interest. So soon as a war in Europe was known to be virtually unavoidable, Titley was instructed to reach an agreement for Danish troops to enter English service. Titley had spoken to both Bernstorff and the king early in 1755, and reported to London that there was no chance whatever of Denmark agreeing to a subsidy treaty for troops to be used at any distance from her own frontiers, though he hoped that Denmark might possibly agree to help defend Hanover. He therefore advised Holdernesse that an offer for troops should only be made if they were to serve in Hanover, and received the prompt reply to conclude a treaty for Danish troops to serve in the British Isles.[2] Denmark naturally

[1] Some of the troubles that beset the joint fleet and particularly the Swedish squadron which is described as ill-found and ill-manned are related in P.R.O., S.P. 95/102, [Gedda] to [Holdernesse], Stockholm, 13 April 1756, and also Moltke Archives, bundle 'Breve fra...Ogier,' Ogier to Moltke, Copenhagen, 7 April 1757, and draft reply by Moltke, 8 April 1757. Ogier, it will be remembered, was the French envoy at Copenhagen.
[2] Holdernesse had ordered Titley in a private letter (B.M., Eg. MS 2694, F. 86, Holdernesse to Titley, 25 February 1755) to approach Bernstorff and the king unofficially. Titley's accounts of his conversations are in P.R.O., S.P. 75/98, Titley to Holdernesse, 22 and 25 February, and 22 March 1755. For the instructions, see Chance, *Diplomatic Instructions, Denmark*, pp. 155ff. The instructions published by Chance were followed by another set of 18 April 1755 which Chance has not printed. These instructions

refused,[1] and she could have done little else even if she had not been determined to remain both neutral and on the side of France. Her neutrality in the coming War was essential if she wanted to reap any benefit from Bernstorff's policy of extending Danish trade, and, rather more important, if she wanted to be certain of surviving intact in the face of likely threats from Russia. Bernstorff had earlier at great expense and at the additional cost of a diplomatic rupture with Spain concluded a series of treaties with Turkey and the Barbary states with the express intention of securing the safety of Danish ships in the Mediterranean against pirate attack so that they could act there as carriers when war broke out, and Danish ships would only be in demand in the Mediterranean if Denmark remained neutral.[2] Loss of neutrality then meant loss of opportunity of Danish trade, and Bernstorff was not the man to neglect any opportunity that would come Denmark's way to profit from war as a neutral. The other consideration which confirmed him in his policy of neutrality was the threat to the Duchies from Peter of Russia. If the Empress Elizabeth should die during the War, an attack on the Duchies could be carried out by Peter more easily than in time of peace and would, Bernstorff realised, receive little if any attention from the guaranteeing powers, France and Britain. Denmark would therefore be extremely unwise to let her troops and her fleet stray far from home. A policy of neutrality alone could ensure that Danish troops would be at the right place if the worst should happen, and Russia attacked the Duchies.

Titley did not brief Cabinet fully enough or early enough on the convulutions of Danish foreign and economic policy. Cabinet therefore did not see why Denmark would and could not hire out her troops as she had done in earlier wars, and Titley was instructed year after year with monotonous regularity to try yet once again to obtain Danish troops either for England herself or later for Prussia. Titley replied that where France had failed before the Reversal

are much more explicit, and Titley is given full powers. See P.R.O., S.P. 75/98, instructions, full powers, and treaty drafts (based on the conventions with Denmark of 1734 and 1739), and covering letter of 18 April 1755.

[1] P.R.O., S.P. 75/98, Titley to Holdernesse, 15 April 1755. It should be noted that Titley did not act on the second set of instructions until early in 1756.

[2] Johnsen, *Norges Historie*, vol. 5, pp. 13f.

of Alliances to make Denmark agree to conclude an alliance with Prussia he could hardly be expected to succeed, and where France had since failed to obtain military or naval aid for herself, England could not hope to be treated any better. Titley might protest at the impossible instructions given him, but he was too loyal not to do his best at Copenhagen and used every argument that he could think of. He harped on the danger to the Protestant religion from an alliance of the principal Catholic powers; on the danger to the Protestant Succession in England if she should lose the War; he assured Bernstorff that England was bound to win and warned him of the black future a country would face that had been on the wrong side.[1] Nothing, of course, could make any impression on Denmark except danger to herself, and she was aware that she might be brought into danger by the proximity of Hanover. Bernstorff had warned England when the Convention of St Petersburg became known that Denmark could not allow Russian troops or naval concentrations in defence of Hanover close to her frontier, an empty threat that received no answer.[2] Russian troops were now in the field though not to defend Hanover. Worse, they might attack Hanover and carry the attack only a little further into the Duchies. Bernstorff, in desperation, tried to meet this threat by

[1] References to treaty offers to Denmark in the State Papers Foreign, Denmark, for the years 1755 to 1760 when the last offer was eventually made, run into the hundreds, and it would be superfluous to cite them all. A selection of arguments used to persuade Denmark to enter into a British alliance may suffice: see P.R.O., S.P. 75/101, Holdernesse to Titley, 28 September 1756, with instructions to use Protestant arguments; and also Dan. S. Arch., T.K.U.A., Engl. B, 106, Rantzau to Bernstorff, 10 August 1756, informing Bernstorff that Cabinet talks of nothing but the danger to Protestantism; and Swed. S. Arch., Anglica 1, Wynantz to Kanslipresidenten, 30 July 1756, to the same effect; see also Säve, *Sjuåriga Kriget*, p. 23, that Maria Theresa regarded the accession of Sweden to the alliance as important as it proved that the War was not being fought against Protestantism; see further on rumours of Jacobite activities P.R.O., S.P. 75/98, Titley to Holdernesse, 5 August 1755, that Jacobites were rumoured to be assembling in Norway for a descent on Scotland; and S.P. 75/107, Goodricke to Holdernesse, 29 September 1758, that Höpken had sent him word of the French proposals to mount an invasion of Scotland from Sweden with the object of raising a rebellion under the Pretender. See also J. S. Corbett, *England in the Seven Years War* (2 vols, London, 1907) vol. 2, pp. 4, 7, 13 and 17ff. on the French plans which were known in England before Höpken passed them on. Goodricke, incidentally, suspected that Höpken had heard that all was known in England and merely gave the information to keep in well with England.

[2] P.R.O., S.P. 75/100, Titley to Holdernesse, 3 February 1756.

obtaining a guarantee of neutrality for Hanover and, when that failed, at least for Bremen–Verden. He succeeded in the end in ridding Denmark of the danger of having to honour her guarantee of that small territory, but neither Titley nor Cabinet had much to do at that time with the affairs of the king's German possessions, which were looked after by the Hanoverian ministers. When Bernstorff, for example, arranged that a Danish intermediary should be used in the negotiations which led to the Convention of Kloster Zeven, Titley was not even informed.[1]

After the Convention of Kloster Zeven was broken and it became clear that Pitt would not allow the war on the Continent to be regarded as separate from the war against France the world over, Bernstorff had to turn again to Titley. He had been concerned since 1756 that an English fleet might sail into the Baltic to assist Frederick II of Prussia by attacking Russian-occupied territory, and possibly also Sweden and her German possessions. Sweden, as has already been noted, was so alarmed over this threat that her neutrality squadron had been recalled for a time in 1757 to guard her Baltic coast. Russia became equally alarmed over the persistent rumours that an English fleet was on the point of sailing for the Baltic to aid Prussia, and as a safeguard against the War being carried into the Baltic concluded in 1758 a convention with Sweden which was represented to Denmark as an extension of the existing Dano-Swedish Armed Neutrality League. A report from an agent in Stockholm that the Russo-Swedish convention had been concluded was received in London within a week of it being signed, and

---

[1] The negotiations which led to Kloster Zeven have been described fully by Corbett, *Seven Years War*, vol. i, *passim*, and from a different angle by E. Charteris, *William Augustus, Duke of Cumberland* (London, 1913), chs 21ff. Nothing of significance has been found that might add to these accounts. The Convention over Bremen-Verden, which is less well-known than Kloster Zeven, and the Danish attempt to arrange for a guarantee of Hanoverian neutrality is in Dan. S. Arch., Engl. C, 264, laid in under date of signatures, Bernstorff–Ogier, 16 July 1757, and appended papers. It appears that the King of Denmark made some difficulties about the Convention, but what they were is not known. Moltke persuaded him to approve it. See Moltke Archives, bundle 'Breve fra...Ogier', Ogier to Moltke, 3 July 1757, and draft reply of 4 July 1757. On Denmark's concern over Hanover, generally, see B.M., Add. MS 6812 (Mitchell Papers), ff. 12–13, Titley to Holdernesse, private, 22 March 1755, that the Danes regarded Hanover as a 'Bulwark to Denmark, on the Side of Germany, and had therefore a real Interest in the Preservation of it'.

Titley reported soon after from Copenhagen that Denmark would not accede to it: her trade was too important to her, and she did not intend endangering it by making the Armed Neutrality Fleet strong enough to seek or even risk a clash with England. Sweden and Russia therefore equipped a joint neutrality fleet in 1758 without Danish participation, and Titley and the agents in Stockholm continued to report very fully on the cruise of the Swedish-Russian squadron in the Baltic. Denmark was continuously pressed to join her Baltic neighbours and consistently refused until, quite unexpectedly, Bernstorff changed his mind in 1760, and the original Danish-Swedish Armed Neutrality League and the subsequent and separate Russo-Swedish League became a joint Danish–Swedish–Russian one. The reason for the Danish change of attitude was a purely political and dynastic one which overrode concern over trade. The perennial Gottorp claims to the Slesvig-Holstein duchies had again been revived, and Bernstorff believed that being a partner with Russia in an extended League would help him in the coming negotiations over the Gottorp claims. Titley was taken completely by surprise when he found out that Denmark had joined with Sweden and Russia in an extended Armed Neutrality League, and even the agents in Stockholm had not sent any warning of what was in the wind. In fact, Titley was so shocked by the Danish accession to the Russo-Swedish convention that he urged his government in near-hysterical terms to bombard Copenhagen and to seize the Danish fleet to prevent it from joining the Russo-Swedish squadron – an interesting anticipation of a later British policy venture. He soon became his normal pacific self again when he realised that Denmark had no intention of being more than a mere signatory to the convention, and that she would not agree to a combined three-power Neutrality Fleet.[1] In the meantime, Russia and Sweden had continued to urge Denmark to become an active member of an extended Armed Neutrality League

[1] The text of the convention is printed in *Danske Tractater 1751–1800*, pp. 172ff. The most pertinent reports are in P.R.O., S.P. 75/103, agent's report [?Count Düben], dated 2 May 1758; and S.P. 75/109, Titley to Holdernesse, private and most secret, 29 April 1760. See also E. Hermann, 'Die Rolle der Seemächte in der Ostsee während des Siebenjährigen Krieges', *Marine-Rundschau*, vol. 45 (Berlin, 1940), pp. 259ff., that neither the Swedish nor the Russian fleets were ever a threat to England as they were practically unseaworthy.

and, to make the invitation appear more pressing the Swedish–Russian fleet appeared near Copenhagen in 1758, anchoring a few miles off the city. This was as bad as having Russian troops manoeuvring close to the Duchies, and Titley was begged for an assurance that England would not provoke a war in the Baltic by sending in a fleet.[1] Cabinet refused to give an assurance, though Frederick II of Prussia had already been persuaded by argument, and a large subsidy, to forego his claim for naval assistance in the Baltic, which would have led to open conflict between England and Sweden as well as Russia. England had no intention of extending the War if it could be helped, but intimated that she was willing to give Frederick other assistance against Sweden.

The assistance that Frederick now asked for was twofold. He wanted to be informed of Swedish military intentions, and to have English help in weakening Sweden by fomenting internal trouble. England was on the surface of things not well placed to oblige him as she had no envoy in Sweden, and her first attempt to send one to Stockholm had ended in failure. England was, as is already known, in touch with affairs in Sweden through the reports sent by Gedda and by de Marteville. An official representative on the spot would have been preferable as he could stir up trouble more easily, and, if the opportunity came, act as an intermediary between Sweden and Prussia. Accordingly, Cabinet picked on a young man who, it thought, might be acceptable at Stockholm where his father was a prominent merchant. The envoy-designate, a Colonel Campbell, was to go to Stockholm without disclosing that he carried credentials, and was to present them only if he was certain they would be accepted. His instructions did not include anything on trade; that could look after itself. From what is known, Campbell believed that it rested with the Swedish Court whether his credentials were accepted, and he would have had a good chance of success if that had been so. The Court, and that meant to all intents Queen Louisa Ulrica, had already in 1755 approached Cabinet through de Marteville for money to help in a *coup d'état*, and had offered to enter into any engagement if England would

[1] P.R.O., S.P. 75/103, Titley to Holdernesse, 19 August 1758. See also Corbett, *Seven Years War*, vol. 1, pp. 152ff.

only supply a few thousand Pounds. That was out of the question at the time as Russia was a guarantor of the Swedish constitution, and an English attempt to interfere in the internal affairs of the country would have led to trouble with Russia if it became known. Cabinet therefore turned a deaf ear to every entreaty, and was not implicated in the attempted *coup d'état* of 1756 which played into the hands of the Hats by making the Court utterly subservient to that party. Cabinet was however still in touch with Louisa Ulrica through its informers at Court, and held out the hope to her that something might be done when circumstances were more favourable. Campbell's appearance in Stockholm and at the Court itself made the queen believe that England had at last become seriously interested in her proposals for a revolution, but it was constitutionally not in her power to accept an English envoy, particularly when he had broadcast all over London, despite instructions to keep his journey a secret, that he was going to Stockholm and intended to remain there as envoy. Campbell had to leave Stockholm,[1] but Cabinet still hoped to succeed in having an envoy accepted by choosing a more discreet man for the mission. The prospective envoy eventually sent was Sir John Goodricke who, as is known, did not get further than Copenhagen. Goodricke was however able to obtain military and political intelligence and was well placed to stir up trouble in Sweden. New agents had been recruited during the short stay in Sweden of the British minister to Russia, Hanbury Williams, who spent some weeks in Stockholm when returning to London from St Petersburg. Among them were some extremely well-placed men.[2] Apart from these agents Goodricke was in touch

---

[1] Campbell's instructions are printed in Chance, *Diplomatic Instructions, Sweden II*, pp. 130ff. Reports about him from London were sent by Wynantz on whom Campbell called before leaving. Wynantz had heard all about his mission well in advance and warned Stockholm. See Swed. S. Arch., Anglica I, Wynantz to Kanslipresidenten, 16, 19 and 26 August, 2 September, and 4 November 1757; and also B.M., Add. MS 6806, f. 217, Mitchell to Holdernesse, Dresden, 26 August 1757, that Campbell's secret mission was the talk of the town. Campbell himself, after reaching Stockholm, was not heard of again in London except through reports from agents who described his every movement. He had forgotten to bring a cypher, and did not dare write *en clair*.

[2] See about Hanbury Williams' stay in Stockholm the report from Gedda in P.R.O., S.P. 95/103, [Gedda] to [Holdernesse], 1 November 1757. Among the agents recruited by Hanbury Williams and later by Goodricke were such well-known men as Count

with Höpken, leader of one of the two main factions in the Hat party who sounded Goodricke about peace terms with Prussia and from time to time passed over information. The queen herself was in direct touch with Copenhagen by messengers and sent yet more information for Goodricke to be transmitted to her brother in Prussia, and continually appealed for funds to help her in further attempts at *coups d'état*. Cabinet, to oblige Prussia, sent at last some small sums without expectation of any plot being successful, and it was not till the Swedish Diet was to meet again in 1760 and money could be employed usefully to bribe deputies that Pitt finally let the queen have £10,000, which in the event turned out to have been spent to little purpose. The smaller sums which had been required for Goodricke's salary and for paying the many agents had most probably been of more use, as the military information for Frederick II which was constantly passed out from Sweden gives the appearance of authenticity. Goodricke had moreover placed himself in a position that allowed him to act towards the end of the Seven Years War as an intermediary between Sweden and Prussia and was of great service to Frederick II.[1]

England was, therefore, doing what she could by diplomacy in Denmark and by intrigue in Sweden to help Prussia and thereby incidentally herself.[2] She obtained information for Frederick II from Sweden and allowed him to remain in touch through his

Düben, Count Wrangel, Baron v. Nölken who after the war came as envoy to London after a short spell at the embassy at Madrid, and various others among whom was a Saxon, probably the Saxon minister at Stockholm, who sent reports about the movements of envoys and at times about their instructions and despatches, and interspersed them with lamentations over any Prussian victory. Louisa Ulrica also sent reports to Goodricke, and had as her own agent in London, the well-known Christopher Springer. The queen was more fortunate in her agents, it seems, than in her messengers who met with every variety of mishap. Reports of agents from Sweden are in P.R.O., S.P. 95/102-, and interspersed among Titley's despatches in S.P. 75/-. Note that the volumes containing these reports are cited in the bibliography of Olof Jägerskiöld, *Hovet och Författningsfrågan 1760-1766* (Uppsala, 1943). Dr Jägerskiöld was unfortunate in finding only one or two reports.

[1] The reports of Goodricke on the Diet of 1760-1, and on his role as an intermediary in peace negotiations etc. are in P.R.O., S.P. 75/108, 110, 111, and 113.

[2] The English diplomatic negotiations with Northern Europe before and early in the war are abstracted in a document of 27 folios in P.R.O., S.P. 75/101, 'Abstract of the Negociations between Great Britain and the Several Northern Courts in 1755 and 1756'. The date is not given, but is about 1756-7. This document provides a valuable background to the diplomacy of the War.

sister Louisa Ulrica with affairs in the enemy's camp; from Denmark she tried to obtain troops for the hard-pressed Prussians and persisted in her attempts despite every rebuff. There was really very little more England could do to assist Prussia, short of declaring war on Russia and Sweden, and Cabinet never even contemplated such a possibility. The rise of Russia to a great power had weakened English influence in the Baltic area, where she found it impossible to prevent Sweden from going to war against Prussia and, once having done so, from continuing her military adventures. As for Denmark, the position was similar: when it came to competing with France for Danish support the best England could hope for was that the Danes would stay neutral, which happened to be in Denmark's best interest and therefore her own chosen policy. The constant attempts to hire Danish troops for Prussia may very well, one suspects, have been no more than a diplomatic manoeuvre to impress Prussia with an English desire to be helpful. At best, Denmark might have considered exchanging some troops for British concessions on neutral trade and for a cast-iron guarantee of assistance in the Slesvig–Holstein dispute, but Britain was not prepared to consider either the one or the other. When the death of the Empress Elizabeth in 1762 brought the issue of the disputed Duchies to a head and Denmark appealed for English aid, she received the reply that England would not meddle in the affair, and Denmark was left to her own devices.[1]

With diplomacy unable to effect to any degree economic or, for that matter, military relations with the Scandinavian countries on which England was dependent during the Seven Years War for essential and irreplaceable supplies of timber and iron, only the merchants were left to uphold English commercial interests. They were successful in continuing to obtain supplies from Sweden and Norway throughout the War, but that was always a chancy business. It could not have been known for certain that war would not interrupt the vital trade with the Scandinavian kingdoms, who were both allied to France. Cabinet, it could be held, should have

---

[1] The best short account of the Russo-Danish confrontation at the accession of Tsar Peter III is by G. Norrie, 'Felttoget i Mecklenburg 1762', *Historisk Tidsskrift* (Copenhagen), 11th series, vol. 6 (1962).

been aware of the dangers of an interruption of essential supplies from Scandinavia – the Swedish iron and pitch and tar embargoes early in the century were sufficient warning – and made at least certain that Russia, the only other, but by itself quite inadequate, source of iron and timber, remained firmly attached to England. Cabinet had of course thought that Russia before the Reversal of Alliances and the subsequent extension of war with France to Europe was a safe ally, but there is no indication whatever that Russia, or for that matter, Sweden and Denmark–Norway were regarded in other than conventional military terms. Questions of supplies of naval stores, of iron for manufactures, of shipping services in time of war were simply not considered. Once war broke out in Europe, England had therefore every possible reason to step carefully in her dealings with every one of the Northern powers. She was not likely to clash with Russia so long as she kept her warships out of the Baltic, and that she was only too happy to do as she could not afford to extend her naval forces any further. Sweden was irrevocably committed to France and at the same time under the sway of Russia. As this was well enough known in London, all Cabinet could do was to hope for the best and trust that Sweden would not act against her own economic interests by going to war with England and thereby denying her the iron of the Swedish mines, while facing as well the destruction of her merchant-fleet with the consequent loss of its earnings as a neutral carrier.

The case of Denmark–Norway was different. The Danish–Norwegian merchant fleet was far larger than the Swedish, and proved invaluable as a neutral carrier for British manufactures, particularly in the Mediterranean. A loss of Swedish ships as carriers and of Swedish iron, even, could be faced: British trade and manufactures would have suffered, and the Admiralty would have had to make unwelcome changes in the iron fittings of men-of-war. The loss of the services of the Danish–Norwegian merchant fleet and of Norwegian timber, however, would have been irreparable. North American timber supplies for ship-building could not in the mid-eighteenth century be extended to make good any such possible losses, and Baltic timber supplies were already stretched to the limit. Despite such vital dependence on Danish–Norwegian supplies and services, England came close to war with the double kingdom over the issue of Danish–West Indian trade. It was sheer good luck that Denmark faced a crisis with Russia just at the time when England began to bring up the Danish West Indiamen, and this crisis helped to hold Denmark back from breaking off relations with England in sheer desperation. The long delay before Cabinet finally dealt with the case of the Danish West Indiamen gives the impression that Cabinet hoped the matter would settle itself, or, more likely, that Cabinet was simply not aware how important it was to the war effort to retain the self-interested goodwill of Denmark–Norway. As it turned out, the crisis was resolved by the commonsense of both British and Danish–Norwegian merchants in reaching a *modus vivendi* and thereby assuring vital supplies of timber and shipping for England. In the last resort, it was due to the merchants rather than their governments that trade in the Northern Seas continued uninterrupted in war as in peace.

Appendix 1:   The Timber-Trade

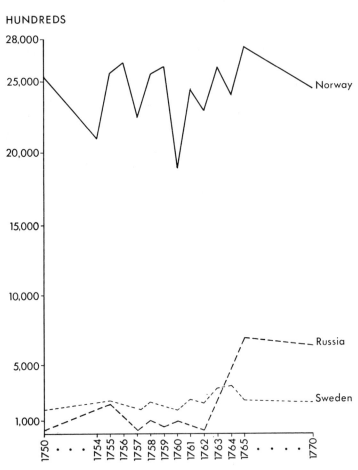

Fig. 1. Imports of ordinary deals into England from all sources, 1750–1770. (The Hundred of deals was of 120 pieces.) From entries in the annual reports of the inspector-general of customs and excise, P.R.O., Cust. 3/50–70.

178

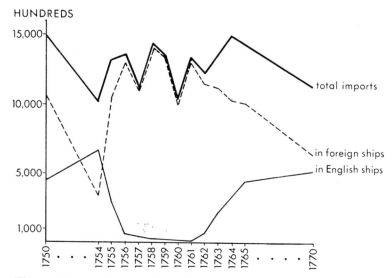

HUNDREDS

Fig. 2. The distribution of shipping in the timber-trade: deal imports into London from Norway, 1750–1770. From entries in the annual reports of the inspector-general of customs and excise, P.R.O., Cust. 3/50–70.

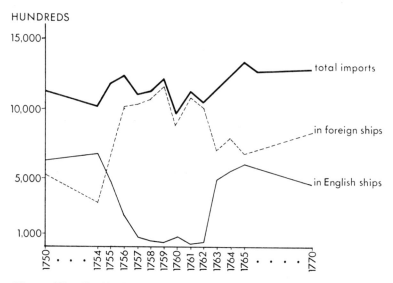

HUNDREDS

Fig. 3. The distribution of shipping in the timber-trade: deal imports into the English out-ports from Norway, 1750–1770. From entries in the annual reports of the inspector-general of customs and excise, P.R.O., Cust. 3/50–70.

179

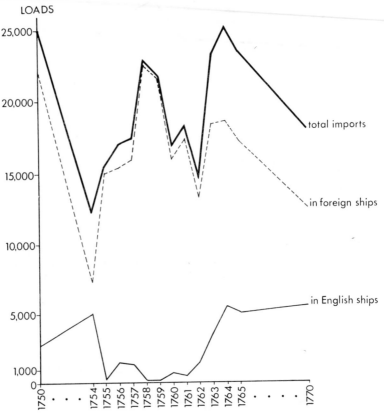

Fig. 4. The distribution of shipping in the timber-trade: imports of 'fir timber' into England from Norway, 1750–1770. (The Load of timber was of 50 cubic feet.) From entries in the annual reports of the inspector-general of customs and excise, P.R.O., Cust. 3/50–70.

TABLE 1 *Imports of masts into England from all sources,* * *1750–1770*

Year	Norway			East Country			Russia			Colonies		
	Great masts	Middle masts	Small masts	Great masts	Middle masts	Small masts	Great masts	Middle masts	Small masts	Great masts	Middle masts	Small masts
1750	258	1721	1789	1468	49	142	0	6	32	128	135	205
1754	90	1411	1402	716	187	443	20	2	60	599	99	194
1755	98	926	1358	1385	259	1147	57	74	114	746	247	393
1756	544	1461	3473	1760	867	1161	14	14	0	329	225	189
1757	28	1407	2112	1305	607	701	23	0	3	34	31	8
1758	40	1791	2000	1091	796	625	138	34	72	312	54	20
1759	39	2285	3434	1026	58	269	869	250	254	202	73	20
1760	60	1566	2007	352	160	55	895	747	583	603	127	58
1761	53	1106	1385	59	35	17	1825	647	342	401	61	48
1762	15	1117	2449	24	17	75	2297	487	622	179	42	80
1763	250	1713	3255	229	133	75	1685	373	414	403	39	3
1764	252	549	697	155	28	148	1832	326	735	515	256	464
1765	18	1832	3255	80	22	162	1365	592	1121	1242	532	977
1770	54	1871	2754	61	72	824	875	473	171	699	581	191

SOURCE: (Masts by number) from entries in the annual reports of the inspector-general of customs and excise, P.R.O. Cust. 3/50–70.
* A few masts were also obtained from Sweden, Germany, and Holland.

TABLE 2   *Timber prices at London, 1757–1770: First and second grade redwood deals measuring 12' × 9" × 2½", shipped from Christiania, Frederickstadt, and Larvik (for the Hundred)*

Year	Christiania deals		Frederickstadt deals		Larvik deals	
	First £ s. d.	Seconds £ s. d.	First £ s. d.	Seconds £ s. d.	First £ s. d.	Seconds £ s. d.
1757	14 15 0	10 0 0	—	—	12 5 0	9 0 0
1758	14 15 0	10 0 0	—	9 0 0	12 5 0*	9 0 0
1759	14 0 0	9 0 0	—	—	—	—
1760	14 0 0	9 0 0	12 0 0	10 0 0	—	—
1761	14 10 0	9 5 0	13 0 0	9 10 0	12 17 6	—
1762	15 0 0	10 10 0	13 15 0	10 10 0	—	—
1763	15 0 0	10 10 0	14 0 0	10 10 0	13 5 0	10 0 0
1764	16 5 0	11 0 0	14 10 0	11 10 0	13 10 0	11 0 0
1765	17 0 0	12 0 0	15 0 0	12 0 0	14 10 0	11 10 0
1766	16 10 0	12 0 0	15 10 0	12 0 0	14 10 0	12 0 0
1767	14 10 0	10 0 0	—	—	14 0 0	10 15 0
1768	15 10 0	10 0 0	—	—	13 10 0	10 10 0
1769	16 0 0	10 0 0	15 0 0	10 0 0	13 10 0	10 0 0
1770	16 10 0	10 10 0	—	—	13 10 0	9 10 0

SOURCE: extracted from Reports, House of Commons, vol. 15, Timber Duties (1835), XIX, appendix 11, pp. 403ff.
* This price agrees with the independent evidence of F. L. Fabricius' list of the price of Larvik timber at London in that year. (See appendix 4, pp. 194–5, and 198.)

TABLE 3 *Cost of importing deals from Christiania to London, 1764 (for the Hundred)*

			£	s.	d.
(a)	First-quality redwood deals, measuring 12′ × 9″ × 2½″	Prime foreign cost	11	0	0
		Freight	2	6	5
		Charges and insurance		11	6
		Import duties	2	1	9
		Total cost	£15	19	8
(b)	Second-quality redwood deals, same dimensions	Prime foreign cost	4	3	3
		Freight	2	6	5
		Charges and insurance		8	0
		Import duties	2	1	9
		Total cost	£8	19	8
(c)	First-quality whitewood deals, measuring 12′ × 9″ × 3″	Prime foreign cost	9	0	0
		Freight	2	15	8
		Charges and insurance		10	9
		Import duties	2	1	9
		Total cost	£14	8	2

SOURCE: extracted from Reports, House of Commons, vol. 15, Timber Duties (1835), XIX, pp. 348f.

Appendix 2:   The Iron-Trade

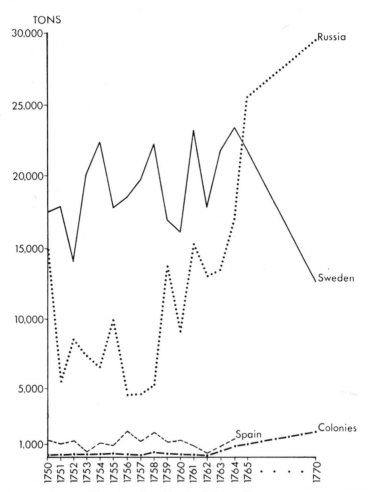

Fig. 5. Imports of bar-iron into England from all sources, 1750–1770, as recorded in the customs ledgers, P.R.O., Cust. 3/50–70. (Note the cautionary remarks on pp. 66f. on imports credited in the customs ledgers to Sweden and Russia.)

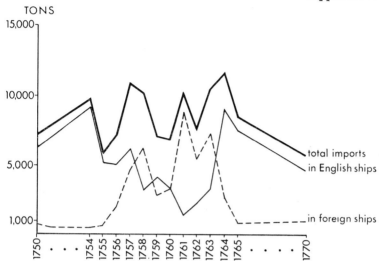

Fig. 6. The distribution of shipping in the iron-trade: bar-iron imported into London from Sweden, 1750–1770, as recorded in the customs ledgers, P.R.O., Cust. 3/50–70.

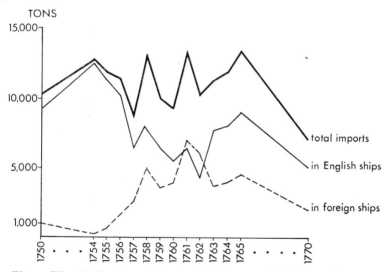

Fig. 7. The distribution of shipping in the iron-trade: bar-iron imported into the English out-ports from Sweden, 1750–1770, as recorded in the customs ledgers, P.R.O., Cust. 3/50–70.

185

TABLE 4 *Imports of bar-iron into England, 1750–70, as recorded in the customs ledgers, P.R.O., Cust. 3/50–70, showing total recorded imports from all sources, imports from Sweden, and the percentage imported from Sweden.* (Rounded off to the nearest ton and percentage.)*

Year	Total recorded imports, in tons	Recorded imports from Sweden, in tons	Percentage imported from Sweden
1750	34,751	17,575	51
1751	26,005	17,859	69
1752	24,613	13,953	56
1753	28,351	20,004	71
1754	30,694	22,424	73
1755	29,321	17,762	61
1756	30,062	18,669	62
1757	26,025	19,769	76
1758	30,341	22,252	73
1759	32,607	17,045	52
1760	27,383	16,328	59
1761	40,735	23,484	58
1762	32,342	17,816	55
1763	36,856	21,708	59
1764	43,210	23,517	54
1765	50,978	21,973	43
1770	45,702	12,725	28

* Note the cautionary remarks on pp. 66f. on imports credited in the customs ledgers to Sweden.

Appendix 3: The Pitch- and Tar-Trade

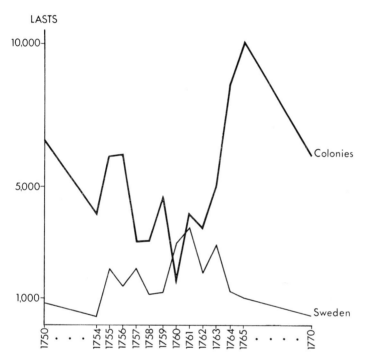

LASTS

Fig. 8. Imports of pitch and tar into England from Sweden and the American colonies, 1750–1770. (The Last was of 12 barrels of *c*. 32 gallons each, or of *c*. 30 cwt dry-measure.) As recorded in the customs ledgers, P.R.O., Cust. 3/50–70.

Appendix 4: Report on the Norwegian Timber-Trade and the Swedish and Norwegian Iron-Trade to England, 1759

Own translation of document in the Norwegian State Archives, Oslo, Ser. Localia, Larvik, 'Underdanigst Rapport Om hwad mig udi Naadigst Instruction af 26de Junii 1758 er befalet at søge oplysning om wed min Naervaerlse i London for saa wit det har waeret mig mueligt, sidinntil derudi at avancere Angaaende den Norske Traehandel til London. London den 6te Februarii 1759 Underdanigst af F. L. Fabricius.'

The writer of this report, F. L. Fabricius, was manager of the Fritsø saw-mills and iron-works of Count Laurvig, the largest land-holder next to the Crown in mid-eighteenth-century Norway. He came to London in the middle of 1758 to study the timber- and iron-trade with a view to increasing shipments from Fritsø, and remained in England until the following year. When writing his report, Fabricius bore in mind that his employer would have no knowledge of commerce, and he therefore went into detail to explain the working of the timber- and iron-trades.

PART I

ON THE TIMBER-TRADE

[*fo 1*] The timber-trade from Norway to London is ordinarily conducted in either of two ways: the timber may be sold in Norway itself on order [of English merchants], or it may be shipped to London for sale there.

Arrangements when selling on order are these: Norwegian merchants at the beginning of the year let their connections here [in London] know at what prices they intend to sell each particular grade and cut of their sawn timber. The price is based on considerations of what is customary at the time, and also on advice received from agents on a shortage or glut in the supply of any type of timber in London. The English merchants then charter English or Norwegian ships to fetch what timber they require from Norway. The Norwegian merchant thus obtains straight-out what price he thought fit to charge without risking anything on shipment, or laying out money on handling costs, export and import duties, and incidentals, which are all paid by the purchaser. He gets as well a commission of generally 2% on the total amount as in such a direct sale he is regarded as the agent of the English merchant. He runs no risks on payment as purchasers are either well-known, substantial people, or have given satisfactory sureties. Payment is generally made by bills sent to Norway, otherwise a bill is drawn so soon as loading is completed.

When shipping timber on his own account to be sold in London, the Norwegian merchant takes care to send such grades as he considers from information received to be most in demand. He must himself bear the risks of the sea, and is responsible for all costs such as freight, duties, and the like, both in Norway and London.

Cargoes shipped on the Norwegian merchant's own account are addressed to one of the Norwegian agents in London. The agent arranges for the timber to be unloaded into barges called 'lighters', and advances money for customs duties, freight, and other charges. Finally, he sells the timber for the best prices that can be obtained. Generally half the amount is paid in cash [*i reede Penge*], and four months' credit is given for the balance. The agent's commission is 2% of the total cost of the shipment. He is, however, not answerable if a purchaser should go bankrupt before having paid a balance still owing, the Norwegian merchant himself bearing that risk. Losses happen very rarely that way as every agent, to get a reputation for dependability and thus obtain business, will have dealings only with substantial people, that is, with people whose bills can be discounted at $\frac{1}{2}$% the month.

[*fo 2*] Notwithstanding the great advantage of selling the timber in Norway itself, rather than shipping it to London for sale, the latter method of trade has become the more general since before

the war [i.e. the Seven Years War]. The war itself has practically stopped direct sale in Norway as English merchants fear losses to their own cargoes through French privateers, but the war is not to blame as direct sales had already fallen off before it. This is largely the fault of the Norwegian merchants themselves. When they found how great the profits in the timber-trade were, they stocked up with more timber than they could afford to hold in store for long without making sales. The English merchants heard of this from agents they had in Norway, and stopped giving orders as they knew that the Norwegians would then be forced to ship the timber themselves in their own vessels. One must fear that they will resort to the same manoeuvre again when the war finally ends. Prices will then come to depend on them [i.e. the English merchants] entirely, while otherwise they would conform to the value that Norwegian merchants are putting on their timber. The English merchants will certainly use that trick unless the Norwegians, by somewhat restricting their large exports, force them to send orders to Norway for cargoes more often than has happened for some time.

When shipments have been ordered directly from Norway, the timber is not inspected for size or grade when it arrives here. The English purchaser has to assume that it is the timber which he ordered. A Norwegian merchant need therefore only be concerned for his reputation to remain as high as is necessary to get orders often. But when the timber is shipped to be sold here, sorting takes place. The cargo is then, straight after arrival, transferred into lighters, which take it after sale at the purchaser's cost to the various timber-yards. There, the timber is sorted or, as it is here called, 'payled' [or, more commonly, 'bracked']. Whatever does not conform in measurement or quality to specification is re-sorted. In the case of deals, Firsts are down-graded to Seconds when they fall short in measurements specified for that type of plank, and they will be classed as rejects if they are uneven in thickness, have rotten patches or are splintered, or are unacceptable because of knotholes and any other faults. If among the Seconds [Fabricius calls that type 'lasts', but 'seconds' was equally often used; both were classed by the Customs as deals] there should be any of too short length or with the above-mentioned faults, then they will also be classed as rejects. Firsts downgraded to Seconds are paid for as Seconds. The price of rejects is very small, and is often fixed by withholding a percentage determined by the number of rejects from the full price of the shipment. But such deductions from the agreed sale price are only made when the amount of faulty timber is unreasonably large.

Timber imported from Norway to London may be divided into six categories: Firsts, Seconds, battens, half-deals, rafters or pailing-board, and ends. The measurements and quality of each category or type should be carefully noted. The first two agree on the whole with the specifications used in Norway for Firsts and Seconds, but as I was particularly concerned to [*fo 3*] get information of use to the Fritsø mills, I shall note what the measurements and qualities of timber from the county of Laurvig [now spelled Larvik when used as a geographical name] should have here in London.

There is no difference in the measurements used at London or Fritsø for Firsts and Seconds. Both are deals of 10 feet or 12 feet. 11-foot deals are regarded at Fritsø as a separate type but in London they count as 12-foot deals. 10-foot deals are in London as at Fritsø from 8 feet 9 inches and up to 11 feet long. Deals of 11 feet and upward are counted as 12-foot deals. Firsts are at least $8\frac{1}{2}$ inches wide, and Seconds are below that width. As the width contributes greatly to the price it is advisable to ship the widest possible deals. Thickness must be exactly to specification as even a small deviation will lead to down-grading. As regards quality, it is considered satisfactory if the timber is free of rot, cracks across the length, too many knotholes, and the like. Above all, the timber must be evenly sawn. If a deal or other type of plank is thicker in one part than another, then the merchant gets a bad reputation, since deals are re-sawn here to a thickness of $\frac{1}{2}$ inch or even $\frac{1}{4}$ inch, and the loss with uneven planks is not only of one or two split-deals, but also in wages, which are very high. Seconds differ from Firsts only in width, and are from 7 to $2\frac{1}{2}$ inches wide. They should otherwise be of the same lengths and nearly the same quality as Firsts. Battens are from 6 to 7 inches wide, and their edges are not sawn, but cut with an axe. Less duty is paid on them than for deals. The wood from which battens are sawn is of the same quality and length as for Seconds.

Half-deals are of the same quality and width as deals, but only 6 to 7 feet long. They pay only half the duty and freight of deals, and it would be of advantage to use for them such wood as cannot be made into deals. Pailing-board is of two kinds, either hewn with an axe into a plank up to 6 feet in length and 4 to 6 inches wide, or it is of the same dimensions as Seconds, battens, and half-deals, but cannot reach the quality required for them. Ends are very short boards, sawn either from stumps or cut down from faulty deals. These last three types of timber are hardly acceptable to merchants, and it does not pay to ship them in quantity, particularly in these days when freights are so high. A few are useful in each cargo as stowage woods, and can be sold to carpenters and small traders. There is no need to give any description of the types of plank sawn from poor quality timber as they cannot be shipped to London without loss. If any of the above mentioned categories [*fo 4*] of sawn timber do not come up to exact specification, their price will suffer at sale, and sometimes a rebate has to be given when faults are only noted on sorting. At all times, though, a merchant shipping any timber not up to specification will get a bad reputation, and his shipments will fetch lower prices.

The above types of sawn timber are all generally exported from Laurvig to London. One cannot well predict which will be the most marketable as that will depend on scarcity and demand. It is therefore best to ask the advice of agents from time to time. One general rule can, though, be given. The duties payable are as high for thin and faulty deals as for wide and thick ones of good quality, while the price differs greatly. London merchants are also good judges of timber whose quality they can assess very exactly. The best advantage is therefore obtained by shipping to London deals of the greatest dimensions and the finest quality. One is also well advised to sort the timber very carefully as some planks not up to specification will make the whole shipment suspect, to the detriment of prices.

In other ports of England where charges are slightly less than in London and where the supervision of customs officers is not so strict, poorer quality timber can be sold to some advantage. The way to set about it, I have been told, is this: the Norwegian shipper sells his cargo on the evidence of the bill of lading without adding import duties to the price. The purchaser undertakes to pay the duties himself on the understanding that some of the shipment is smuggled ashore. He thus avoids paying the full duties, and can therefore afford to pay more for the timber than it is worth. In those ports, where timber imports are not so large as in London, one is also not so particular about it [i.e. the quality].

Apart from the expenses incurred in Norway through the sorting, preparing, and loading of timber, and through export duties, the following charges have to be borne by the Hundred [that is, 120 pieces] boards exported to London:

Freight – this is assessed from all ports in Southern Norway on the basis of 10-foot 'Christiania deals'. They are 1¼ inches thick, ten dozen to the Hundred, and no distinction is made between Firsts and Seconds. Deals of greater length or thickness pay more in proportion to cubic contents. Freights have risen very greatly during the war. The rate from Laurvig which used to be 15s. to 17s. [per Hundred Christiania Deals] has risen since the beginning of the war to an average of £1 8s. Freight is higher from places like Drammen and Christiania where deals are sawn wider, and loading is more difficult and takes longer.

[*fo 5*] *Duties* in England are equally high on all sizes of deals up to 20 foot long, without regard to their being fir or spruce, to their thickness, length, or quality. They are,

for the Hundred deals, to London, in Norwegian ships – £1 11s. 4½d. or Rd.7 81sk.
for 120 battens –   7s. 10½d. or Rd.1 92¼sk.
for 120 half-deals –   15s. 8¼d. or Rd.3 88½sk.
for 120 pailing-board –   2s. 2d.   or   52sk.
for 120 ends –   10s. 1½d. or Rd.2 51sk.

The duties are a shilling in the Pound lower when timber is imported in English ships. Other charges are 1s. 6d. or 36sk. for scavage and portage per Hundred deals, and lower in proportion for the other types of timber. This payment is to the Lord Mayor of London alone, and not demanded in other English ports. [Fabricius was mistaken. Similar charges were made elsewhere.]

There are also some minor clearance expenses for papers, clerks, and the like which amount to about 7*d.* or 8*d.* per Hundred deals, and less in proportion to duties on the other types.

Lighter Freight is paid to have the timber taken from the ship to the merchants' yards, and is charged to the vendor. It comes to 1*s.* per Hundred 1½-inch-thick boards, without regard to width and length, and is proportionately higher for thicker boards.

Agent's Fee is 2% of the total sale price.

Insurance on timber from Norway to England cannot be exactly assessed as it will depend on circumstances. It should not be higher than 1¾% if taken out in London, and can often be obtained for 1%.

Finally, one must consider the loss on bills of exchange which one is given for balances due. It is, though, only a loss occasionally, and a profit may at times be made. Up till now, the difference in value between Danish [Norwegian] and English money has not been above 3%, English money being of less value in Norway than in England.

I have not heard of any other charges to detract from the profit on timber here in England. I do not think there are any unless one counts a small tip here and there which is of little consequence. The charges are the same in peace or war except for freight.

[*fo 6*] I shall now give my report on London timber-prices in the past and the present time. I have done my best to find out about them, but merchants generally like to keep such matters dark and it was very difficult to get satisfactory information...I was able, however, to make these conclusions on prices in the past: Deals have generally never fetched so low a price that Norwegian merchants who acted prudently suffered loss. On the contrary, they have ordinarily made a good profit since export from Norway to England has grown over the years despite a rise in prices of sawn timber in most districts. Prices up to 1748 were, I know, generally lower than they have been since. They rose that year because the dearth of deals was so great that Norwegian merchants, particularly in Drammen and Christiania, saw fit to raise prices by 6*s.* to 8*s.* the Hundred when taking orders for shipment. This higher price has been maintained through the attention to their business by agents

here, and through the agreements of merchants in the principal ports in Norway. Neither fluctuations in demand nor the increase in shipments could affect the high price, and it brought great profit to Norwegian merchants when freights were half of what they are now, and the cost of timber lower.

My information on prices in England at the present time, and on Laurvig timber in particular has been more detailed...One can conclude that timber from the Fritsø sawmills, after all expenses are deducted, is sold with a reasonable profit despite the present excessive freight rates...

[*fo 7*] Timber which is not acceptable in the English market and cannot be sold at home or in Denmark must be shipped to France where I hardly believe a great profit can be made, particularly at this time when trade both to and from France is practically ruined by the enormous privateering activities of the English.

There is no need to anticipate any lowering of prices as they have remained at their present level throughout the war despite the heavy shipments from Norway last year. The English continue to live practically as well as before the war, and there is as much money among the people as in peace-time. The timber-trade will become even more profitable when the war ends, as freights will fall. The consumption of timber will also become greater as many landlords who now desist from building because of the high taxes on windows and income, will then start building again. Further, it should be possible to bring direct sales of timber on orders received from England under way again after the war. There is the danger, though, that Norwegian merchants might push the English too far and lead them to increase their imports from the Baltic and their colonies in America. They could do that the easier as the last government had already tried to foster the timber-trade with the plantations by allowing duty-free imports from there [Fabricius refers to the Act of 1720]. The English admit, however, that Norwegian timber is much better than that from the Baltic or the colonies, and cannot be done without for some purposes. Moreover, trade with those places meets with many difficulties and requires much capital, and one need therefore not fear too greatly that it will become a danger unless the Norwegians let their greed overstep all bounds (*medmindre de Norske drive deres Begierlighed alt for laengt over grendserne*)...

I submit a list of the most prominent merchants dealing in Norwegian timber. I know them all personally and can say that they are esteemed, substantial, and reliable people with whom one can deal with the greatest confidence. As to the agents handling timber, I have come to know them so well that I can give a list [*fo 8*] of them all and add to it an estimate of their character which I have gone to great trouble to have confirmed.

Johan Collet [a Norwegian] merits to be placed first for his great acumen and his honesty, and also for the services given to his countrymen and to the trade of Norway. He used his great resources to keep up prices by giving merchants here unusually long credit. He also allowed his acquaintances in Norway to draw on him well beyond the balances due to them. His death [lately] was therefore a great loss to the Norwegian people. He left, after £50,000 had been paid to his heirs, an estimated £100,000 to his executor.

Claus Heede [Heide], Mr Collet's executor, was left that sum on condition that he carry on the business. He had already directed it during Mr Collet's last years, and is an efficient, honest, and well-intentioned man. One may well conclude that he will follow his late principal in being the best and most trustworthy agent.

Jens Peterson, a Norwegian, is a substantial and efficient man who understands the trade well. He had next to Mr Collet the greatest number of commissions, but could never earn the same high reputation by such disinterested actions as Mr Collet's.

John Rigg is an Englishman of good fortune who owns a large cloth manufactory from which he sends much to Norway. He takes on Norwegian timber commissions. He is a useful and courteous man who has the reputation of treating his principals well and honestly, and therefore several large saw-millers in Norway have given him their business...

James Norman, an Englishman, has also for some time had a number of commissions from Norway, particularly from Councillor Poul Vogt of Christiania, and from Lars Smith's widow at Drammen. He is, however, also a timber-merchant, and I do not know how far he can therefore be trusted with keeping up prices. I have been told that he is no friend to the Norway trade, and is very active in increasing the Baltic and American trade.

There are one or two others in London apart from these four agents, who are given commissions by Norwegian merchants. One is a Holstein confectioner by the name of Ehlers, but the dealings of these small people are few and their knowledge of the trade so slight that they harm rather than help it.

Of further information that I have obtained, I wish to add the following as it would help to increase profits on our timber from Fritsø, especially if it were to be shipped on own account. Every particular district in Norway has in this country a reputation for producing one grade or type of timber in which it excels all other districts. Spruce timber from Laurvig has so far not been well thought of here, while our fir timber [*fo 9*] is regarded as passable. Every effort should therefore be made to obtain as much fir as possible for our saw-mills. As to spruce, care must be taken to mill as little as possible of lowland growth because timber from the low-lying regions is in bad repute for its tendency to splinter and for the difficulties carpenters have in planing it. The Laurvig sawmills would show a better profit on their shipments to London if more 12-inch boards could be produced and thereby escape the competition of Drammen and Christiania which ship mainly 10-inch deals. Better still would be shipments of 14- and 16-inch boards for which even the otherwise useless spruce timber from the lowland forests might be used. How profitable it might be to ship greater lengths can be seen from the experience of Skien whose long deals fetch prices quite out of proportion to their length although the quality of their wood is not anywhere near the same as that from the Laurvig sawmills...

[Fabricius continues to make suggestions about the most suitable cuts for the London market.]

Finally, deals from our sawmills must be well finished off. The ends should be well charred, the surface should be smooth, and, above all, the thickness must be even throughout. Many places, and particularly Christiania and Drammen, have a better reputation here for their produce than Laurvig because deals are evenly sawn.

This is all I have been able to find out about timber shipped from Norway to England. There may possibly be some tricks of the trade that one does not get to know about unless one is a shipper oneself. These finer points could best be discovered by sending here a trial shipment which, if not too large, should involve one in neither much work nor any loss. I would certainly recommend taking that course. I shall, however, not let up pursuing my inquiries if my recommendation is not approved, and should be able to find out more next April when Norwegian timber-ships come again into London, though I might by then have obtained some further information by other means...

[*fo 10*. The report on the timber-trade concludes with a list of London timber-merchants and of London price-currents for Laurvig timber during the past season.]

PART 2

ON THE IRON-TRADE

[*fo 11*] A great amount of bar-iron is imported into England, and especially into London, not only from Sweden, but also from Russia and Spain. Some comes from Norway, but so far not in as large quantities as from the other exporting countries.

Russian iron is bought in St Petersburg and other Russian towns by the agents of the Russia company, and shipped by them on their own account to England. It is not so well thought of as Swedish iron as it is regarded as being rather hard and cold-short.[1] Spanish iron is generally imported in Spanish ships. It is exceedingly soft and somewhat red-short, and can therefore not be satisfactorily worked without being blended with a harder iron.[2] It then gives a strong and tough grade of iron particularly suitable for anchors. The greatest quantity of iron imported, though, comes from Sweden. The organisation of the Swedish iron-trade is the same as that of the Norwegian timber-trade. The iron is either ordered in Sweden by English merchants on their own account, and carried by ships

[1] Cold-short iron is brittle in the cold state, and red-short iron brittle when red-hot and therefore hard to work.
[2] An English writer of the period differed from this opinion, and described Spanish iron as a hard iron. See Ashton, *Iron and Steel*, p. 238, n. 2.

they have themselves chartered, or it is sent to market here by the Swedes.

Most of the Swedish iron imported into London is shipped on English account. The reason for this is, that the merchants who contract to deliver iron to government departments, to the different trading companies and to other public concerns, are settled in this city and order what they require. The greatest consumption of iron for building and naval construction is in and around London, and London is therefore the best market in the whole of England. Trade to Bristol, Liverpool and Hull, which are next to London the best markets, is carried on more generally by Swedish merchants shipping on their own account. Shipments to London are generally from Stockholm and Öregrund, while to the outports they are mainly from Gothenburg.

Iron from Norway is mostly shipped from Frederikshald, Christiania, the Fargesund Customs Station, and from Ahrendahl. The greater part of the iron shipped from the first two ports is Swedish, but neither Swedish iron imported to England via Norway, nor Norwegian iron is regarded as being of such good quality as that from Stockholm and Öregrund which is preferred to all other.

The dimensions of Swedish iron bars shipped to the outports are not known to me, but I have seen for myself, or have it on good authority, that Swedish iron is imported into London as round, square, and flat bars. The dimensions of each sort may be seen from the appended list on which I have also noted the forge marks of the most highly regarded makers. Norwegian iron shipped to London consists largely of flat bars 2 to $2\frac{1}{2}$ inches wide and $\frac{1}{2}$ inch thick. It comes mainly from the Fossum, Bolwig, Eegeland, Hassel and Dinnemarken works, and passes in England, together with Swedish [*fo 12*] iron shipped via Norway, through the hands of Norwegian agents living here who accept it on the same terms as timber...[Fabricius then repeats information on the handling of timber already noted above. In the following paragraph, he mentions that iron is always quoted by the ton; gives the current duties on iron; and notes incidental charges borne by the shipper which are identical with those encountered in the timber-trade.]

Freight for iron shipped from Stockholm and nearby ports has to the best of my knowledge during the present war been 30*s.* the ton, and from Gothenburg generally 23*s.* the ton. Freights from Norway have been lower as the amount of iron ordinarily carried from there in any one ship is no greater than what can be stowed conveniently among its main cargo of timber; freights can therefore be obtained at 18*s.* to 19*s.* the ton. As to agent's commission, the course of exchange, and insurance premiums, I wish to refer to my earlier observations on the timber-trade, as these are the same for both iron and timber excepting only insurance from Stockholm which is likely to be higher by ¾% to 1% than from Norway.

Iron from different countries is regarded as being of different quality, and prices reflect this belief. Spanish iron is held to be the worst. It is hard to work unless blended with other grades, and its price is therefore the lowest, having been last summer [1758] only £15 to £16 the ton. Russian iron is meant to be somewhat better, but too hard. It can be made more malleable by blending. Its price [*fo 13*] has generally been £16 to £17 the ton. The Norwegian iron which has so far been imported is also not very highly regarded, and brought last summer £17 10*s.* to £18 the ton. I know of one instance when Councillor Löwenskiold's iron was sold last October for £17 11*s.*, but £18 may generally be obtained when three months' credit is given. Some of the Swedish iron is in no better repute than Norwegian, particularly that shipped via Norway, and some of the Gothenburg shipments. Most of the iron coming from Stockholm and Öregrund, however, is meant to be of better quality than any other, and has therefore with the best Gothenburg iron brought last summer £19 to £23 the ton, the price within that range depending on the shape into which it had been forged.

The price difference between Swedish and Norwegian iron is due to the strong preference given to the former which is so marked that the Admiralty will not accept any of the latter for government dockyards. I have enquired into it among iron-merchants and in particular among smiths who, I found, are absolutely convinced that Norwegian iron is far too hard, and that most of it is cold-short; also, that it requires more stone-coal for working than Swedish iron, and loses more by oxidation. Shipwrights and sailors further insist that Norwegian iron can be proved by experiment to be far more magnetic than any other, and their fear of it affecting the compass will hardly allow it to be used in ship's work. I regret that I have not enough knowledge of mineralogy to say whether this can be so, or whether there is some other explanation.

I must admit that the Swedish iron I have myself seen here, particularly that of Stockholm and Öregrund, has generally been smoother and more accurately worked than Laurvig bars which are in those respects better than most other Norwegian iron I have seen. Despite the insistence in England that the above-noted bad characteristics are more prevalent in Norwegian than in Swedish iron, I hardly think this the case . . .

[*fo 14.* In a concluding paragraph, Fabricius asks that iron samples from Laurvig should be sent with the next timber shipment. He had arranged with an iron-merchant to have them thoroughly tested, and hoped that a market would be found. Iron would show a profit even if only £18 were obtained, and this should be borne in mind if iron prices in Norway and Copenhagen were to fall. The tests to be made on Laurvig iron might show that it had none of the faults imputed to Norwegian iron, or, if it did indeed have any, advice could be obtained on how to remedy them. Appended to the report is a table giving the dimensions of the best Swedish bar-iron seen by Fabricius in London. Round-iron was from $\frac{3}{4}$ to $1\frac{1}{2}$ inches in diameter; square bars measured from 2 to 9 inches square in section; and flat bars were 7 to 12 inches wide, and $\frac{3}{8}$ to $\frac{3}{4}$ inches thick. Eighty different dimensions for square and flat bars are listed. The forge marks of fifteen makers are also noted.]

Appendix 5: The emigration of British workers to Scandinavia

The loss to English as much as the gain to foreign manufacture by the emigration of skilled workers led in 1719 to the first of a series of Acts[1] to prevent their settling abroad. Both Denmark, Norway and Sweden recruited British artisans, and Titley noted in 1737 that the Danish Board of Trade (Kommerskollegium) employed agents in England for the purpose. One such recruiting agent was a ribbon-weaver, Wilkins. He brought to Copenhagen a whole boat-load of silk-workers, who had been told that they were to be taken to Yorkshire. Wilkins had been assisted in England by one Becket, 'a man of some Substance', who was given a royal pension for his part in the affair. Several of the silk-weavers called on Titley in Copenhagen and asked for his help in returning to England. Another group of woollen-workers who had been 'deluded' by one William Dyke into coming to Denmark later made the same request, and Titley intended to pay their passage home out of his own pocket.[2] The Board of Trade in London was already concerned over the drain of workers to Denmark where several woollen mills and brass foundries had been staffed with them,[3] and the Attorney-General was instructed to report on means to stop further losses of artisans to Denmark.[4] He replied that workers did not leave the country on their own initiative, but through abduction or when led by agents promising high wages. The only available remedy lay in a stricter application of the law against 'seducing' them.[5]

[1] 5 Geo. I, c. 27, 'Act to prevent the Inconveniences arising from seducing Artificers in the Manufactures of Great Britain into Foreign Parts'.
[2] B.M., Egerton MS 2695, Titley papers, diary, entries of 14 August and 16 September 1737.
[3] P.R.O., S.P. 75/137, Board of Trade reports on manufactures in Denmark, 17 December 1736 and 5 October 1737.
[4] Ibid., S.P. 44/129, Harrington (Northern Secretary of State] to Attorney-General, 25 October 1737.
[5] Ibid., S.P. 75/137, report of Attorney-General, 2 November 1737.

As the existing Act was ineffectual in preventing the emigration of artisans, the remedy was seen in 1750 in passing another Act providing for greater penalties.[1] Yet within three years, Titley had to report that three London glass-blowers were petitioning the king of Denmark for permission to erect a glass-works in Denmark. They would bring with them the necessary equipment and capital if they were given a monopoly of manufacture. Titley had intercepted the man who was to present their petition, but knew that sooner or later it would reach the king and be granted. Newcastle, he hoped, would be able to stop their desertion.[2] Titley's vigilance was to no effect. In a despatch of 1760 he noted that the 'Manufacture of Ordinary Glass, set up some years ago in Norway, was chiefly supplied with Hands from England', and a week later gave the news of an edict of which he had just heard, prohibiting the import of glass into Norway as the factory there could supply all the demand for it. That new prohibition, he reported, affected only England, which alone had supplied Norway with glass.[3]

At least some of the English workers in the Norwegian glass-works had been recruited by one Morten Waern, who came to England in 1754 to study crystal-glass manufacture.[4] He was arrested when found to be arranging passage to Norway for seven craftsmen, fined £3,500, and imprisoned in Newgate until he could pay the fine.[5] The Danish envoy, Rantzau, interceded for him with Newcastle, but had no success. Rantzau's secretary, Hanneken, then took the matter in hand. He engaged a lawyer who found 'six necessitous Englishmen of easy conscience' prepared to swear for a consideration that they each possessed £1,000, and would stand bail for Waern in that sum. Waern was released, and fled to France. The lawyer hoped to repeat the manoeuvre for the glass-workers themselves who also had been imprisoned. The commotion was great when Waern's flight was discovered, but by then, Hanneken

[1] 23 Geo. II c. 13, 'Act for the Effectual punishing of Persons convicted of seducing Artificers in the Manufactures of Great Britain or Ireland out of the Dominions of the Crown'.
[2] P.R.O., S.P. 75/96, Titley to Newcastle, 17 November 1753.
[3] P.R.O., S.P. 75/109, Titley to Holdernesse, 29 March and 8 April 1760.
[4] A. Polak, 'English connections in Norway's old glass-industry', *Apollo* (July 1952).
[5] Dan. S. Arch., T.K.U.A., Engl. B, 105, Rantzau to Bernstorff, 22 August 1755

concluded his reports, he had already shipped another group of seven to Norway, of whom the authorities had not known.[1]

English artisans were even taken as far afield as the Danish West Indies, to which, it was reported, they 'had been seduced from England by one Skerrit, conveyed to the Island of St Croix claimed by the Crown of Denmark and detained there'.[2] Cosby, Titley's assistant at Copenhagen in 1764 and 1765, gave this verdict on Danish efforts to establish manufactures with English workers: the Danes, he wrote, 'are extremely intent on the Establishment of Manufactures here and spend very large sums with this in view but hitherto without much success, for all the Articles they make are so extremely dear and Bad that they wou'd not be consum'd if it was not for the strict prohibition of importing goods...Instead of encouraging the breeding of Cattle and Agriculture the natural sources of wealth to this Country which are at the lowest Ebb they give their whole attention to debauching Artisans from England which for many reasons can never answer.'[3]

Sweden was interested both in obtaining artisans and in getting her own craftsmen to discover manufacturing secrets in England itself. Wynantz, the Swedish chargé d'affaires in London until 1758, was given instructions accordingly. He was to recruit English workers[4] and to assist Swedish artisans working in England who were paid an allowance by their government. A Swedish shipwright was actually imprisoned after he had attracted attention by making models of warships, and was examined by the Secretary of State himself. He was finally released, and Wynantz arranged for him to return to Sweden.[5] Swedish ordnance-workers, who had already travelled in Germany and France, were in England between at

[1] Dan. S. Arch., T.K.U.A., Engl. B, 105, Hanneken to Bernstorff, 22 August and 26 September 1755. Own translations. The magistrate who had allowed bail was accused of having been too lenient, lost his appointment, and later migrated to Denmark or Norway. See *ibid.*, 108, Bothmer to Bernstorff, 19 June 1758.

[2] Journal of Commissioners for Trade and Plantations, 1764–7. Letter from governor of the Leeward Islands, read on December 1753.

[3] P.R.O., S.P. 75/118, Cosby to Sandwich, 23 February 1765.

[4] Swed. S. Arch., Diplomatica, Anglica I, Kanslikollegium to Wynantz, 1 August 1757.

[5] *Ibid.*, Wynantz to Kanslipresidenten, 21 January 1755, 12 July and 19 August 1757.

least 1749 and 1756 and drew their allowance from Wynantz.[1] On other occasions, Wynantz was asked to help some Swedish artisans to obtain information on metal-casting[2] and to assist an English miner who had returned to recruit friends for employment in Sweden.[3]

English workers in Sweden were numerous. The well-known English ironmaster, Samuel Garbett, reported in 1764 that the Swedes were constantly trying with success to entice workers and also manufacturers to settle in their country.[4] Garbett's partner, John Roebuck, set himself to watch such moves, and could soon give detailed information on a group of workers under a foreman, who were to leave for Gothenburg with foundry equipment.[5] He was thanked for his information, which had led to immediate action being taken against their leaving the country.[6] A while later, Roebuck was asked to get information on a suspected scheme involving another group of iron-workers and equipment. The scheme, he reported,[7] was indeed afoot, and the man behind it was the naturalist, Dr Solander: 'his address is the British Museum, Bloomsbury Square, London'.

[1] *Ibid.*, Brev till W. från Kanslikollegium o.a., Krigskollegium to Wynantz, 18 July 1749, 23 July 1755 and 22 March 1756.
[2] *Ibid.*, Manufakturkontoret to Wynantz, 26 June 1755.
[3] *Ibid.*, Manufakturkontoret to Wynantz, 2 April 1757.
[4] Calendar of Home Office Papers, 1760–5, pp. 420f., entry 1359, Garbett to Stanhope, 26 June 1764.
[5] *Ibid.*, pp. 414f., entry 1339, John Roebuck to [?], 2 June 1764.
[6] *Ibid.*, p. 417, entry 1347, Lovell Stanhope [Under-Secretary, Northern Department] to Roebuck, 6 June 1764.
[7] *Ibid.*, p. 517, entry 1818, Stanhope to Roebuck, 3 July 1765, and p. 601, entry 1919, Jas Farquharson (for Roebuck) to William Burke, 19 July 1765.

Bibliography

MANUSCRIPT SOURCES

A. PUBLIC RECORD OFFICE, LONDON

(*a*) *State Papers, Foreign:*

Denmark, ref. S.P. 75, vols 93 to 118 (1750–65) and vol. 137 (supplementary).

Volumes 93 to 103, 105, 106, 109, 112, 114, 116, 117, and 137 contain instructions to and despatches from British envoys to Denmark–Norway; consular reports; miscellaneous papers; and intelligence reports on Sweden. Volumes 104, 107, 108, 110, 111, 113, and 115 contain instructions to and despatches from Sir John Goodricke, British envoy to Sweden; intelligence reports; miscellaneous papers; and information on the abortive mission to Sweden of Colonel Campbell in 1757.

Sweden, ref. S.P. 95, vols 102, 103, 106 to 108, 133, and 134 (1750–80).

Intelligence reports from Sweden on internal politics, privateering, and trade; miscellaneous papers.

Foreign entry books, ref. S.P. 104, vols 8 and 9 (1761–3)

Précis books of letters received and sent by Secretaries of State, Northern Department. The entries are not complete.

News letters, ref. S.P. 101, vol. 93

Intelligence reports from Sweden, and miscellaneous papers. 1761–3.

Foreign Ministers in England, ref. S.P. 100, vols 1, 65 and 70

Memorials, and answers to them, from Danish and Swedish envoys in England.

Royal letters, ref. S.P. 102, vols 5 and 6 (Denmark), and vol. 57 (Sweden).

Correspondence between the British, and Danish and Swedish royal families

Treaties, ref. S.P. 108, bundles 35 and 518.

Anglo-Danish treaty of 1670, and Anglo-Swedish treaty of 1661. Originals.

Archives, Denmark, ref. S.P. 105, vol. 1.

Transcripts for use of Sir John Goodricke of Journal of Swedish Diet, 1760–2, and of the resolutions of the Diet's Secret Committee. The transcripts were obtained through intelligence agents, and a comparison of extracts with the originals in the Swedish State Archives showed no discrepancies.

Various, ref. S.P. 109, vols 68 to 76.

Précis books of correspondence by Departments of State, 1756–64.

Supplementary, ref. S.P. 110, vol. 85.

Under-Secretaries' entry books, Northern Department, 1760–6. Contain précis letters of informal nature to Titley.

Hamburg and Hansa Towns, ref. S.P. 82, vol. 79 (1762).

Intelligence reports on Denmark and Sweden by British agent in Hamburg.

Russia, ref. S.P. 91, vols 62, 65 and 66 (1756–8).

Reports on Danish and Swedish policy by British envoy to Russia.

Holland, ref. S.P. 84, vol. 507 (1765).

Reports on contraband trade.

(*b*) *State Papers, Domestic:*

George III, ref. S.P. 37, vol. 16.

Trade report on Denmark–Norway.

Secretaries' letter books, ref. S.P. 44, vols 129 (1737), and 134 to 139 (1749–71). These volumes are indexed in manuscript (contemporary), Ind. 8913.

Economic information through letters to and from Secretaries of State.

Naval, Orders in Council, ref. S.P. 42, vol. 140 (1756–82).

Contraband trade and neutral rights.

(*c*) *Foreign Office Records*

Great Britain and General, ref. F.O. 83, Law Officers' Reports, vol. 2279.

Reports on neutral rights in Seven Years War.

King's letter books, ref. F.O. 90, vols 8 to 10 (Denmark) and vols 66 and 67 (Sweden).

Ministerial and consular patents and instructions, and credentials and revocations of foreign envoys.

(*d*) *Admiralty Records*

Secretary's Department, in-letters, ref. Ad. 1, letters from consuls, vols 3833 to 3836.

Intelligence reports and some scattered information on trade, 1751–67.

Ibid., letters from Custom House, vol. 3866.

Information on smuggling from Scandinavia, 1757–80. Neutral rights, 1748–67.

Ibid., letters from Secretaries of State, vols 4120 to 4126.

Neutral rights; consular letters from Norway referred to Admiralty; orders to fleets.

Ibid., Secret letters, vol. 4352.

Intelligence and commercial reports.

Secretary's Department, out-letters, ref. Ad. 2, Secret Orders and Letters, vols 1331 and 1332.

Neutral rights and contraband trade 1745–78.

(*e*) *High Court of Admiralty Records*

Sentences in Prize Cases, ref. H.C.A. 34, vols 37, 40 and 42.

Records of Danish and Swedish ships that had been taken prize, 1756–63.

f) *Colonial Office Records*

Original correspondence, Board of Trade, ref. C.O. 388, vols 46 to 55, and vol. 95 (1754–66).

Surveys of Anglo-Danish trade, and miscellaneous economic information.

Board of Trade, entry books, ref. C.O. 389, vols 30 and 31 (1739–67).

Information on Anglo-Swedish trade.

Board of Trade, statistics, ref. C.O. 390, Custom House receipts, vol. 9.

Statistics on Anglo-Scandinavian trade.

Board of Trade, minutes, ref. C.O. 391, vols 62 to 72.

Information on trade, particularly in the last volume.

(g) *Board of Trade Papers*

Miscellania, ref. B.T. 6, vol. 185.

An annotated copy (contemporary) of Whitworth's *State of the Trade of Great Britain in its imports and exports* (see below, 'Contemporary Works').

(h) *Custom and Excise Records*

Ledgers of imports and exports, England (customs ledgers), ref. Cust. 3, vols 50 to 70.

Trade statistics, 1750–70.

Ledgers of imports and exports, Scotland (customs ledgers), ref. Cust. 14, vol. 1*a* and 1*b*.

Trade statistics for Scotland, 1755–70.

(i) *Chancery Masters' Exhibits*

Jackson v. Nemes, ref. C. 104, bundles 141–5 (unsorted).

Letter books and accounts of the Russia merchant William Heath, who also traded to Denmark. 1726–70.

(j) *Treasury Papers*

African Companies, ref. T. 70, Accounts, vol. 1205.

Contains some information on trade with Scandinavia.

Miscellania various, ref. T. 64, vols 276*a* and 276*b*. These volumes are indexed in manuscript, Ind. Engl. 3. T. 49.

Returns of imports and exports of special commodities.

(k) *Court of Bankruptcy Records*

Order Books, ref. B. 1, vol. 39 (1761–2).

Entry of bankruptcy of the London agent of the Swedish State Bank.

(*l*) *Exchequer Papers*

King's Remembrancer, port books, ref. E. 90, vols 366, 368, 370, 373, 375.

Port books of Hull, 1748–66.

(*m*) *Gifts and Deposits*

Chatham papers, ref. P.R.O. 30/8, bundles 20, 40, 51, 80, and 88.

Letters and memoranda from and on Denmark and Sweden.

B. BRITISH MUSEUM, LONDON

Egerton MSS 2694 and 2695.

Titley papers, correspondence and diary.

Egerton MS 2696.

Gunning papers. Reports on Danish trade.

Egerton MS 1755.

Bentinck papers. Correspondence from Titley and Goodricke.

Additional MSS 6805, 6806, 6807, 6812, 6814, 6815, 6817, and 6829.

Mitchell papers. Correspondence of Titley and Goodricke with Mitchell and Holdernesse.

Additional MSS 35425, 35480, 35482, 35483, 35484, and 35485.

Hardwicke papers. Correspondence of Titley and Goodricke with Lord Hardwicke, Sir Robert Keith and others. Reports on Swedish trade.

Additional MS 15956.

Anson papers. Assessment of danger from a combined Danish–Swedish fleet.

Additional MS 14035.

Board of Trade papers. Danish and Swedish trade.

Additional MS 38387.

Liverpool papers. Trade with Norway.

Additional MSS 32824, 32825, 32846, 32848, 32849, 32851, 32855, 32864, 32876, 32877, 32889, 32896, 32897, 32935, and 32936.

Newcastle papers. Correspondence, reports, and Cabinet memoranda on the Scandinavian powers.

c. CAMBRIDGE UNIVERSITY LIBRARY, MSS DEPARTMENT
(On temporary deposit)

Minutes of the Russia Company, 1734–56, and *ibid.*, 1756–78.
Accounts of the Russia Company, 1734–83.

Information by British consuls in Denmark, on British merchants, on trade, and finance.

d. CUSTOM HOUSE, KING'S LYNN

Letter books, 1754–66.

Timber and iron tallies.

Customs organisation, trade, and smuggling.
Ship-movements and cargoes.

e. DANISH STATE ARCHIVES (*Rigsarkivet*), COPENHAGEN

Tyske Kancellis Udenlandske Afdeling, Special Del. (abbreviated T.K.U.A., Sp. Del.) England B, Gesandtskabs-Relationer, bundles 103–14.

Despatches and private letters from Danish envoys and consuls in England 1752–65.

T.K.U.A., Sp. Del., England C, Gesandtskab-Arkiver, bundles 260–7, and 274.

Instructions to envoys in England; legation archives; drafts of despatches; consular papers; reports on trade, shipping and neutral rights; letters patent.

T.K.U.A., Sp. Del., Frankrig B, Gesandtskabs-Relationer fra Grev Wedel-Friis, 1758. Bundle 103.

Despatches and papers from Danish envoy in France on diplomatic issues and neutral rights.

T.K.U.A., Sp. Del., Frankrig A II, bundle 17, Akter og Dokumenter vedr. det politiske Forhold til Frankrig, 1757 to 1770.

Diplomacy, finance, and neutral rights.

T.K.U.A., Sp. Del., Rusland B, Gesandtskabs-Relationer, bundles 85 and 86.

Despatches from Danish envoy at St Petersburg on his relations with the British envoy there.

T.K.U.A., Sp. Del., Rusland C, Gesandtskabs-Arkiv, bundles 172 and 174.

Instructions to Danish envoy in Russia and his correspondence with envoys in England and France.

T.K.U.A., Sp. Del., England A
II, bundle 30.

Trade and financial relations with England, and intercepted despatches, 1752–69.

T.K.U.A., Sp. Del., England A,
II, bundle 31 *b*.

Consular correspondence from Great Britain.

T.K.U.A., Sp. Del., England A,
III, bundles 42 and 43.

Correspondence and documents on Danish–Norwegian ships brought up by British warships and privateers, and on British ships taken into Norwegian harbours by French privateers, 1732–64.

T.K.U.A., Almendilig Afdeling,
bundle 430.

Martin Hübner's letters from England on trade and neutral rights to Bernstorff, and instructions to him.

T.K.U.A., Almendilig Afdeling,
Realia og Handelssager, bundle
428.

Trade with Great Britain.

Danske Kancelli, Indlaeg til
Vestindiske Sager.

Trade of Danish colonies with England.

General Told Kammer, Relationer og Resolutioner ang. Vestindien og Guinea, 1760–5.

As above.

Rentekammerets Vestindisk-Guinisk Renteskriver-Kontor:
Kongelige Resolutioner vedr. Vestindien og Guinea, 1759–60, bundles 154–8.

As above, and including papers on smuggling, and on finance.

Rentekammeret, Københavns Civiletats-kontors Kopiprotokoll, 1748–50, and 1750–2.

Commercial information.

Rentekammeret, Kopiprotokoll for Aalborg og Viborg Stifters Kontor, 1756–8.

Commercial information.

Rentekammerets Relations og Resolutionsprotokoll (Dansk) 1757.

Commercial information.

Rentekammerets Relations og Resolutionsprotokol, Norsk, 1758.

Trade with Norway, and finance.

Generalmagasinet, 1760, nr. 633, 36.

Report on British imports into Norway.

Asiatisk Kompagni, Inden- og Udenlandske Breves Copie-Bog, 1753-9.	Trade with Denmark–Norway, and movements of bills of exchange.
Admiralitets og General-kommissariets Collegium, Kongelige Resolutioner, 1760-2.	Neutral rights.
Protocol over de fra Sø-Etatens Kriegs-Cancellie expederede Kongelige Resolutioner, Patenter, og Ordres. (For years 1759-60, and 1760-1.)	Neutral rights.
Søetatens Generalkrigsretsager 1762, Protocol og Documenter; Sagen Søkrigsprokurøren med Kommandørkaptejn H. L. Fisker, 1762.	Neutral rights.
Sundtoldsreignskaber, 1761-3.	Sound Toll Registers.

F. PROVINCIAL ARCHIVES FOR SJAELLAND (*Landsarkivet for Sjaelland m. v.*), COPENHAGEN

Notarial Protokoller (For the years 1749-77).	Trade, and movements of bills of exchange.

G. DANISH BUSINESS ARCHIVES (*Erhversvsarkivet i Aarhus*), AARHUS

Kiøbenhauns Grossereres Protokol, 1759-74.	Reports on the course of British bills of exchange.

H. DANISH ROYAL LIBRARY (*Kongelige Bibliothek*), COPENHAGEN

Wasserschleben Arkiv, Nye kgl. Samling, no 700.	Currency exchange rates, Denmark–Norway and England.

I. THE PRIVATE ARCHIVES OF THE COUNTS MOLTKE AT BREGENTVED CASTLE, SJAELLAND, DENMARK

These Archives are not open to search, and an exception was made in this case. They yielded valuable information through letters to Count Adam Gottlob Moltke from Titley and others, and through Count Moltke's preserved draft replies. Official papers were also found and threw much light on commercial matters. The various MSS used are cited in footnotes.

War and Trade in Northern Seas

J. SWEDISH STATE ARCHIVES (*Riksarkivet*), STOCKHOLM

Diplomatica, Anglica I; Svenska sändebuds skrivelser till K. M:T, Kommissionssekretareren Arnold Wynantz' brev till Kanslipresidenten, 1747–58. (9 volumes and bundles).

> Despatches from Swedish chargé d'affaires to President of the Chancery (i.e. chief minister). These are very full, and often informal.

Ibid., Brev till Kanslikollegium, 1748–58 (8 volumes and bundles).

> Despatches to the Chancery (council of ministers), complementing the above, particularly on trade matters.

Ibid., Wynantz' Koncept, 1748–58 (14 bundles).

> Drafts of despatches, and memoranda.

Ibid., Brev till Wynantz från kanslipresidenten och kanslitjaenstemaen, 1747–58 (1 bundle).

> Instructions, and miscellaneous documents.

Ibid., Brev till Wynantz från kanslikollegium och andra ämbetsverk i Sverige, 1747–58 (1 bundle).

> Instructions, generally on trade matters and neutral rights.

Ibid., Brev till Wynantz från svenska beskickningar och konsuler (1 bundle).

> Letters from Swedish envoys and consuls, generally on trade.

Ibid., Brev till Wynantz från myndigheter och enskilda samt strödda beskickningshandlingar.

> Letters on commercial matters.

Diplomatica, Anglica II, Strödda Handlingar. Handlingar ang. Kaperier (1 bundle).

> Trade, and neutral rights.

Diplomatica, Hollandica I, Brev till Preis från svenska beskickningar från London (1 bundle).

> Correspondence of Wynantz with Swedish envoy in Holland.

Utrikes Expeditions Registratur, 1756 (1 bundle).

> Trade and neutral rights.

Ämnesserier: Handel och Sjöfart. Ser. II, Handlingar rörande Utrikeshandel, nr 9 (1 bundle).

> Trade with Great Britain. Rich in commercial correspondence.

Ibid., ser. III, Handlingar rörande handeln i allmänhet. nr 26 (1 bundle).

> Trade and neutral rights.

Enskilda Samlingar: Arkivfrag-ment: Arkivbildare: Kommer-seråd Frans Jennings Corre-spondance.

Merchants' letters and accounts.

K. LUND UNIVERSITY LIBRARY. MSS DEPARTMENT

De la Gardieska Samlingen: Historiska Handlingar: Adolf Fredrik de la Gardie: Oecono-mica: Jämförelse mellan sven-ska Ostindiska kompaniet och utlandska innrättningar af sam-ma slag, 1757.

Comparison of Swedish with English financial practice.

L. GOTHENBURG PROVINCIAL ARCHIVES (*Landsarkivet i Göteborg*), GOTHENBURG

Göteborgs Stads Räkenskap Bö-ker m.d. Verificationer, 1725, 1750, 1775.

Gothenburg port books.

M. UPPSALA UNIVERSITY LIBRARY, MSS DEPARTMENT

MS F. 367. Neutralitet till Sjös: Baron Ungern-Sternbergs bref-vexsling, 1756–60.

Official despatches not in the State Archives, drafts of des-patches, and private letters from Swedish envoy to Den-mark on the Armed Neutrality and neutral rights. Also, re-ports on his conversations with Goodricke.

MS F. 386: Brev till Sir John Goodricke.

A collection of private letters to Goodricke from Newcastle, Hardwicke, Holdernesse, Brit-ish envoys and others. This collection had been bought in England at a private sale.

N. NORWEGIAN STATE ARCHIVES (*Riksarkivet*), OSLO

Serie Localia: Hedrum, Holme-strand, Lardal, Larvik.

Anglo-Norwegian trade.

Serie Privatarkiver; nr 65: Lauritz Smith Kopibøker 1740–4, and 1755–66.

Copy-books of correspondence and accounts of an Anglo-Norwegian merchant trading with England.

Serie Privatarkiver; nr 67: James Bowman, Porsgrund 1707–39.

Copy-books and miscellaneous papers of an English merchant trading from southern Norway mainly with England.

Serie Personalia, nr 38. a. 2, Thomas Fearnley.

Copy-book of an English merchant in Norway, 1753–69, containing his own copies of about 1,000 business and private letters, memoranda and accounts.

Serie Toldbøger; Bergen. 1756, 1760, 1763.

Bergen port books.

O. BERGEN CITY ARCHIVES (*Statsarkivet i Bergen*)

Byfoged og Byskriver i Bergen: Notarial protokoll nr 2, 1762–71.

Notarial archives, containing trade and financial information.

PRINTED SOURCES

A. TREATIES, AND CASE AND STATUTE LAW

(*a*) *Great Britain:*

An Abridgement of Penal Statutes...to 1786. Ed. W. Addington. 3rd ed., London, 1786.

British and Foreign State Papers, London, 1841–.

Historical Manuscripts Commission, House of Lords Manuscripts, New Series, 4, pp. 401ff., Anglo-Danish Treaty of 15 July 1701.

Reports of Cases determined by the High Court of Admiralty, 1758–1774, coll. Sir W. Burrell. Ed. R. G. Marsden. London, 1885.

Reports of Cases determined in the High Court of Admiralty, 1745–1859. Ed. E. S. Roscoe, vol. 1. London, 1905.

Prize Papers, Lords Commissioners of Prizes, Case of the Sankt Jacob: appellant's case and appendix, respondent's case and appendix, 1757.

Public Acts and Books of Rates, Charles II to George III.

(*b*) *Denmark–Norway:*

Danmark–Norges Traktater 1523–1750, med dertil hørende Aktstykker.
Ed. L. R. Laursen. Copenhagen, 1907–.

Danske Traktater. Udgivet paa Udenrigsministeriets Foranstaltning.
Copenhagen, 1882.

Chronologisk Register over Kongelige Forordninger og Aabne Breve, 1670–1775. Ed. J. H. Schou. Copenhagen, 1777–.

Rescripter, Resolutioner og Collegial-Breve for Kongeriget Norge. Ed.
J. A. S. Schmidt. Christiania, 1847–.

Kongelige Rescripter, Resolutioner og Collegial-Breve for Norge. Ed. F. A.
Wessel Berg. Christiania, 1841–.

*Kommercekollegiets, Rentekammerets og Generaltoldkammerets Ordres,
Missiver og Reskripter.* (These are preserved in the Danish State
Archives, and comprise edicts on commerce and trade not bound
in with the following.)

Kongelige Forordninger og Aabne Breve. In contemporary editions,
preserved in the Danish State Archives.

(*c*) *Sweden:*

Utdrag utur alle ifrån den 7 dec. utkomne publique handlingar. Ed. R. G.
Modée. Stockholm, 1742–.

*Svenskt Allmänt Författningsregister för Tiden från År 1522 till och med
År 1862.* Ed. N. H. Quiding. Stockholm, 1865.

Kungl. M:ts Förordningar. In contemporary editions, preserved in the
Swedish State Archives.

B. GOVERNMENTAL AND PARLIAMENTARY RECORDS, AND THE
LIKE

Calendar of Home Office Papers, 1760–5, London, 1878.
Journal of the Commissioners for Trade and Plantations, 1740–. London,
1932–.
Journals of the House of Commons.
Reports of the House of Commons.
The London Gazette.
*Tabeller over Skibsfart og Varetransport gennem Øresund 1661–1783, og
gennem Storebaelt 1701–1748.* Ed. N. E. Bang and K. Korst. Copen-
hagen, 1930–45.
Göteborgs Handel och Sjöfart 1637–1920. Historisk-Statistisk Översikt.
Ed. Ivan Lind. Gothenburg, 1923.

War and Trade in Northern Seas

Tableau des Droits et Usages de Commerce relatifs au Passage du Sund.
Ed. T. A. de Marien. Copenhagen, 1776.
Saxby, H. *The British Customs.* London, 1757.

C. NEWSPAPERS

Gentleman's Magazine, 1753.
Lloyd's Evening Post, 1759.
Whitehall Evening Post, 1759.
London Chronicle, 1762.

D. AUTOBIOGRAPHICAL RECORDS AND EDITED DIPLOMATIC DESPATCHES

Asseburg, Freiherr A. F. v. der. *Denkwürdigkeiten.* Berlin, 1842.
Bernstorffsche Papiere. Ed. Aa. Friis. Copenhagen, 1904–13.
Bernstorff. *En Brevvexling mellem Grev J. H. E. Bernstorff og Hertugen af Choisoul.* Ed. P. Vedel. Copenhagen, 1871.
 Correspondance Ministerielle du Comte J. H. E. Bernstorff. Ed. P. Vedel. Copenhagen, 1882.
British Diplomatic Instructions: Denmark, 1689–1789. Ed. J. F. Chance. Camden Soc. Publication. London, 1926.
British Diplomatic Instructions: Sweden, 1721–1789. Ed. J. F. Chance. London, 1928.
Buckingham, John, Earl of. *Despatches and Correspondence from the Court of Catherine II of Russia, 1762–1765.* Camden Soc. Publication. London, 1900–2.
Grafton, Augustus, Duke of. *Autobiography.* Ed. Sir W. Anson. London, 1898.
Historical MSS Commission, 10th Report, App. 1: Weston-Underwood MSS London, 1885.
 11th Report, App. 7: Duke of Leeds MSS. London, 1883.
Höpken, A. J. von. *Skrifter.* Ed. C. Silfverstolpe. Stockholm, 1890–3.
Keith, Sir Robert Murray. *Memoirs and Correspondence.* Ed. Mrs. Gillespie Smith. London, 1849.
Lynar Graf R. F. zu. *Hinterlassene Staatsschriften und andre Aufsätze.* Hamburg, 1793–7.
 Zur Geschichte der nordischen Politik im achtzehnten Jahrhundert. Oldenburg, 1873.
Rapport de la Légation de France à Copenhague, Correspondance Consulaire Relatifs à la Norvège, 1670–1791. Ed. O. A. Johnsen, vol. 1, *1670–1748*, Oslo, 1934. [I am grateful to Professor Johnsen for having allowed me to consult the unpublished MS of vol. 2.]

Recueil des Instructions Données aux Ambassadeurs et Ministres de France.
Vol. 2: *Suède*, ed. A. Geffroy. Paris, 1885. Vol. 8; *Russie*, ed. A. Rambaud. Paris, 1890. Vol. 13; *Danemark*, ed. A. Geffroy. Paris, 1895.
Waldegrave, James, Earl of. *Memoirs from 1754 to 1758.* London, 1821.
Yorke, P. C. *Life and Correspondence of Philip Yorke, Earl of Hardwick.* Cambridge, 1913.

WORKS BY CONTEMPORARY OR NEAR-CONTEMPORARY AUTHORS ON TRADE, FINANCE, AND LAW

Baldwin, S. *A survey of the British customs.* London, 1770.
Beawes, W. *Lex mercatoria rediviva.* 2nd ed., London, 1761.
[Canzler, J. G.], *Mémoires pour servir à la Connaissance des Affaires Politiques et Economiques du Royaume de Suède jusqu'à la fin de la 1775ème année.* Londres [?], 1776.
Chalmers, G. *An Estimate of the comparative strength of Britain.* London, 1782.
Cross, A. L. (ed.). *Eighteenth Century Documents relating to the Royal Forests, the Sheriffs, and Smuggling: Selected from the Shelburne MSS in the William L. Clements Library.* New York, 1928.
Essay on the Increase and Decline of Trade in London and the Out-Ports. Anon. London, 1749.
Gee, J. *The Trade and Navigation of Great Britain Considered.* New ed., London, 1767.
Gunnell, W. A. (ed.). *Sketches of Hull Celebrities.* Hull, 1876.
Holberg, Ludvig, *Danmark og Norges Beskrivelse.* Copenhagen, 1729.
Hübner, Martin. *De la Saisie des Bâtimens Neutres.* The Hague, 1759.
Jars, M. C. *Voyages Métallurgiques,* vol. 1. Paris, 1774.
Liverpool, Charles Jenkinson, Earl of. *Discourse on the Conduct of the Government of Great Britain in respect of Neutral Nations.* 2nd ed., London, 1759.
McCulloch, J. R. *Dictionary... of Commerce and Commercial Navigation.* New ed., London, 1869.
McPherson, D. *Annals of Commerce, Manufactures, Fisheries and Navigation,* 4 vols. London, 1805.
Madison, James. *Examination of the British Doctrine which subjects to capture a Neutral Trade not open in time of war.* London, 1806.
Magens, N. *Essay on Insurances.* London, 1755.
[Magens, N.] *The Universal Merchant.* Translated by W. Horsley. London, 1753.

M[agens], N. *Farther Explanations of some particular subjects.* London, 1756.

M[allet], P. H. *Forme du Gouvernement de Suède.* Copenhagen and Genève, 1756.

Marriot, James. *The Case of the Dutch Ships Considered.* 2nd ed., London, 1759.

Oddy, J. J. *European Commerce...detailing the Produce and Manufactures of Russia, Prussia, Sweden, Denmark, and Germany.* London, 1805.

[Pontoppidan, E.] *Oeconomiske Balance eller Uforgribelige Overslag paa Danmarks naturlige og borgerlige Formue.* Copenhagen, 1759.

Postlethwayt, M. *Universal Dictionary of Trade and Commerce.* 4th ed., London, 1774.

Postlethwayt, M. *Great Britain's Commercial Interest Explained and Improved.* 2nd ed., London, 1759.

Pufendorf, Samuel von, *De Jure Naturae et Gentium.* (Carnegie Endowment edition.) London, 1934.

State of Trade in the Northern Colonies considered. Anon. London, 1749.

Stockley, E. *The earnest address of E. S....to the Legislature, for the Public Good.* Hungerford-Market, 1759.

Three Reports of the Select Committee appointed by the Court of Directors ..., on the Export trade...laid before...the Privy Council (n.d., n.p., [1793]). Pamphlet in Cambridge University Library, class mark Ddd. 25. 170.

Vattel, E. de. *Le Droit de Gens ou Principes de la Loi Naturelle.* (Carnegie Endowment edition.) Washington, 1916.

Warden, D. B. *On the Origin...Nature, Progress and Influence of Consular Establishments.* Paris, 1813.

[Whately, Thomas]. *Trade and Finances of the Kingdom.* London. 1766.

Whitworth, Sir Charles. *State of the Trade of Great Britain in its imports and exports.* London, 1776.

WORKS BY LATER AUTHORS

A. GENERAL

The works listed in this section deal mainly with politics, diplomacy, war, institutions and law. Works dealing more specifically with economic affairs are listed separately in section B.

Adair, E. R. *The Exterritoriality of ambassadors in the sixteenth and seventeenth centuries.* London, 1926–9.

Albion, R. G. *Forests and Sea Power – the Timber Problem of the Royal Navy, 1652–1862.* Harvard, 1926.

Anderson, R. C. *Naval Wars in the Baltic in the Sailing-Ship Epoch, 1522–1850.* London, 1910.

Arnheim, F. 'Beiträge zur Geschichte der nordischen Frage in der zweiten Hälfte des 18. Jahrhunderts', *Deutsche Zeitschrift für Geschichtswissenschaft*, 2, 5 and 8. 1889, 1891, and 1892.

Atherley-Jones, L. *Commerce in War.* London, 1907.

Barthélemy, E. de. *Histoire des relations de la France et du Danemarc sous le ministère du Comte de Bernstorff, 1751–1770.* Copenhagen, 1887.

Basye, A. H. *The Lords Commissioners of Trade and Plantations, 1748–1782.* New Haven, 1925.

Bayer, F. 'Fra Martin Hübners Rejseaar, 1752–1756', *Historisk Tidsskrift*, 7th series, 5. Copenhagen, 1904–5.

Bisschop, W. R. *The Rise of the London Money Market.* London, 1910.

Boye, Th. *De vaebnede Neutralitetsforbund.* Kristiania, n.d. [1912].

Brandt, O. 'Das Problem der Ruhe des Nordens im achtzehnten Jahrhundert', *Historische Zeitschrift [Sybel's]*, 140, 1929.

Bugge, A. and Steen, S. (eds). *Norsk Kulturhistorie*, vol. 3. Oslo, 1938.

Cannan, E., *see* Smith, Adam.

Carlquist, G. *Carl Frederick Scheffer och Sveriges politiska förbindelser med Danmark, åren 1752–1765.* Lund, 1920.

Chance, J. F. *George I and the Northern War, 1709–1721.* London, 1909.

'List of English Diplomatic Agents and Representatives in Denmark, Sweden and Russia, and of these Countries in England, 1689–1762' in Firth, C. H., *Notes on the Diplomatic Relations of England with the North of Europe.* Oxford, 1913.

The Alliance of Hanover, London. 1923.

Charteris, E. *William Augustus Duke of Cumberland.* London, 1913.

Cumberland and the Seven Years War. London, 1925.

Clark, G. N. *The Dutch Alliance and the War against French Trade, 1688–1697.* London, 1923.

'Neutral Commerce in the War of the Spanish Succession and the Treaty of Utrecht', *British Year Book of International Law, 1928*.

Conway, Sir Martin. *No Man's Land: A history of Spitsbergen.* Cambridge, 1906.

Corbett, J. S. *England in the Seven Years War.* 2 vols, London, 1907.

Cunningham, W. *The Growth of English Industry and Commerce.* Cambridge, 1882.

Dorn, W. L. 'Frederick the Great and Lord Bute', *Journal of Modern History*, 1, 1929.

War and Trade in Northern Seas

Dorn, W. L. *Competition for Empire, 1740–1763.* New York and London, 1940.

Eyck, E. *Pitt versus Fox.* London, 1950.

Fabricius, K. *Holland–Danmark, Forbindelser mellem de to Lande gennem Tiderne,* ed. Hammerich, L. L. and Lorenzen, V. 2 vols, Copenhagen, 1945.

Fayle, C. E. 'Deflection of Strategy by Commerce in the Eighteenth Century'. In *Royal United Services Journal,* 68. 1923.

Foster, G. J. *Doctors' Commons; its Courts and Registries.* London, 1868.

Friis, Aa. *Bernstorfferne og Danmark, 1750–1835.* 2 vols, Copenhagen, 1903–19.

Friis, Aa., Linvald, A., and Mackesprang, M. *Danmarks Historie,* vol. 3. Copenhagen, 1942.

Fulton, T. W. *The Sovereignty of the Sea.* London and Edinburgh, 1911.

Gerhard, D. *England und der Aufstieg Russlands.* Berlin, 1933.

Gidel, G. *Le Droit International Publique de la Mer.* vol. 3. Paris, 1934.

Hammerich, L. L. *see* Fabricius.

Hatt, G. *see* Vahl.

Hatton, R. M. 'Scandinavia and the Baltic', In *The New Cambridge Modern History,* vol. 7, ed. J. O. Lindsay. Cambridge, 1957.

Heckscher, E. F. *Mercantilism,* transl. M. Shapiro. 2 vols, London, 1935.

Hermann, E. 'Die Rolle der Seemächte in der Ostsee während des Siebenjährigen Krieges', *Marine Rundschau,* 45 (3 articles), Berlin, 1940.

Hildebrand, E. *see* below Stavenow.

Hill, C. E. *Danish Sound Dues and the Control of the Baltic.* Duke University Press, 1926.

Holm, E. *Danmark–Norges Historie under Frederik V, 1746–1766.* Copenhagen, 1897–8.

Horn, D. B. *Sir Charles Hanbury Williams and European Diplomacy, 1747–1758.* London, 1930.

(ed.) *British Diplomatic Representatives, 1689–1789,* Royal Hist. Soc., 1932.

Hovde, B. J. *The Scandinavian Countries, 1720–1865.* 2 vols, New York, 1948.

Jägerskiöld, O. *Hovet och Författningsfrågan, 1760–1766.* Uppsala, 1943.

Jensen, Hans. *Dansk–Norsk Vekselvirkning i det 18. Aarhundrede.* Copenhagen, 1936.

Jensen, Magnus. *Norges Historie fra 1660 till Våre Dager.* Oslo, 1949.

Jessup, P. C. *The Law of territorial waters and maritime jurisdiction.* New York, 1927.

Jessup, P. C., and others. *Neutrality, its History, Economica, and Law.* Vols 1 and 2. New York, 1935–6.

Johnsen, O. A. *Norges Historie*, vol. 5 (1746–1813). Kristiania, 1914.

Jørgensen, E. *Historieforskning og Historieskrivning i Danmark indtil Aar 1800.* Copenhagen, 1931.

Judges, A. V. 'The Idea of a Mercantile State', *Transactions, Royal Hist. Society*, 4th series, 21, 1939.

Kent, H. S. K. 'The Historical Origins of the Three-Mile Limit', *American Journal of International Law*, 48, 1954.
'The Background to Anglo-Norwegian Relations', *The Norseman*, 11, no. 3, 1953.

Kulsrud, C. J. *Maritime Neutrality to 1780.* Boston, 1936.

La Cour, V. *Mellem Brødre. Dansk–Norsk problemer i det 18. Aarhundredes Helstat.* Birkerød, 1943.

Lindsay, J. O. (ed.), *see* Hatton, R. M., *and* Robson, E.

Lindsay, J. O. *Trade and Peace with Old Spain, 1667–1750.* Cambridge, 1940.

Linvald, A., *see* Friis, Aa.

Lipson, E. *Economic History of England.* 2nd ed., London, 1934.

Lodge, Sir Richard. *Great Britain and Prussia in the Eighteenth Century.* Cambridge, 1923.

Lorenzen, V., *see* Fabricius, K.

Mackesprang, M., *see above*, Friis, Aa.

McLachlan, J. O. (Mrs J. O. Lindsay). 'The uneasy neutrality – a study of Anglo-Spanish disputes over Spanish ships prized', *Cambridge Hist. Journal*, 6. 1938.

Mahan, A. T. *The Influence of Sea Power on History, 1660–1783.* 12th ed., Boston, 1896.

Maiander, H. (ed.). *Sveriges historia genom tiderna.* Stockholm, 1947–8.

Malmström, C. G. *Sveriges Politiska Historia från Konung Karl XII.s Död till Statshvälfningen 1772*, vols 3–6 (1741–72). 2nd ed., Stockholm, 1893–1901.

Meyer, C. B. V. *The Extent of Jurisdiction in Coastal Waters.* Leiden, 1937.

Moffit, L. W. *England on the eve of the Industrial Revolution.* London, 1925.

Mootham, O. H., 'The Doctrine of Continuous Voyage, 1756–1815', *British Year Book of International Law, 1927.*

Namier, Sir Lewis. *The structure of politics at the accession of George III.* London, 1929.

Norrie, G. 'Felttoget i Mecklenburg 1762', *Historisk Tidsskrift*, 11th series, 6. Copenhagen, 1960–2.

223

War and Trade in Northern Seas

Olsen, A. *Danmark–Norge i det 18. Aarhundrede.* Copenhagen, 1936.
Pares, R. *War and Trade in the West Indies, 1739–1763.* Oxford, 1936.
Colonial Blockade and Neutral Rights 1739–1763. Oxford, 1938.
Piggott, Sir Francis. 'Sea Power, Armed Neutralities, and President Wilson', *The Nineteenth Century*, 81. 1917.
'Ship Timber and Neutrality', *Quarterly Review*, 236. 1921.
Raested, A. *Kongens Strømme; Historiske og folkeretlige undersøkelser angaaende sjøterritoriet.* Kristiania, 1912.
La mer territoriale – études historiques et juridiques. Paris, 1913.
Rashed, Z. E. *The Peace of Paris, 1763.* Liverpool, 1951.
Richmond, Sir Herbert. *Statesmen and Seapower.* Oxford, 1946.
Robson, E. 'The Seven Years War', *The New Cambridge Modern History*, vol. 7, ed. J. O. Lindsay. Cambridge, 1957.
Roscoe, E. S. *Lord Stowell: His Life and the Development of English Prize Law.* London, 1916.
A History of the English Prize Court. London, 1924.
Studies in the History of the Admiralty and Prize Courts. London, 1932.
Rydberg, S. *Svenska studieresor till England under frihetstiden.* Uppsala, 1951.
Satow, Sir Ernest. *The Silesian Loan and Frederick the Great.* Oxford, 1915.
A Guide to Diplomatic Practice. 2 vols, London, 1917.
Säve, Th. *Sveriges Deltaganda i Sjuåriga Kriget, Åren 1757–1762.* Stockholm, 1915.
Schäfer, A. *Geschichte des Siebenjährigen Krieges.* 3 vols, Berlin, 1867–1874.
Senior, W. *Doctors' Commons and the Old Courts of Admiralty.* London, 1922.
Smith, Adam. *The Wealth of Nations*, ed. E. Cannan. 2 vols, London, 1930.
Sprinchorn, C. 'Ett bidrag till den väpnade neutralitetens historia i norden'. *Historisk Tidskrift*, 1. Stockholm, 1881.
Stavenow, L. *Sveriges Historia till Våra Dager*, ed. Hildebrand and Stavenow, vol. 9, *Frihetstiden. 1718–1772.* Stockholm, 1922.
Steen, S., *see* Bugge.
Sutherland, L. S. 'The Law Merchant in England in the 17th and 18th centuries', *Transactions, Royal Hist. Society*, 4th series, 17, 1934.
Thomson, M. A. *The Secretaries of State, 1681–1782.* Oxford, 1932.
Trevelyan, G. M. *English Social History*, illustrated ed., vol. 3. London, 1951.
Turner, E. R. *The Privy Council, 1603–1784.* 2 vols, Baltimore, 1927–1928.

Vahl, M. and Hatt, G. *Jorden og Menneskeliv*, vol. 4. Copenhagen, 1927.
Vedel, P. *Den aeldre Grev Bernstorffs Ministerium*. Copenhagen, 1882.
Waddington, R. *La Guerre de Sept Ans*. 5 vols, Paris, 1899–.
Walker, Wyndham L. 'Territorial Waters: The Cannon Shot Rule.' *British Yearbook of International Law, 1945.*
Walpole, Horace. *Memoirs and Letters*, ed. Mrs P. Toynbee. 16 vols and supplement, London, 1903–26.
Ward, A. W. *Great Britain and Hanover. Some Aspects of the Personal Union.* Oxford, 1899.
Wiegner, M. *Die Kriegskonterbande in der Völkerrechtswissenschaft und der Staatenpraxis*. Berlin, 1904.
Williams, Basil. *William Pitt, Earl of Chatham*. 2 vols, London, 1913.
The Whig Supremacy, 1714–1760. Oxford, 1945.
Wilson, Charles. *England's Apprenticeship 1603–1763*. London, 1965.

B. ECONOMICA

Although some of the works in this section contain other matter, their use for this study has been mainly on questions of trade and finance.

Ashton, T. S. *Iron and steel in the industrial revolution*. 2nd ed., Manchester, 1951.
Ashton, T. S. and Sykes, J. *The Coal Industry of the Eighteenth Century*. Manchester, 1929.
Baasch, E. *Holländische Wirtschaftsgeschichte*. Jena, 1927.
Barnes, D. G. *A History of the English Corn Laws 1660–1846*. London, 1930.
Behre, Göran. 'Ostindiska Kompaniet och Hattarna. En storpolitisk episode 1742', *Historisk Tidskrift*, 2nd series, 29. Stockholm, 1966.
Beveridge, Sir William. *Prices and Wages in England*, vol. 1. London, 1939.
Bisgaard, H. L. *Den danske Nationaløkonomi i det 18. Aarhundrede*. Copenhagen, 1902.
Bobee, L. 'Den Grønlandske Handels og Kolonisations Historie indtil 1870', *Meddelelser om Grønland*, 55, no. 2. Copenhagen, 1936.
Brakel, S. van. 'Schiffsheimat und Schifferheimat in den Sundzoll-registern', *Hansische Geschichtsblätter*, 21. 1892.
Bro-Jørgensen, J. O. *Forsikringsvaesenets Historie i Danmark indtil det 19. Aarhundrede*. Copenhagen, 1935.
Industriens Historie i Danmark, Tiden 1730–1820, ed. Axel Nielsen. Copenhagen, 1943.
Brønsted, J., *see* Rasch, Aa., *and* Vibaek, J.
Bugge, A. *Den norske Traelasthandels Historie*. Skien, 1925.

Bull, E. and Sønstevold, V. *Kristianias Historie*, vol. 3. Oslo, 1936.

Campbell, J. *A Political Survey of Great Britain*. 2 vols, London, 1774.

Cawston, G. and Keane, A. H. *The Early Chartered Companies*. London, 1898.

Chance, J. F. 'England and Sweden in the time of William III and Queen Anne', *Engl. Hist. Review*, 26. 1901.

Christensen, A. E. 'Der handelsgeschichtliche Wert der Sundzollregister', *Hansische Geschichtsblätter*, 1934.

Christelow, A. 'The Economic Background of the Anglo-Spanish War of 1762'. *Journal of Modern History*, 18. 1946.

Christie, W. H. (ed.). *Genealogiske Optegnelser om Slaegten Christie i Norge 1650–1890*. Bergen, 1909.

Clark, G. N. *Guide to English commercial statistics, 1696–1782*. London, 1938.

Cole, W. A., *see* Deane, P. and Cole, W. A.

Davis, Ralph. *The rise of the English shipping industry in the seventeenth and eighteenth centuries*. London, 1962.

Deane, P., *see* Mitchell, B. R. and Deane, P.

Deane, P. and Cole, W. A. *British Economic Growth 1688–1959*. 2nd ed., Cambridge, 1967.

Eagley, R. V. 'Monetary Policy and Politics in Mid-Eighteenth Century Sweden', *Journal of Economic History*, 29, no. 4. 1969.

Essén, A. W. *Johan Liljencrantz som Handelspolitiker – Studier i Sveriges handelspolitik 1773–1780*. Lund, 1928.

Fahlström, J. M. *The history of a Gothenburg House of Merchants*. Privately published by Ekman & Co., A–B., Gothenburg, n.d. [1952].

Falbe-Hansen, V. A. and Scharling, V. *Danmarks Statistik*. 5 vols, Copenhagen, 1887–.

Fell, A. *The early Iron Industry of Furness and District*. Ulverston, 1908.

Findlay, J. A. *The Baltic Exchange, 1744–1927*. London, 1927.

Furber, H. *John Company at Work*. Harvard, 1951.

Gatty, A. *Sheffield past and present*. Sheffield, 1873.

Glamann, K. 'Studier i Asiatisk Kompagnis Økonomiske Historie, 1732–1772', *Historisk Tidsskrift*, 11th series, 2. Copenhagen, 1949. 'The Danish Asiatic Company, 1732–1772,' *Scandinavian Economic History Review*, 8. 1960.

Hamilton, H. *The English brass and copper industries to 1800*. London, 1926.

Heaton, H. *The Yorkshire Woollen and Worsted Industries*. Oxford, 1920.

Heckscher, E. F. *Ekonomi och Historia*. Stockholm, 1922. *Ekonomisk-historiska Studier*. Stockholm, 1936.

'Un grand chapitre de l'histoire du fer: le monopole suédois', *Annales d'histoire économique et sociale*, 4, nos 14 and 15. 1932.

'Den svenska kopparhanteringen under 1700 talet', *Scandia, Tidskrift for Historisk Forskning*, 13, pt 1. 1940.

Sveriges ekonomiska historia från Gustav Vasa, part I, 1 and 2, *Före Frihetstiden*. Stockholm, 1935.

Sveriges ekonomiska historia från Gustav Vasa, part II, 1 and 2, *Det moderna Sveriges grundläggning 1720–1815*. Stockholm, 1949.

De svenska penning-, vikt-, och måttasystemen, 3rd ed., Stockholm, 1942.

'Utvecklingen av den svenska järnhandteringen och dess export', *Järnkontorets Annaler för År 1919*. Stockholm, 1919.

'Multilateralism, Baltic Trade and the Mercantilists', *Economic History Review*, 2nd series, 3, no. 2. 1950.

Hildebrand, K. G. 'Foreign Markets for Swedish Iron in the Eighteenth Century', *Scandinavian Economic History Review*, 6. 1958.

Johnsen, O. A. *Norwegische Handelsgeschichte*. Jena, 1939.

Johnsen, O. A. and others. *Larviks Historie*, vol. 1. Kristiania, 1923.

Tønsbergs Historie, vol. 2. Oslo, 1934.

'Les relations commerciales entre la Norvège et l'Espagne dans les temps modernes', *Revue Historique*, 165. Paris, 1930.

Keane, A. H. *see* Cawston.

Kennedy, W. *English Taxation 1640–1799*. London, 1913.

Kent, H. S. K. 'The Anglo-Norwegian Timber Trade in the Eighteenth Century', *Economic History Review*, 2nd series, 8, no. 1. 1955.

King, W. C. T. *History of the London Discount Market*. London, 1936.

Kjaerheim, S. 'Norwegian Timber Exports in the Eighteenth Century. A Comparison of Port Books and Private Accounts', *Scandinavian Economic History Review*, 5. 1957.

Koht, Halvdan. 'Les répercussions de la conquête sur la politique scandinave', *Revue Historique*, 164, 1930.

Lloyd, G. I. H. *The Cutlery Trade*. London, 1913.

Lorange, K. *Forsikringsvesenets historie i Norge inntil 1814*. Oslo, 1935.

Mitchell, B. R. and Deane, P. *Abstract of British Historical Statistics*. Cambridge, 1962.

Morse, H. B. *The Chronicles of the East India Company trading to China 1635–1834*. 5 vols, Oxford, 1926.

Murray, J. J. 'Baltic Commerce and Power Politics in the Early Eighteenth Century', *Huntington Library Quarterly*, 6, no 3. 1943.

'Memoirs on the Swedish Tar Company', *Huntington Library Quarterly*, 10, no 4. 1947.

Nielsen, Axel. *Dänische Wirtschaftsgeschichte*. Jena, 1933. *See above* Bro-Jørgensen.

Polak, A. 'English connections in Norway's Old Glass-industry', *Apollo, a Magazine of the Arts*. London and New York, July, 1952.

'Storbritannia og Norge', *Nordsjøkulturen – Britisk Kunsthåndverk (i Norge) 1650–1850*. Norway (n.p.), 1955.

Price, J. M. 'The Rise of Glasgow in the Chesapeake Tobacco Trade 1707–1775', *William and Mary Quarterly*, 3rd series, no. 2. April, 1954.

Ramsay G. D., 'The Smugglers' Trade', *Transactions, Royal Hist. Society*, 5th series, 2. 1952.

English overseas trade in the centuries of emergence. London, 1957.

Rasch, Aa. 'Dansk Ostindien 1777–1845', in Brønsted, J. (ed.), *Vore Gamle Tropekolonier*, vol. I. Copenhagen, 1952.

Dansk Toldpolitik 1760–1797. Aarhus, 1955.

Rasch, Aa. and Sveistrup, P. P. *Asiatisk Kompagni i den Florissante Periode 1772–1792*. Copenhagen, 1948.

Rees, J. F. 'Phases of British Commercial Policy in the Eighteenth Century, *Economica*, 14. June, 1924.

Rosman, H. and Munthe, A. *Släkten Arfwedson: Bilder ur Stockholms Handelshistoria*. Stockholm, 1945.

Samuelsson, K. *De stora köpmanshusen i Stockholm, 1730–1815*. Stockholm, 1951.

'International Payments and Credit Movements by the Swedish Merchant-Houses, 1730–1815', *Scandinavian Economic History Review*, 3. 1955.

Schäffer, D. 'Die Sundzollrechnungen als internationale Geschichtsquelle', *Internationale Wochenschrift für Wissenschaft, Kunst und Technik*, 1. 1907 (2 articles).

Schlote, W. *Entwicklung und Strukturwandlungen des englischen Aussenhandels von 1700 bis zur Gegenwart*. Jena, 1938.

Schovelin, J. *Fra den Danske Handels Empire*. 2 vols, Copenhagen, 1899–1900.

Schreiner, Johan. 'Et problem i norsk handel', *Historisk Tidsskrift*, 43. Oslo, 1964.

Scrivenor, H. *A Comprehensive History of the Iron Trade*. London, 1841.

Sinclair, G. A. 'The Scottish Trader in Sweden', *Scottish Historical Review*, 25.

Söderberg, T. *Försäkringsväsendets historia i Sverige inntil Karl Johanstiden*. Stockholm, 1935.

Steen, Sverre. *Kristiansands Historie, 1741–1814*. Oslo, 1941.

Stråle, G. H. *Alingsås Manufakturverk*. Stockholm, 1884.

Sutherland, L. S. *A London Merchant, 1695–1774*. London, 1933.

Sveistrup, P. P., *see* Rasch, Aa. and Sveistrup, P. P.

Sveistrup, P. P. and Willerslev, R. *Den Danske Sukkerhandels og Sukker-produktions Historie*. Copenhagen, 1945.

Tveite, S. 'The Norwegian Textile Market in the 18th Century, *Scandinavian Economic History Review*, 17. 1969.

Vaughan, W. *Tracts on Docks and Commerce*. London, 1839.

Vibaek, J. 'Dansk Vestindien 1755–1848', in Brønsted, J. (ed.), *Vore Gamle Tropekolonier*, vol. 2. Copenhagen, 1953.

Westergaard, W. *The Danish West Indies under Company Rule*. New York, 1917.

Willerslev, R., *see* Sveistrup.

Wilson, Charles H. *Anglo-Dutch Commerce and Finance in the Eighteenth Century*. Cambridge, 1941.

'Treasure and Trade Balances – the Mercantilist Problem', *Economic History Review*, 2nd series, 2, no 2. 1949.

'Treasure and Trade Balances – Further Evidence', *Economic History Review*, 2nd series, 4. 1951.

Worm-Müller, J. S. (ed.). *Den Norske Sjøfarts Historie*, vol. 1. Kristiania, 1923.

Wright, C. and Fayle, E. *A History of Lloyd's*. London, 1928.

Index of Statutes

12 Car. II c. 6 (book of rates), 11
1 William and Mary, c. 12 (bounty act), 94 n. 7
3 and 4 Anne c. 10 (naval stores), 9, 12, 81 n. 3
9 Anne c. 6 (coal trade), 100 n. 4
12 Anne c. 9 (coal trade), 100 n. 4
5 Geo. I c. 11 (naval stores), 81 n. 5
5 Geo. I c. 27 (enticement of artificers), 202
8 Geo. I c. 12 (naval stores), 12, 81 n. 5, 195
8 Geo. I c. 15 (export duties), 92 n. 1
11 Geo. I c. 7 (book of rates), 11
2 Geo. II c. 35 (naval stores), 81 n. 5, 82 n. 1
9 Geo. II c. 35 ('Act of Indemnity'), 116, 118
19 Geo. II c. 36 (naval stores), 48 n. 3
23 Geo. II c. 13 (enticement of artificers), 203
23 Geo. II c. 29 (iron trade), 10, 61 n. 1
30 Geo. II c. 16 (iron-trade), 61 n. 3
32 Geo. II c. 25 ('Privateering Act'), 148
5 Geo. III c. 43 (drawback, Faeroe Islands), 119 n. 4
24 Geo. III c. 38 ('Commutation Act'), 125 n. 2
50 Geo. III c. 77 (book of rates), 11

General Index

Aardahl, Årdal, 14 n. 1
Aberdeen, 18
Acts of Parliament, *see* Index of Statutes
Admiralty, 132, 134 n. 3, 136; convoy committee, 29, 36; iron supplies of, 76f.; timber supplies of, 40, 48, 138f.; *see also* Admiralty Courts; convoys in wartime; ships, men-of-war; prize of war; marque, letters of
Admiralty Courts, 4, 83 n. 2, 86, 139, 144f., 147, 151 n. 1, 153, 155, 157; *see also* Admiralty; contraband; privateers; prize of war
Adolphus Frederick, king of Sweden, 163
Ahrendahl, Arendal, 199
Altona, 89 n. 1
Amsterdam, 74, 122 n. 3, 129
Armed Neutrality League of 1756: convention, 132, 135–7, 146, 167, 170f.; neutral maritime zones, 137, 150 n. 1, 166; Neutrality Fleet, 134, 136f., 146, 167, 171; and France, 131, 134, 137, 141, 146, 165; and Holland, 134 n. 3, 151f.; and Russia, 134 n. 3, 146, 149, 166; *see also* contraband; conventions; Denmark–Norway; Doctrine of Continuous Voyage; Free Ships Free Goods principle; Rule of the War of 1756; Sweden
arms trade, 131f.
Armstrong, John, carpenter and builder, 44 n. 4
artisans, enticing and kidnapping of, 24, 202–5

Baker, George, builder, 44 n. 4
Baltic trade: in fish, 94; freights, 81 n. 1; merchants in, 18f.; neutrality in Seven Years War, 36f., 137, 150 n. 2; shipping, 66f., 78 n. 2, 94, 98, 137, 161; textiles, 107f.; timber, 44f., 54; *see also* iron-trade, timber-trade
barter trade, 57f., 65, 74, 95

Bergen: copper mines, 14; British consul at, 26f., 119, 126; Scottish trade with, 56; and smuggling trade, 115, 119, 126; trade of, 15, 84, 89f.
Bernstorff, Baron J. H. E. von, Danish statesman: Armed Neutrality League, 134 n. 3, 135f., 142f., 146f., 166f., 170f.; consular appointments, 25f.; defence of Hanover, 169f.; neutral rights, 159–61; privateering, 148; Slesvig-Holstein dispute, 164; West Indies trade, 151–7
Bestuchev-Ryumin, Aleksyei, Russian Grand Chancellor, 164
bills of exchange: on Amsterdam, 51, 74, 122; in Denmark, 122f.; on London, 31, 50f., 74f., 122; in Norway, 194; on out-ports, 51; in Sweden, 76; *see also* exchange and exchange rates
Blackburn, Thomas, Liverpool timber-merchant, 46
blockades: of French coast, 131, 150; of Prussian coast, 150
Blount, Richard, London iron-merchant, 64 n. 4, 69 n. 4, 73 n. 4, 74, 78, 123
Board of Trade, 12, 19 n. 3, 21 n. 3, 31f., 132, 202
bonding facilities and rights, 64; in Denmark, 17, 91, 102, 107f.; in England, 19, 52; in the Faeroe Islands, 119; in Norway, 16, 91, 107; in Sweden, 91
Borré and Fenger, Copenhagen merchants, 30 n. 2, 122 n. 2
Bothmer, Count Hans Caspar von, Danish envoy in London: activities, 23f., 142 n. 2, 144; privateering, 148, 153, 158; West Indies trade, 153–5
Bowman, James, English agent and merchant in Porsgrund, Norway, 95
brandy and brandy-trade: excise on, 125; methods of smuggling, 78, 114f., 126; quantities, 115; seizures by English customs, 115

Bremen, 81

Bristol, 18, 27, 61, 77, 104, 199

Brown, John and David, Copenhagen financiers and merchants, 33

Bute, John, Earl of, Secretary of State and First Lord of the Treasury, 141

Campbell, Lt-Col Robert, envoy-designate to Sweden, 21, 172f.

Canada, 85; *see also* timber-trade

Canton, 117, 123f.; *see also* tea-trade

Cattegat, Kattegat, 36; *see also* Armed Neutrality League of 1756

Channel Islands: consuls in, 27; smugglers' mart, 118, 121; *see also* tea-trade

Charitable Corporation, 14 n. 1; *see also* copper-trade

China, trade with, 5, 7; *see also* Canton; Macao; tea-trade

Christiania, Oslo, 15f., 33, 35, 50 nn. 4, 5 (freight), 109, 193, 196f.

Christiansand, Kristiansand, 15f., 30; *see also* timber-trade

Clifford and Sons, Amsterdam financiers and merchants, 122 n. 3, 124 n. 2

coal-trade, 21 n. 3, 97, 99–101; with Copenhagen and Baltic, 17, 33, 37 n. 6; 100; with Norway, 15, 57f., 90, 100; smuggling, 100f.

coffee-trade, 102f.

Colchester, 115

Collett, Johan (John), Norwegian timber-merchant in London, 32, 52, 53 n. 5, 196

commercial agents and factors, 30, 32f., 49f., 52f., 73f., 188f., 194, 198–200; *see also* Bowman; Collet; Fabricius; Fearnley; Heide; Pederson; Spalding and Brander

commercial edicts and regulations: Danish–Norwegian, 6–9, 12, 15 n. 1, 16f., 46, 89–91, 93, 98, 109, 203; Swedish, 5 nn. 2 *and* 3, 6, 8, 11, 33, 70–2, 78f., 83 n. 2, 89–91

commercial statistics, assessment of, 90–3, 95–7, 99, 102, 105–10, 112f.; *see also* Custom House; smuggling

consuls and consulage, 18 n. 9, 25–31; approbation of foreign consuls, 28; deputies and vice-consuls, 27, 103; duties, 25f., 29, 38, 96 n. 4, 103–5;

fees, 26, 29; nationality issue, 28f. 33; *see also* Dobrée; Falck; Fenwick; Mulderup; Muylman; von Passow; Tigh; Wallace

contraband, 2, 4f., 26 n. 3, 36, 144; arms, 131; dried, salt and fresh fish, 139f.; iron, 78; pitch and tar, 83, 84 n. 1, 137 f.; provisions de bouche, 139; salt beef, 85f., 139; timber 138f., 149

conventions: of Armed Neutrality (of 1691 and 1692), 165 n. 4, (of 1756), 140ff., (of 1780), 159; of St Petersburg (1755), 165, 166 n. 2; on Bremen-Verden (1757), 164, 170; of Kloster-Zeven (1757), 170; Franco-Danish (of 1758), 164; Russo–Swedish (of 1758), 170f.; *see also* treaties

convoys in wartime: British 4, 26, 29, 36–8, 79, 83, 136f.; Danish, 136f.; Dutch, 136f., 139 n. 1; Swedish, 136; *see also* Fighting Instructions for warships; privateers; ships, men-of-war

Copenhagen: Baltic trade, 17, 107; bombardment of suggested, 171; bonding of goods, 102, 107; British trade, 17, 107; Mediterranean trade, 158f.; smuggled goods, 109, 112; tea-trade, 118, 122; West Indies trade, 152–6; *see also* Baltic trade; Denmark–Norway; East India Companies

copper-trade, 14, 87f.

Cosby, Alexander, minister-resident in Denmark, 13 n. 1, 17 n. 6, 106, 129, 204

Cottin and Co., Danish merchants in London, 24

Crop, A. J. and Co., Amsterdam merchants and financiers, 51

Custom House, procedure and frauds, 114–18, 125; in bar-iron-trade, 65–7, 70; in tea-trade, 115; in textile-trade, 106f., 110; in timber-trade, 45–8, 54; in tin-trade, 99f.; in tobacco-trade, 103–6; *see also* smuggling

Dannemora, 67f.; *see also* iron-trade

Denmark–Norway: relations with France, 137f., 142f., 150f., 156f., 160, 162f.; with Holland, 160; with Prussia, 162; with Russia, 157, 171; with Sweden, 138, 140, 157, 165, 172; *see also* Slesvig-Holstein dispute

Drammen, 33, 35, 50 n. 4, 193, 196f.; *see also* timber-trade

Dobrée, Isaac, Gurnsey merchant and Danish consul, 28f.; *see also* smuggling; tea-trade

Doctrine of Continuous Voyage, 149, 151, 153–6; *see also* Rule of the War of 1756; Armed Neutrality League of 1756

Düben, Count C. W., Swedish politician and British agent, 173 n. 2

Dundee, 18; *see also* Scotland

Dunkirk, 116; *see also* smuggling

dye- and spice-trades, 101f., 163

Dyke, William, labour recruiting agent, 202; *see also* artisans

East Country, 39, 46, 63, 65–7, 84f., 109; *see also* timber-trade

East India Companies: Danish (Asiatic Co.), 7, 112, 114, 123, 125, 127, 129; Dutch, 113 n. 1, 114, 117, 123, 125; English, 6, 112f., 120, 125 n. 2; French, 113 n. 1, 114, 123, 125; Ostend, 112, 114; Prussian, 117; Swedish, 6, 112, 114, 117, 120–3, 125, 127; interlopers, 6, 112, 117

Eastland Company, 34

Elbe river and region, 3 n. 2, 14, 39

Elizabeth, empress of Russia, 175

Elsinore, *see* Sound, the

espionage
 commercial and industrial, 23f., 103–5; *see also* artisans, *and under* consuls
 military and naval, 26, 119, 131 n. 1, 132f., 136; *see also* Düben; Gedda; Höpken; de Marteville; Nölken; Springer; Wrangel

exchange and exchange rates: with Denmark–Norway, 15 n. 4, 17 n. 2, 50f., 123, 124 n. 4, 194, 200; with Sweden, 72, 123, 124 n. 4, 125 n. 1; *see also* bills of exchange

export duties, re-export duties, and bounties: British, 19, 92f., 110, on coal, lead and tin, 97, on coal and tin, 99f., on tobacco, 104; Norwegian, on timber, 50; Swedish, on iron, 79

Fabricius, F. L., Norwegian factor, 49 n. 4, 188–201

factors, *see* commercial agents

Faeroe Islands, 118f.; *see also* bonding facilities and rights

Falck, Bernard, Danish consul in Falmouth, 27f.

Falmouth, 27

Fargesund, Farsund, 199; *see also* timber-trade

Fearnley, Thomas, English merchant and factor in Christiania, 18 n. 5, 32f., 42 n. 4, 47, 49 n. 4, 54, 74, 108–10, 119 n. 3

Fenwick, Nicholas, English merchant and consul at Elsinore: appointment as consul, 25f.; shipping agent, 33, 109 n. 5

Fighting Instructions for warships, 136f.; *see also* convoys in wartime; ships, men-of-war

Finch, Edward, British envoy to Sweden, 11 n. 1

Finlay, Robert (also Finlay and Co., and Jennings and Finlay), Stockholm merchant, 75

Finmarken, Finnmarken, 15 n. 1

fish-trade, 14, 19, 21 n. 3, 86f., 93f., 98, 139f.; *see also* contraband

Fludyer, Samuel and Thomas, London financiers and cloth manufacturers, 33 n. 2

Flushing, 118; *see also* smuggling

Fox, Henry (Lord Holland), Secretary of State, 141; *see also* Armed Neutrality League

France: alliance with Denmark, 142f., 156, 163–5; navy, 86; neutral rights, 151f., 156f.; and Prussia, 163; and rice-trade, 102; and Russia, 164, 166; and Slesvig-Holstein dispute, 164f.; and Sweden, 165–75; and tea-trade, 113 n. 1, 114, 120f.; trade, with Denmark–Norway, 48, 101, 138f.; with Sweden, 59 n. 1, 74, 101; with colonies, 101, 102 n. 3, 150f., 153; war-time and coastal shipping, 110f., 143f., 149f.; *see also* Armed Neutrality League; Denmark; Sweden; privateers; contraband; prize of war

Frederick V, king of Denmark, 154, 163, 170 n. 1

Frederick II, king of Prussia, 133, 163, 170, 172, 174; *see also* Prussia

Freckeshald, Fredrikshald, Halden, 16, 109, 199; *see also* timber-trade
Free Ships Free Goods principle, 135f., 140–3, 153, 157–9; *see also* Armed Neutrality League
Fritsø, 188ff.; *see also* Fabricius; iron-trade; timber-trade

Garbett, Samuel, English ironmaster, 65, 70, 204
Gedda, Baron Karl ('Wilkinson'), Swedish agent in British service, 75 n. 2, 133, 172
George II, 154, 164
Germany, 120f., 170, 204
glass: manufacture in Denmark, 203; in Norway, 203f.
glassware-trade, 8, 24, 99; enticement of artisans, 203f.; exports to Denmark–Norway, 20 n. 1, 97, 99; Norwegian import-duties, 20 n. 1
Glückstadt, 3
Goodricke, Sir John, British envoy to Sweden: and Armed Neutrality League, 142; career, 20f., 173; commercial intelligence, 75f., 77; military and naval intelligence, 158, 173f.
Gothenburg: espionage in, 132; general trade, 18, 90; illicit tea-trade in, 113, 116, 118f., 120–2; iron from, 69, 74, 200; as privateering base, 26, 79, 147
Gottorp claims, *see* Slesvig-Holstein
grain and foodstuffs, trade in: butter and cheese, 57, 90, 96f.; flour and grain, 15, 57, 58 n. 1, 94–6, 110; ginger-bread, 96 f.; hops, 90; malt, 90, 94–6, 110; potatoes, 90, 96f.; salt beef, 85f.; smuggling of grain, 95f.; *see also* contraband; Custom House
Grill, C. and C., Stockholm merchants and financiers, 31 n. 4
grindstones, trade in: 97f.
Gunning, Robert, minister-resident at Copenhagen, 13 n. 1
Guy Dickens, Col Melchior, British envoy to Sweden, 20, 36

Halden, *see* Fredrickshald
Hamburg, 75
Hanbury Williams, Charles, envoy to Russia, 173; *see also* espionage

Hanning, tea-smuggler, 116
Hanover, defence of, 162, 164, 167, 170; *see also* conventions
Hardman, John, Liverpool merchant, 19 n. 1
Harrington, Lord, Secretary of State, 10, 12 nn. 5–7
Haworth and Stephenson, Hull merchants, 32, 35 n. 3, 42 n. 4, 47, 57, 109
Heide or Heede, Claus, Danish timber-merchant in London, 32, 52f., 119 n. 5, 196
hemp and flax, trade in, 14, 85, 87, 90; *see also* naval stores
Holdernesse, Robert Earl of, Secretary of State: on Armed Neutrality League, 135, 137, 140f., 167; on privateers, 143f.; quarrel with Count Rautzau, 23; on West Indies trade, 152–4
Holland: and Armed Neutrality of 1756, 134 n. 3, 140f., 146; in Seven Years War, 134 n. 3, 136, 139 n. 1, 146, 149; tea-trade, 113 n. 1, 114f., 116, 120f.; trade with Britain, 57, 63, 84, with Norway, 15, with Sweden, 59 n. 1, 74, with West Indies, 150–4, 157 n. 3; *see also* Doctrine of Continous Voyage; Rule of the War of 1756; Free Ships Free Goods principle; conventions
Holland, John, and Holland and Co., Hull timber-merchants, 47f., 51 n. 3, 57
Höpken, Anders Johan von, Swedish statesman and British agent, 61f., 169 n. 1
Hübner, Martin, German–Danish jurist, 159f.; *see also* Armed Neutrality League
Hull, 18, 32, 51 n. 6, 57, 68, 70, 73, 77, 109, 199; *see also* iron- and timber-trades
Huntsman, Benjamin, English steel-converter, 73

import duties, 110; British, on bar-iron, 9, 31 n. 1, 61f., 70f., 77, 199, on tea, 113, on timber, 41 n. 4, 42, 50, 191–5, on tobacco, 104; Danish–Norwegian, on glass, 20 n. 1, on tea, 113f., on textiles, 106f.; Swedish, on tea, 113, on textiles, 106; *see also* pitch- and tar-trade import licences in Scandinavia: for hardware, haberdashery, and millinery, 90f., 99; for sugar, 102; for textiles, 106

India: trade with, 5, 7, 76 n. 4; war in, 131

insurance, *see* marine insurance

Ireland: Danish troops for, 162; iron-imports, 64

Iron Bureau (Jernkontoret), 35, 71, 75, 79; *see also* iron-trade

iron-trade, 59–79, 198–201
   in bar-iron: Baltic, 63, 65; colonial, 59, 61f., 184; German, 63; Norwegian, 14, 16, 63, 65, 74, 198–201; Russian, 9, 11, 34, 57, 63, 65f., 79, 184, 198; Spanish, 59f., 63, 198, 200; Swedish, 9, 11, 14, 18, 21 n. 3, 33f., 61, 63–5, 74, 184–6, 198–201; cost, credit, and prices of bar-iron, 71–6, 79, 200f.; dimensions of bar-iron, 69f., 73, 199, 201; import duties on bar-iron, 9, 31 n. 1, 61f., 70f., 77, 199; re-export of bar-iron, 67; for Royal Navy, 76f., 199–201; uses and properties of, 67–9, 76f., 198, 200f.
   combinations of merchants and iron-masters, 34f., 61f., 77
   insurance in, 72f., 78, 200
   iron as ballast, 65
   iron production: colonial, 10, 59, 61f., 76f.; English, 60f., 64, 71, 76f.; Norwegian, 199–201; Russian, 60, 79, 198; Swedish, 18, 36, 59f., 79, 198–201
   pig-iron, 62f., 76
   shipping in, 198–200
   smuggling and frauds in, 64–7, 70
   statistics of, 59f., 62–4, 66–8, 184–6
   steel, 68, 73f., 70 n. 3
   and war, 59, 78f., 103; in Seven Years War, 62–4, 69 n. 2, 78f., 103, 175f., 198–201
   see also Iron Bureau

ironmongery, trade in, 57, 63, 90, 97, 99

Isle of Man: 104f., 118f., 120; *see also* Custom House; smuggling; tea-trade

Isselin and Co., Copenhagen merchants, 24 n. 2, 122 n. 2

Jennings, Frans, Stockholm merchant, 64 n. 4, 69 n. 4, 73 n. 4, 75f., 78, 123; *see also* Finlay

Jennings and Finlay, Stockholm merchants, 33f., 35

Kattegat, *see* Cattegat

King's Lynn, 15 n. 6, 56, 96

Knyphausen, baillage of, 163 n. 3; *see also* France; Prussia

Korn, Jens, Copenhagen merchant, 51 n. 3

Kragerø, 56 n. 5

Kristiansand, *see* Christiansand

Landscrona, fortification of, 165

Larvik, Laurvig, 16, 50 n. 4, 188ff., 201; *see also* iron-trade; timber-trade; Fabricius

Laurvig, Count, Norwegian landowner, 49, 188

lead, trade in, 57, 97, 99f.

leather and skins, trade in, 14, 21 n. 3, 57, 74, 85, 87, 93

Leeds, 18

Lindegren, Anders and Carl (Charles), Swedish merchants in London, 31, 73

Liverpool, 18f., 46, 53f., 77, 99, 104, 199; *see also* salt-trade

livestock, trade in, 97, 126f.

Lloyd's Coffee House, 37; *see also* convoys in wartime; marine insurance

London: as money market, 75, 129; Scandinavian merchants in, 31f.; as smugglers' market, 115, 121, 124; trade, with Baltic, 54, 98, with colonies, 34, 61, with Norway, 16, 34f., 54–7, 89, 188–98, with Sweden, 18, 61f., 74, 76f., 96, 198f.; trade statistics of, 178–85

Louisa Ulrica, queen of Sweden, 133, 172, 173 n. 2, 174f.; *see also* espionage, military and naval; Sweden

Macao, 117; *see also* tea-trade

Magens, Nicholas, Danish merchant, financier, and author in London, 23

Maister, William, British merchant in Stockholm, 34 n. 3

Mandahl, Mandal, 16; *see also* timber-trade

marine insurance, 50, 78, 129, 157; brokers in London, 148, 194; of iron cargoes, 72f., 78, 200; of timber cargoes, 50, 52, 194

marque, letters of, 4, 158; *see also* contraband; prize of war; privateers
Marshall, Newcastle timber-merchant, 57
Marteville, L. de, Dutch envoy at Stockholm and British agent, 133, 172
Mediterranean trade, 23, 81; and war, 24, 27, 128, 147, 151, 158f.
miscellaneous goods, trade in, 14 nn. 5–6, 57f., 78, 89–91, 93; *see also* smuggling; textile-trade
Moltke, Count Adam Gottlob, Danish statesman, 86, 129 n. 3, 152, 154, 162f.
most favoured-nations rights, 4, 12, 17, 140f.
Mulderup, Christian, Norwegian timber-merchant and consul in Scotland, 30f.
Münchhausen, Philip Adolf von, Hanoverian minister in London, 154
Muylman, Henry, merchant and Danish consul in London, 25, 29f.

naturalisation, commercial advantages of, 31 n. 1, 32, 33
naval stores, *see* hemp and flax, trade in; iron-trade; pitch- and tar-trade; sailcloth, trade in; timber-trade
Newcastle, Thomas Duke of, Secretary of State and First Lord of the Treasury, 21f., 23 n. 2; intercedes for seized Danish ships, 46, 96, 119 n. 5; and West Indies trade, 154
Newcastle-on-Tyne, 14 n. 1, 77, 98; *see also* iron-trade; shipping; timber-trade
Nölken or Nolcken, Baron G. A., Swedish politician and diplomat, and British agent, 173 n. 2
Norcliffe, R., Hull merchant, 15 n. 3
Norman, James, London timber-merchant, 34 n. 5, 196f.
North American colonies: iron exports to, 67, 76 n. 4; masts from, 44; merchants, 34; pitch and tar from, 40, 80–2, 85; tea-trade, 118, 121; and war, 131

Ogier, Jean-Francois, French envoy in Denmark, 146 n. 2, 167 n. 1

Öregrund, 18, 199, 201; *see also* iron-trade
Oslo, *see* Christiania
Ostend, 118; *see also* smuggling

Parker, William, English timber-merchant and builder, 12 n. 3, 44 n. 4
Passow, Christian Albrecht von, Danish consul in London, 30, 104, 119 n. 5
passport, *see* ship's passport in war
Pederson or Petersen, Jens, Norwegian timber-merchant in London, 31 n. 1, 32, 33 n. 2, 52, 196
Peter of Holstein-Kiel, later Tsar Peter III of Russia, *see* Slesvig-Holstein dispute
Pewterers' Company, 99
piracy, 143f., 148, 159; *see also* privateers
pitch- and tar-trade, 9, 14, 15, 34, 74, 80–5, 176, 187; colonial, 80–5, 187; duties, 84 n. 2; legislation on, 81; merchants in, 84; monopoly in, 80f.; Norwegian, 15 n. 6; prices, 81f.; re-export, 81; Royal Navy, 81–3; shipping, 84; statistics, 187; *see also* Acts of Parliament; contrabrand; smuggling
Pitt, William, Earl of Chatham, 20, 132, 140f., 142f.; on privateering, 144 n. 1, 148f.; on West Indies trade, 154
Pontoppidan, Erik, Danish author and divine, 109, 112
Porsgrund, Porsgrunn, 16; *see also* timber-trade; Bowman
Portugal, 59 n. 1, 81, 98f.
privateers, privateering: English, 38, 85 n. 5, 86, 127f., 136, 139, 141 n. 3, 143–5; French, 26f., 36, 79, 83, 128f., 146f., 190; Prussian, 68 n. 3, 127f., 158; Swedish, 150 n. 1; in West Indies, 151; Privateering Act (of 1759), 148f.; profits, 145, 148, 151, 156; ransoming of prizes, 144f.; syndicates, 148f., 153; *see also* marque, letters of; piracy; prize of war
prize courts, *see* Admiralty Courts
prize of war, 2, 4, 27, 30 n. 2, 32 n. 6, 79; French edict on, 37 n. 5; ransoming of prizes, 144f.; sale of, 146f.; *see also* Admiralty Courts; contraband; privateers

Prussia, 131, 133; in Seven Years War, 127, 142, 163, 166; 168f., 170, 172–5; *see also* privateers

Rantzau, Count Cai, Danish envoy in London: and Admiralty Courts 144f.; Armed Neutrality League, 135, 140–3; quarrel with Holdernesse, 23
rice-trade, 102
Riga, 46, 54, 66; *see also* timber-trade; Baltic trade
Rigg, John, timber-merchant and textile manufacturer, 196
Robinson, John, British envoy in Sweden, 81 n. 2
Roebuck, John, English ironmaster, 64, 70, 204
Rosenkrantz, Iver Eriksen, Danish politician, 46
Rule of the War of 1756, 149–56; *see also* Doctrine of Continuous Voyage; Armed Neutrality League
Russia: and England, 166, 174f.; and France, 164, 166; and Sweden, 165–75; trade, 9, 32, 34, 57, 84f., 87, in iron, 63, 67, 176, in tea, 121, in textiles, 109, in timber, 40, 44, 176; *see also* Denmark; France; Sweden; treaties; conventions
Russia Company, 25, 29, 34 n. 1, 37 n. 2, 57, 198; *see also* consuls

sailcloth-trade, 84
St Croix, St John, and St Thomas, *see* West India Company, Danish
St Petersburg, 66, 71, 79 n. 4
Sandwich, Earl of, Secretary of State, 77
salt-trade, 7, 8 n. 1, 19, 58 n. 1, 92 n. 2, 97–9, 110, 163; *see also* smuggling
Scotland: Baltic shipping, 105; export, of coal, 100f., of fish, 194; import, of iron, 64, of linens, 92 n. 2, of pitch and tar, 84, of stockfish, 87, of timber, 39, 46f.; tobacco-trade, 105; smuggling, 96, 100f., 126 n. 3; *see also* coal-trade; shipping
Seven Years War: effect, on balance of trade, 127f., on French trade, 100f., on iron-trade, 175f., on Mediterranean trade, 24, 128, 158f., on money and credit, 53, 75f., on shipping, 36,

55 n. 3, 69 n. 2, 127–9, on tea-trade, 123f., on timber-trade, 16 n. 3, 175f., on tobacco-trade, 105; Jacobite issue in, 169 n. 1; Protestant issue in, 169; *see also passim*
Sheffield, 73, 77
ship-building, 11, 43f., 82f., 130
ships
  men-of-war: British 44 n. 3, 131, 134 (Keppel's squadron), 145, 147, *Antelope* (Capt. Webb), 143 n. 3; Danish, *Groenland* (Capt. Fisker), 158f.; Dutch, 136f., 139 n. 1; Swedish, 136; *see also* Armed Neutrality League; convoys in wartime; Fighting Instructions; privateers; prize of war
  merchantmen: *Agnes and Jannet*, 15 n. 5; *Eenrom*, 145; *Friendship*, 90; *Gode Christian*, 151 n. 1; *Good Intent*, 15 n. 5; *Henriette*, 56 n. 2; *James and Catherine*, 15 n. 5; *John and Mary*, 15 n. 6, 56 n. 5; *John and Rachel*, 56 n. 5; *Lark*, 90; *Lynn*, 18 n. 8; *Margrath and Arbroath*, 15 n. 5; *Mitchel and Polly*, 15 n. 5; *Providence*, 56 n. 5; *Rex Sveciae*, 117 n. 2; *Den Ringende Jakob*, 145; *St Croix Packet*, 151 n. 1; *Trenne Brødre*, 89f.
shipping
  English, 8, 10, 100, 103, 127, 129f.; in Baltic trade, 17, 26, 36–8, 46, 66, 137f.; in colonial trade, 102f.; in Mediterranean trade, 128, 158f.; in Norwegian trade, 14, 15, 35, 54–8; in Russian trade, 36–8; in Swedish trade, 26, 64, 69–71, 78, 83, 130; to and from London, 35, 38, 54–6; to and from out-ports, 38, 54–7, 77f., 103; to and from Scotland, 15, 58, 64 n. 2, 100f.
  foreign: Danish–Norwegian, 16, 37, 54–7, 127f., 130f., 176f., 188ff.; French, 148f.; Swedish, 8, 37, 64 n. 2; 69 n. 2, 78f., 83, 127–9, 131, 138, 176
  British and foreign: freight rates, 12, 41, 45 n. 1, 65f., 71, 78; in timber-trade, 189f., 192ff.; tonnage in iron-trade, and timber-trade, 78; in war, 26f., 36–8, 44, 54–6, 64 n. 2, 78f., 83,

shipping (*cont.*)
  101–3, 127–31, 144f., 176f., 190, in Seven Years War, 36–8, 48 n. 5, 50, 83, 127–30, 193–5, 199f.
  see also Admiralty; Mediterranean trade; privateers; ships; Sound; timber-trade
ship's passport in war, 2, 4, 25, 144
Skien, 16, 197
Slesvig-Holstein dispute, 89 n. 1, 163–5, 171, 175
Smith, Lauritz or Lars, English merchant in Drammen. 33 n. 2, 196
smuggling, 21 n. 3, 23f., 38, 74, 89, 148; of bar-iron, 64–7, 70; of brandy, 78, 114f., 125f.; of coal, 100f.; of copper, 87; of glass, 99; of grain and food-stuffs, 95–7; of ironmongery, 97, 99; of livestock, 97, 126f.; of salt, 98f.; of sugar, 102; of tea, 112–29; of textiles, 107–10; of timber, 46–8, 57, 192f.; of tin, 99f.; of tobacco, 103–6, 110, 115, 119 n. 4; of wool, 127; *see also* trade statistics: separate trades; Custom House; Heide, Wallace
Smyth, Edward, English timber-merchant, 51 n. 1
Solander, Daniel Charles, botanist and Swedish agent in London, 205
Solly, E., English timber-merchant, 43 n. 2
Sound, the: bonding of goods at, 17, 102, 107; consuls at, 25f., 96 n. 4; convoy station, 36f., 83; neutrality of, 131; passage of, 3, 78 n. 2, 96, 98; toll, 16f., 20 n. 2, 25, 98; *see also* Baltic trade; shipping
Spain: iron exports to Britain, 59f., 198, 200; iron imports from Sweden, 59; pitch and tar imports, 81; salt-trade, 98f.; shipping in war-time, 141, 146, 149
Spalding and Brander, Swedish merchants and financiers in London, 22 n. 2, 31, 73
Spieker, Johan, Swedish merchant in London, 32
Spooner, A., English iron-merchant, 18 n. 2
Springer, Christoffer, Swedish merchant and political agent in London, 22f., 173 n. 2

Stacy, John, English merchant, 57 n. 2
steel, *see* Huntsman; iron-trade
Stockholm, 18, 132f.; *see also* Sweden; iron-trade; shipping
Stockholm Tar Company, *see* pitch- and tar-trade
Stromboe, G., Norwegian merchant, 42 n. 4, 51 n. 6
sugar-trade, 7, 23, 102
Sunderland, 43 n. 2
Swallow, British merchant and consul in St Petersburg, 79 n. 4
Sweden: political parties, 5, 135, 165f., 172, 175; relations, with Denmark, 138, 140, 165, 172, with France, 160, 162, 165–7, 176, with Prussia, 162, 166f., 172, 174f., with Russia, 165f., 170, 172f., 176; *see also* iron-trade; timber-trade
Sykes, Joseph, Hull iron-merchant, 68

tea-trade, 112–29, 74; dealers, in Copenhagen, 122, in Channel ports, 120f., in England, 116f., 119 n. 1, 120f., 124, in Gothenburg, 121f.; prices and profits of, 113, 115f., 117 n. 4; smuggling methods in, 114f., 119–21; statistics of, 115–18, 119 n. 1, 120 n. 3, 124; types of tea imported, Bohea, 113, 116f., Hyson and Singloe, 113; and war, 130; *see also* Canton; China; Custom House; East India Companies; Macao; smuggling
territorial waters, 2, 4, 36f., 131, 147; *see also* Armed Neutrality League
textile-trade
  cottons, linens, and silks, 15 n. 5, 90, 92 n. 2, 93, 109, 117, 122
  woollens, 8, 15, 74, 91, 106–11; export, to Denmark, 7 n. 8, 106–10, to Norway, 57, 106–10, to Sweden, 106, 110f.; smuggled goods in Copenhagen shops, 109; smuggling, methods, 109f., statistics, 107f., 110; types of cloths exported, 107f.; *see also* smuggling
textiles, woollen, manufacture of: in Denmark, 6f., 89 n. 1, 108, 110, 163; in England, 57, 107f.; in Sweden, 5, 110, 127; *see also* artisans

Thurot, Capt. Francois, French privateer, 79, 83

Tigh, Robert, British consul and merchant at the Sound, 25

timber: articles and implements, 85; bracking of, 49, 54, 190; for domestic building, 44f.; prices of, 35, 41, 45 n. 1, 48–50, 53, 182f., 190–5; production, of Norway, 16, 40–2, 49, 190, of Russia, 40, of Sweden, 40, 47; seasoning of, 52; redwood (red deal, yellow deal), uses of, 40f., in warship construction, 43f.; whitewood (white deal), uses of, 40f., 43

timber-trade, 39–58, 11f., 14f., 32f., 103, 178–83, 188–98

with Baltic, 44f., 54

capital and credit in, 51–4, 189, 196

cargoes: Baltic spruce, 39, 197; Baltic pine, 46f.; barrel staves, 39; battens, 191f.; fir baulks, 39; fir deals, 35, 39–45, 188–98; firewood, 45; masts, 39, 43–5, 181; oak, 3, 40, 45f., 50 n. 6, 57; wainscot boards, 50 n. 6, 56 n. 2, 57 n. 6

customs frauds in, 45–8, 54

import duties in, 41 n. 4, 42f., 50, 189, 191–5

insurance, 50, 52, 194

merchants and agents, 30, 32f., 35, 49, 54, 57, 188ff.; in London, 189f., 196f.; in Norway, 35f., 42 n. 4, 49, 51 n. 6, 188–98; in outports, 192f., combinations of merchants in, 35f., 188–90

with North America, 40f.

of Scotland, 39, 46f.

in Seven Years War, 138f., 149, 175f., 178–83, 188–98

smuggling in, 46–8, 47, 192f.

statistics of, 39 n. 3, 41, 44, 178–83

tin-trade, 97, 99f.

Titley, Walter, British envoy in Denmark, 12, 21; advises bombardment of Copenhagen, 171; assistance to English artisans, 202f.; espionage, 132f., 136; on exchange rates, 123; on Neutrality League, 138, 142, 146f., 170f.; on privateering, 148; on Slesvig-Holstein dispute, 164; on trade and trade disputes, 12, 17,

19f., 93f.; on treaty negotiations, 162f., 167–9; on West Indies trade, 152, 154–7

tobacco-trade, 8, 103–6; with Copenhagen and Baltic, 17; smuggling, 103–5, 110, 115, 119 n. 4

Tønsberg, 16; *see also* timber-trade

Tottie, Charles and William, Scottish merchants in Stockholm, 34

trade reprisals as policy measures, 13, 22 n. 3, 136f., 166; *see also* commercial edicts and regulations

treaties: Anglo-Danish (of 1670), 1–4, 6, 12, 46, 140f., 144; Anglo-Dutch (of 1674), 12, 140f.; Anglo-Russian (of 1734), 9f.; Anglo-Swedish (of 1661), 1f., 11, 140f., (of 1700 and 1720), 140 n. 2, 144; Franco-Danish (1742) 142f., 156, 163; of Utrecht (1713), 137; of Westminster (1756), 164, 166; *see also* conventions

Trondheim, 15, 84; *see also* timber-trade

Tuite, Nicholas, British merchant in Danish West India trade, 23f.

Uhthoff, Henry, Swedish merchant in London, 32

Vogt, Poul, timber-merchant in Christiania, 49 n. 3, 196

Waddington, English timber-merchant, 42 n. 4

Waern, Morten, Danish labour-recruiting agent: 203f.; *see also* artisans; glass trade

Wallace, Alexander, British merchant and consul in Bergen, 26f., 109 n. 5, 119, 126

Walpole, Sir Robert, 116

Walter, Abraham, tea-smuggler, 116

War of the Austrian Succession, 38, 86

War of the Spanish Succession, 81

Warburton, H., English timber-merchant, 12 n. 3, 40 n. 4, 42 n. 5, 57 n. 1

West India Company, Danish, produce and trade of, 3, 5, 7, 27, 32, 102, 150, 177; *see also* Armed Neutrality League; Doctrine of Continuous Voyage; Holland; Rule of the War of 1756; West Indies

West Indies, trade of, 23, 67, 150; *see also* West India Company
Whitby, 43 n. 2
Wilder and Co., Copenhagen merchants, 30 n. 2
'Wilkinson', *see* Gedda
Wilson, Samuel, tea-smuggler, 116, 117 n. 4
wool-trade, 128; *see also* smuggling
Worster, Samuel, British merchant in Stockholm, 34 n. 3
Wrangel, Count A. J., Swedish statesman and British agent, 173 n. 2

Wynantz, Arnold, Swedish diplomat in London: and Armed Neutrality, 135, 138, 140f., 143f.; duties, 21f.; on English iron industry, 61f.; entice-ment of English artisans, 204f.; Prize Courts, 144f., recall, 23
Wynantz, Francis, Swedish merchant in London, 22, 38

Yarmouth, 51 n. 6, 115
Yorke, Sir Joseph, envoy at the Hague, 21